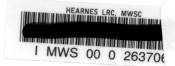

Parish Nursing

Parish Nursing

PROMOTING WHOLE PERSON HEALTH WITHIN FAITH COMMUNITIES

EDITED BY
PHYLLIS ANN SOLARI-TWADELL
MARY ANN McDERMOTT

SAGE Publications
International Educational and Professional Publisher
Thousand Oaks   London   New Delhi

For information:

SAGE Publications, Inc.
2455 Teller Road
Thousand Oaks, California 91320
E-mail: order@sagepub.com

SAGE Publications Ltd.
6 Bonhill Street
London EC2A 4PU
United Kingdom

SAGE Publications India Pvt. Ltd.
M-32 Market
Greater Kailash I
New Delhi 110 048 India

Printed in the United States of America

Library of Congress Cataloging-in-Publication Data

Main entry under title:

Parish nursing: Promoting whole person health within faith
communities / edited by Phyllis Ann Solari-Twadell and Mary Ann
McDermott.
    p. cm.
   Includes bibliographical references and index.
   ISBN 0-7619-1182-0 (cloth: acid-free paper)
   ISBN 0-7619-1183-9 (pbk.: acid-free paper)
   1. Parish nursing. I. Solari-Twadell, Phyllis Ann. II. McDermott,
Mary Ann.
   RT120 .P37 1998
   610.73′43—ddc21   98-25454

99 00 01 02 03 04 05 7 6 5 4 3 2 1

Acquiring Editor:	Dan Ruth
Editorial Assistant:	Anna Howland
Production Editor:	Wendy Westgate
Editorial Assistant:	Nevair Kabakian
Typesetter/Designer:	Christina M. Hill
Cover Designer:	Candice Harman

Contents

I. PARISH NURSING
An Overview of the Practice

II. PARISH NURSING
A Collaborative Practice

III. PARISH NURSING
Context for the Practice

IV. PARISH NURSING
Challenges to the Practice

Foreword

In the late 1960s and early 1970s I had the opportunity, as a faculty member of the University of Illinois College of Nursing, to participate in one of the Wholistic Health Centers developed by Granger Westberg in a church setting. Over the past 30 years, I have had the opportunity to see the ideas of whole person health develop from the early church-based family practice models to the current growing movement of parish nursing. As a program director and vice president of the Kellogg Foundation in more recent years, I have followed the development of parish nursing through a number of projects we have had the privilege to support. This compendium of chapters related to parish nursing provides a comprehensive overview of both the underlying philosophical and pragmatic issues of establishing parish nursing in a wide array of contexts. As we at the Kellogg Foundation focused our programming upon community-based models for health services delivery, we became increasingly convinced of the power of *community* as a positive influence on the health and well-being of people, and often, at the center of the community, was the church: the institutional hub around which the community was organized. Through the years, the development of parish nursing has resulted in the church becoming an increasingly important force influencing the health and well-being of people.

Granger Westberg, the driving force behind the whole person health movement, describes in his chapter on the historical development of parish nursing how "the role of parish nursing is basically a reaching out for more whole-person ways of ministering to people who are hurting." In many ways, that captures the essence of nursing, whether it be in hospital or community settings. Nurses through the ages have been the bridges between people and medical care systems. In parish nursing, nurses are bridges between people in the congregation, the church with its healing mission, and the medical care providers—physicians, dentists, hospitals, managed care systems, and a wide array of allied health providers. Time after time, nurses have emerged as the "glue" that holds things together, but we keep forgetting that lesson, and somehow we can't find a way of "fitting things" together so that support for the glue becomes as important as any of the individual pieces. In many ways, our current medical care system is one gigantic jigsaw puzzle, with each of the pieces magnificent in its detail and its sophisticated technologi-cal underpinnings. What good does it do to have magnificent pieces if they don't come together in a discernible pattern around the real health needs of people?

Westberg notes that in the early evaluation of the Wholistic Health Centers, the evaluators determined that one of the most important factors in their success was that the nurses employed in the clinics spoke two languages: "the language of science and the language of religion. The nurses were acting as translators." The role of nurse as translator is key to the success of parish nursing and, indeed, of nursing as a whole. Helping the person understand his or her physical condition, whether ill or well, and assisting that individual to take control of the management of his or her health is of primary importance. However, with our concentration upon the wonders of technology and our ability to "fix" things, too often attention is focused upon the wrong things. It is commonly assumed that building more health centers, bringing better technological equipment into communities, and bringing medical doctors into these practice settings will improve the health of people. Time after time, the evidence shows that this does little. We as a society have become fixated upon the medicalization of a whole array of problems: Attention-deficit children, depression, fatigue, obesity, wrinkled skin—all are viewed as medical problems to be solved with a pill or a potion. People needing only an understanding ear come to the doctor's office, to be given 8 minutes of time and most likely a prescription that will do little to address their underlying problems. No one in our society has time to listen, and certainly listening is not a reimbursable service in the world of medical care management.

While the strength of parish nursing comes from the ability to bridge the worlds of medicine and religion and link to people, that also constitutes one of its greatest potential weaknesses. Where is the base of support for maintenance and further development of parish nursing? One of the most difficult challenges facing nursing in general and parish nursing in particular is the question of reimbursement for listening to people and being the glue to hold the whole system together around the needs of patients. One of the central problems described in this book is that of getting church finance committees to allocate money to parish nursing. Should the churches be the source of payment? Much of the parish nurse movement has been dependent upon nurses volunteering time and providing services. While volunteers are certainly important, parish nurses are just able to scratch the surface of the needs of people. Without a stable source of support for the adminis-tration of a parish nurse program, the effective use of volunteers is limited in addressing the comprehensive needs of the parish. Should the source of support for parish nurses be from the health care system? While the nurse is working to bring the pieces together around the needs of the patient, and thus facilitating the work of the system as a whole, it is highly unlikely that in our current frenzy to control costs (through the most ineffective ways), the effectiveness of parish nurses would be recognized in the form of financial support. What are people willing to pay out of their own pockets? If they do pay for parish nurses and demand them as part of the church budget, are they then not in competition with the churches themselves over revenue streams?

In a capitalistic society, with societal institutions vying with one another for financial survival, there is little room for support of the bridges, or the societal glue, which holds things together. Parish nurses are at the center of this societal dilemma. While this book demonstrates the valuable societal role that parish nurses can play in a wide array of contexts, will there be sufficient societal support to maintain and expand this movement over time? While there is overwhelming evidence that getting members of a community together to focus upon solving common problems is a powerful way of effectively managing these problems, few of our resources are directed toward this end. Yet we continue, as a society, to pour more and more money into the "sophisticated" approaches while ignoring ways of mobilizing communities to take charge.

Parish nurses, with their links to people, churches, and health providers, need to make highly visible the value of the work they are doing and openly address the issues related to long-term sustenance of this important movement. By mobilizing the church to fulfill its mission of being a healing force, parish nurses can assist in bringing wholeness to fragmented people and society. To do so, however, churches must embrace this as a legitimate part of their function rather than as an "add-on."

Parish nurses in a wide array of settings are reaching out to people who are hurting; they are joining with the church in its mission of healing. We hope that the church will embrace this movement and form a nurturing environment, that this book will become a widely used resource to expand this movement, and that churches, whatever their denomination, may join together in making this a more humane and caring society.

Helen K. Grace, R.N., Ph.D., F.A.A.N.
W. K. Kellogg Foundation
Battle Creek, Michigan

Introduction

Unfortunately, most readers of this book will be nurses and pastors.

Now that I have your attention, given that crabby opening line, let me say what I mean by that opening word "unfortunately." Certainly, it does not imply lack of respect for members of the nursing and clergy professions. They are key to the development of the parish nurse concept and to realizing it. And—now let me use the second person—*you* nurses and nursing educators, *you* ministers and priests who have this book before your eyes, may not represent a congregation of the "converted." This means that the authors of this book do not assume they are only "preaching to the converted."

You may be only half converted. That is, if you are a nurse, you are almost certain to be tantalized by the vision of parish nursing offered here, but you may immediately lose heart when you picture how hard it is to realize the role. Again, you may be only half converted as a pastor because, although you will see at once where this concept fits into the theology and mission of a congregation, you may have a hard time summoning energies to add "one more thing" to the complex institution to which you minister. Your table and agenda are full.

Yet, I am convinced in both cases that you will be convinced by the arguments, inspired by the vision, and informed by the practical details of this book. The worry is that neither you nurses nor you pastors, without whose support the parish nurse project will get nowhere, will be lonely, apparently self-interested promoters. "Unfortunately," you cannot carry it by yourself. Now let me drop the second-person language and start talking also to other readers who, one hopes, might be looking over your shoulder or might respect your recommendation.

Fortunately, this *is* a book for, say, finance committees and stewardship committees of congregations. Pastor Granger Westberg, in his lucid and memorable account of how the parish nurse program was invented, tells how he worked his way around congregations, making the case. All went well until he reached the finance committee. There the trouble started. How can an item costing $17,000 or more be fit into a congregational budget? In his story, they are not villains but realists. Some of his best friends, and mine and yours, are no doubt on finance and stewardship committees, or should be. They simply know how hard it is to get busy congregations and their members to give priority to something new.

One could say that the parish nurse program is a great money saver, but that does not work well because most members will never know it. A young politician doing some apprentice or intern work for a United States senator once told me of his work on a piece of legislation. As I recall it, the law would simply seek to enforce the demand that freight trains come equipped with a certain kind of flashing strobe light which would serve as a warning to cars approaching crossings. From studies made in the states which enforced and did not enforce such laws, it was estimated that about 20 lives would be saved every year. "Unfortunately, those 20 people will not ever know that this law, and the action by this senator, saved their lives, but, still, their lives will be saved."

There is no doubt, no doubt at all, that a parish nurse will similarly save people money. They help teach *preventive* medicine, which is the least expensive form of care there is. Through their counseling, their referrals, their "brokering" and "fixing," there is no doubt that they will help individuals, insuring agencies, and governments save money in a time of health care financing crisis. One could verge on the point of overselling by reminding readers that healthy congregates have more woman- and man-hours to give through their congregations to the service of others and that the parish nurse program will help keep more of them healthy. But I use the fiscal theme here at the beginning only to symbolize the fact that there are large potential audiences for this book and to express the hope that it reaches them.

Why make such a fuss about the locale for this recently developed form of service? Why focus on the congregation, when, historically, people have connected through the nursing profession with hospitals, visiting nurse programs, or home care—but not with places that have steeples and domes, altars and high steps, which made things hard for people in wheelchairs? Why?

Some years ago, while writing about health and medicine in our part of the Christian tradition, I interviewed the presiding bishop of a denomination in that tradition. What advice could he give to someone who has just been given medical bad news? His answer: "My advice is that the person should have been an active member of a vital congregation for quite a few years." Meaning? Meaning that when misfortune comes, it is important to be part of a community of care. A congregation enfolds one in intercessory prayer— loving one's neighbor on one's knees. A good congregation provides care and casseroles, rides to clinics, and cards for the beside table. It represents a gathering of people who have heard and keep on hearing the word of the Healer, who are busy interpreting the message of wholeness in a world of brokenness. By their own stumbling words, halting actions, and only sometimes distracted thoughts, they help the person who is ill come to terms with some of his or her problems, to cope, and, in a way, to transcend them on the pilgrimage to triumph.

So the congregation is important. It will become more so as people realize its vital role in a time when health care in traditional institutions is simply beyond the range of more and more people, in a time when expenses grow. Not too long ago, a veteran physician who cares for aged people told me that he visited his 90-year-old father daily in a Jewish senior citizens' home. This physician can afford the best of care, and he provides it, for a man whose dignity is threatened along with his memory, which fails him thanks to a disease. "I have to say," said this Jewish physician, "that for all the professionals in his range, the person who treats my father as a dignified and worthy human being, and who seems to get some response, is a young black aide who probably will tell you she does that for him because she loves Jesus." The doctor went on to use that as an illustration of a resource in the believing community. "You folks spend too much time working on the religious angle in hair-raising, urgent, sudden health care crises—like 'Shall we pull the plug?' Religion has most to offer in terms of long-term care, of sustained relations, where year in and year out people have to be motivated to take care." Congregations exist for that, and the parish nurse program helps them realize such care intelligently.

In a way, the invention of the parish nurse concept is part of several revolutions going on before our eyes but hard to define and grasp.

First, it is part of a revolution in the understanding of health and medicine. For two centuries we had been moving, usually unwittingly but sometimes wittingly, into accepting the model—as jargon has it, "paradigm"—that believed only conventional science could cure. Invest enough in research, make enough discoveries, develop enough professionals, build enough institutions, spend enough money, show enough awe, and such science would take care of our problems.

Today, that model or paradigm is very much in question, not least among many scientists, researchers, discoverers, professionals, institution builders, and appropriators. They are coming to recognize that humans have or are "healing systems," which come into positive effect only when they are seen in the context of the larger systems around them. Westberg reminds us that the parish nurse program was nurtured initially by a hospital that believes in human ecology. Believing thus, it promotes the idea that we humans have to be seen in the delicate web and fibers of our context, which includes God, nature, others, and the self.

Of course, the search for a new paradigm can lead to many devices or prescriptions that can delude and misuse people. Some uses of the term "holistic," for instance, are connected to ideas that connect the individual to the universe, its forces and energies, in such a way that the individual is "part of God" or "becomes God" or is offered complete transcendence of suffering and care. Often, this goes by the code word "New Age" holistic care. Without needing to contend that nothing good comes from disciplines connected with such an approach, we can observe its limits. People do keep suffering, falling ill, and dying in spite of their beliefs of that sort—or, for that matter, their belief in the God beyond the gods who is the Creator, the Healer, the One who cares and weeps with us on the path to fulfillment.

The parish nurse concept is born in an entirely different context of "whole person" care. It knows that in congregations people hear messages and try to realize them, messages directed to a world in which hate and misery, limits and pain, doubt and despair threaten almost as much as love and joy, boundary-breaking and pleasure, faith and hope are promised and realized.

Not many seasons ago, I presented an essay by a Christian neurosurgeon to a secular group of physicians, humanists, and social scientists. He told what the service of "Christ crucified" meant to him when he interpreted his vocation, his life in respect to patients. Of course, the author reminded readers, he stayed within the bounds of his profession and kept the physician's convenant that one keeps in a pluralist society. That is, while he may use "invasive" techniques in brain surgery, he is not "invasive" in respect to patients' belief systems, not disruptive of their patterns, not ready to be distracted from what they have sought by coming to him. It was a nice, important distinction, without which he could not function and help in healing.

One of the participants in the group spoke up in response. I suppose one who wanted to stereotype him would call him a latter-day Marxist social scientist. That is, he uses Marxist techniques of social analysis to call into question the professions and structures of our society. (He does have a good mind, and does not offer Marxian therapy, simply "socialized" care at this late date.) But he spoke up for others in the group when he said he hoped that the surgeon was not engaging in a new version of the body-mind distinction. That is, when this Christian deals with the body, he is nothing but a scientist, and when he deals with the mind, his mind, he is a believer. Without spelling out *how,* this professor said he hoped *that* the physician was more whole person oriented. He should use his faith to engage in critical analysis of how his profession works and through what institutions he works and toward what end they are all directed.

This is not the place to follow up on what all that means and can mean. It is the place to remind ourselves that, in even the most apparently remote corners of "scientific" and "academic" life, thoughtful people are giving second thoughts to the place of faith in the provision of health care. It may take a few minutes to work such people around to understanding the vital role of congregations in the ecology of the lives of half of America. It may take a few hours to help them come to see the promise of the parish nurse program in respect to that role. This book will certainly help in such tasks.

Most readers, however, are not going to be Marxist sociologists, scientific skeptics, secularists whose spiritual imaginations have atrophied (if they were ever given a spiritual vision at all). Most readers will be nurses and pastors, church committees and, one hopes, theologians, people whose vision has not yet been caught. They are people for whom constraints of time and money will be in the front of the mind but in whose hearts the Holy Spirit, who "calls, gathers, and enlightens" the congregation, is also active.

One of the great advantages of parish nurse work, in contrast to that of the neurosurgeon in a high-tech hospital or the employee in a tax-supported institution, is that nurses work in a context where certain meanings are allowed to be developed explicitly. Theologian James Fouler has written on the two languages of pluralist society. On one level, out of respect for each other, in a spirit of tolerance and deference, to keep civil peace, we do not always "unload" the whole focused theme of our beliefs. Often we may feel that those beliefs could be of direct aid to someone else. Still, the rules of the game call for some holding back. For example, one doesn't enter into an interfaith dialogue and then suddenly change the rules of the game midway and try to pounce on partners with pitches for conversion.

At the same time, says Fouler (I am rephrasing a bit), sometimes this situation makes us feel as if we are biting our tongues, choking to hold back what we might utter, holding our breaths, or stepping cautiously because we know there is a particular story, a special language of faith, a distinctive grasp of God's grace, which would be of greater aid than the language we would elsewhere use.

The parish nurse program works chiefly in congregations or communities where a certain language of faith is ready at hand. This does not mean that the nurse becomes a preacher or has to be an explicit teacher or a theological expert. It means that she or he knows that one's individual faith story is privileged and not only can be brought up but is expected to have its place. It means that the nurse works in an ecology of meanings and care that asks her to draw on that message of grace and the practices and habits it encourages.

One of the rules of etiquette for writers of introductions is that they should not give the plot away. There were many times, as I read this manuscript, that I wanted to steal more than the single Westberg story of his encounters with finance committees, to lure readers on, but these authors can and do speak for themselves. One of my marginal notes on the manuscript of a practical essay in this book—and there are several—is "these authors think of everything." This is "how to" literature of a high order. Maybe what makes it all hold together is that it is also "why to" literature. We have needed that and will need it if we accept the "risk" about which Westberg speaks and dreams. We might risk helping discover and invent something new in human care at a time of great need, when hearts grow faint but the message of God in Christ does not.

Rev. Martin E. Marty, Ph.D.
University of Chicago

Preface

This book represents the work of many. Several of the authors are pioneers. Others offer their perspective, passion, and expertise in forwarding the ongoing development of parish nursing. The editors, through their relationships with the chapter authors, intend to address those who are interested in learning more about the concept of parish nursing. This book could be used as a text for parish nursing coursework, as well as introductory reading for health professionals, clergy, and lay leaders of congregations. The content should be of interest to any nurse interested in innovative, community-based practice.

The concept of parish nursing is not new. Deaconesses and other religious men and women worked as part of the early church, nurturing health and healing. However, it was only in 1984 that Rev. Granger Westberg, who first had the idea of parish nursing, approached Lutheran General Hospital in Park Ridge, Illinois about initiating a pilot parish nurse program. Six nurses in six churches representing different denominations began to implement Westberg's vision. Thus a portion of the writing reflects the influence of this Illinois experience. In spite of this Midwest Christian beginning and the brief time period, parish nurses can be found internationally, serving both Christian and non-Christian faith communities.

Terminology and language present a challenge. The gathering place for faith communities has many titles. Congregation, church, parish, temple, synagogue, and mosque are but a few of the names that identify these gathering spaces. The roots of parish nursing grow from a Christian perspective, and the text reflects this dynamic. There is no intent to ignore, exclude, diminish, or deny any faith, beliefs, traditions, or orientation. The term "parish nursing" was the name given by Rev. Granger Westberg to describe this concept. From a historical and societal perspective, other names, such as "congregational nurse" or "pastoral nurse," are used today. These titles represent the intent of parish nursing. The pronoun *she* is used when referring to the parish nurse, as the overwhelming majority of individuals serving in this role are female.

At the inception of parish nursing, the concept of the congregation as a health place was not well understood; however, there was a willingness to experiment and resources available to dedicate to pioneering this program. Today, with an emphasis on healthier

communities, there is better understanding of and openness to the role of the congregation in health and the contribution of parish nursing. Unfortunately, increased demands
on dwindling resources strain dedication to the growth and support of this program. Lack
of documentation systems and research inhibit understanding of the outcomes and true
value of parish nursing to the transformation of health care delivery.

This book is divided into four sections. Part I addresses the unique modern-day
history of parish nursing. Included are chapters that represent several perspectives: that
of Rev. Granger Westberg, who had the original idea; that of those who have had the
privilege of working very closely with him throughout the ongoing development of the
movement; and that of those who have pioneered this role in various geographic and
cultural settings. In Part II, parish nursing is discussed as being most effective when
health ministry is intricately woven into the corporate life of the faith community. For
this to occur, the parish nurse must understand that the congregation is a workplace where
the mission of health and wellness gradually unfolds through the collective gifts and
work of all parties. This second section is dedicated to these basic understandings. Part
III highlights the parish nurse's work with multiple dimensions of life, nursing practice,
and knowledge bases. This section of the book explores some of these important
considerations. For the continuous learner, the chapters in Part III provide only highlights of each subject area, identifying a framework for more in-depth study. Part IV
speaks to the challenges that are present in these early stages of the development of parish
nursing: the expansion of the parish nurse concept internationally, areas for future study,
and questions yet unanswered. The ongoing integrity of this practice will depend on
client consideration, continuous dialogue, creative thinking, and the grace of God.

There are a number of acknowledgments to be made. The editors first of all want to
thank Rev. Granger Westberg for his creativity, tenacity, and inspiring leadership. The
initial administrative leadership for the pilot of this program from Lutheran General
Hospital needs to be recognized for their spirit of openness to the Westberg vision:
George B. Caldwell, former President and Chief Executive Officer; Rev. L. James Wylie,
Vice President of Church Relations; and Rev. Larry Holst, Director of Pastoral Care.
Special acknowledgment is given to Anne Marie Djupe, R.N.,C., M.A., who was the first
Director of Parish Nursing Services for Lutheran General HealthSystem. Anne Marie
was a treasured colleague and friend; she died in 1995. Appreciation is given for the
current support provided to the International Parish Nurse Resource Center of Advocate
Health Care, the successor organization to Lutheran General HealthSystem. Through
this vehicle many of the relationships undergirding the development of this text were
worked out. Particular thanks are given to Richard Risk, President and Chief Executive
Officer, and Rev. L. James Wylie, Senior Vice President for Religion and Health, of
Advocate Health Care for their endorsement of the vision and their commitment to parish
nursing. The editors express their gratitude to each of the contributors who were so
generous in sharing their knowledge and experience. Special thanks go to Annette
Mariani, Rusty McDermott, Denise Dowling, and Audrey Munger for their patience and
persistence in typing and meeting deadlines as well as their dedication to parish nursing.
Thanks also go to Sage Publications for believing in this project.

There are also some individual acknowledgments to be made. Phyllis Ann Solari-
Twadell expresses her gratitude to her daughter and son-in-law, Kim and David Kuhl-
man, and her stepson and his wife, Eric and Anne Twadell, for their love, encouragement,

and support. Ann expresses her ongoing appreciation to her mother, Phyllis Solari, and her deceased father, Archie J. Solari, for the opportunities they provided for her. In addition, Ann acknowledges the contributions her brothers Joseph and Robert Solari have made to her life. She thanks John S. Klein and Rev. John Keller for the gracious direction they provided to her. Individually, she is grateful for the teaching and guidance provided by Rev. L. James Wylie. Her contribution to this work is dedicated in thanksgiving for the life, love, and support of her late husband, Stephen Lacombe Twadell.

Mary Ann McDermott thanks her husband Dennis and her children, Dennis, Michael, Sarah, and William, for facilitating her interest in the parish nurse role. She thanks her former dean, Dr. Julia Lane; her present dean, Dr. Shirley Dooling; and her colleagues at Loyola University School of Nursing, particularly Ida Androwich and Mary Lynch, who were essential in the initial development of the program at St. Ignatius Parish, and to the faculty, students, pastors, and parishioners who have continued to make the program flourish. She is delighted to have been affiliated with the former Lutheran General Health Care System as a member of the system and hospital governance and current involvement in the governance of Advocate Health Care. She was a member of the previous Advisory Committee of the National Parish Nurse Resource Center.

Finally, we want to thank all parish nurses past and present who have worked hard preserving this role in their faith communities. May God bless you all!

Phyllis Ann Solari-Twadell, R.N., M.S.N., M.P.A.
International Parish Nurse Resource Center
Park Ridge, Illinois

Mary Ann McDermott, R.N., Ed.D.
Marcella Niehoff School of Nursing
Loyola University of Chicago

I

PARISH NURSING

An Overview of the Practice

1

The Emerging Practice
of Parish Nursing

Phyllis Ann Solari-Twadell

Parish nursing is a health promotion, disease prevention role based on the care of the whole person and encompassing seven functions. These functions are integrator of faith and health, health educator, personal health counselor, referral agent, trainer of volunteers, developer of support groups, and health advocate. This nursing role does not embrace the medical model of care or invasive practices such as blood drawing, medical treatments, or maintenance of intravenous products. It is a professional model of health ministry using a registered professional nurse. The focus for the practice is the faith community and its ministry (McDermott & Burke, 1993).

Philosophy of Parish Nursing

Study of the *Philosophy for Parish Nursing* (see Appendix A) provides an excellent way to respond further to the question "What is parish nursing?" (Solari-Twadell, McDermott, Ryan, & Djupe, 1994). A philosophy is a particular system or set of beliefs about the nature of something. It serves as a compass for identifying the meaning, important elements, and development of the phenomena under discussion: in this case, parish nursing.

The first key statement in the philosophy is "Parish nursing holds the spiritual dimension to be central to the practice. It also encompasses the physical, psychological, and social dimensions of nursing practice." This statement indicates how the time of the nurse is to be spent. It calls the nurse to tend to the whole person but to pay special attention to the spiritual dimension of the individual. This being the focus of the role, it begins to shape the knowledge and skills required by a nurse practicing in this role. The pastoral dimensions of nursing care are emphasized, with particular attention to the spiritual maturity of the nurse. This begins to distinguish the practice from the traditional community health nurse and to set the parameters of the role.

The second key statement is "The parish nurse role balances knowledge with skill, the sciences with theology and with the humanities, service with worship, and nursing care functions with pastoral care functions. The historic roots of the role are intertwined with those of monks and nuns, deacons and deaconesses, church nurses, traditional healers, and the nursing profession itself." The implications of this statement are that balance is a key concept for the parish nurse. It emphasizes how the nurse in this role will need to balance self-development, self-care, and caring for others. Also emphasized is the way in which the parish nurse has feet in religion and medicine, in faith and health, and in the arts and sciences. This statement alludes to the fact that even if this nursing role is new for this time, it has deep roots in many faith traditions. It also calls attention to the parish nurse's need for ongoing professional development.

The third key statement reads "The focus of practice is the faith community and its ministry. The parish nurse, in collaboration with the pastoral staff and congregational members, participates in the ongoing transformation of the faith community into a source of health and healing. Through partnership with other community health resources, parish nursing fosters new and creative responses to health concerns." This statement implies that, unlike traditional nursing, in which the client is an individual, and also unlike community health nursing, in which the client is an external community, the parish nurse's client is primarily the faith community. The parish nurse is not intended to be an "appendage" ministry for the congregation; she functions as part of the congregation's ministerial team. Integral to the life and work of the faith community, the parish nurse interfaces with all the committees and groups in the faith community. Integration and collaboration are primary terms that are inherent to this practice. Through this ministry, the congregation begins to be linked to other agencies, services, and programs through-out the external community in ways never anticipated. Just as the parish nurse program connects, it also is intended to be a catalyst for change within the faith community. The parish nurse program mirrors the dynamic nature of health and encourages the corporate health of the congregation to reflect the ever changing health and healing mission of the faith community.

The fourth key statement reads "Parish nursing services are designed to build on and strengthen the capacities of individuals, families, and congregations to understand and care for one another in the light of their relationship to God, faith traditions, themselves, and the broader society. The practice holds that all persons are sacred and must be treated with respect and dignity. In response to this belief, the parish nurse assists and empowers individuals to become more active partners in the management of their personal health resources." This statement highlights a partnership relationship with those being served. The parish nurse is not considered the expert but the facilitator, counselor, educator, referral source, developer, trainer, and advocate. The care of the whole person is defined "in the light of their relationship to God, faith traditions, themselves, and the broader society." The parish nurse is called to assist the parishioner in learning new attitudes and skills to make it possible for parishioners to be better health consumers. This is a most important function. With all the fast-paced changes in health care, the consumer often gets confused and lost. Interfacing with a health system often demands new and different attitudes, as well as skills, on the part of the consumer. Who will help consumers clarify their personal definition of health, values they have related to health, and how to live these values out in a society that often provides conflicting messages? If not the church, who? Finally, this statement calls for a recognition of the sacred nature of the person and the value of being in service to another.

In the fifth key statement, "The parish nurse understands health to be a dynamic process that embodies the spiritual, psychological, physical, and social dimensions of the person. Spiritual health is central to well-being and influences a person's entire being. Therefore, a sense of well-being and illness may occur simultaneously. Healing may exist in the absence of cure." This statement emphasizes that the concept of health means different things to different people. It is important, then, to clarify with individuals what is meant when the term health is used. Health changes, sometimes gradually, subtly, over time, and sometimes dramatically, quickly. Again, the spiritual nature of health is emphasized, along with the fact that one may be spiritually well and physically ill. This is in concert with the understanding that a person may not be able to be cured of his or her disease, but healing may occur in his or her life.

Once the nature of the parish nurse role is understood, it is clear that to introduce traditional nursing tasks as a part of this role would leave no time to develop the client relationship within which the spiritual, emotional, and psychosocial aspects of the individual can be explored; spend the necessary time to "multiply the ministers" in training volunteers; or develop support groups to reach groups of like-minded people in the congregation.

Models of Organizational Frameworks for Parish Nursing

In 1984, when Granger Westberg approached Lutheran General Hospital to investigate this institution's interest in piloting parish nursing, he had an organizing framework in mind (Djupe, Olson, & Ryan, 1994). This framework included a contractual arrangement between a hospital and a congregation or multiple congregations, a paid position for the nurse that included employment by a health care institution and reimbursement by the congregation for the nurse's salary, a prescribed selection process for the nurse, and ongoing continuing education and supervision by the hospital for the parish nurse (Holst, 1987). As parish nursing has continued to grow across this country and internationally, different kinds of organizing frameworks have emerged to fit the needs of the faith communities and communities at large. Each of these organizational frameworks is designed to facilitate the actualization of the parish nurse role. Appendix B includes tables that identify the discriminating features of the four basic models of organizational frameworks.

For the purposes of this chapter, the term *institution* is meant to include a hospital, health care system, home care agency, long-term care facility, health maintenance organization, school of nursing, a community coalition that has incorporated, public health department, hospice, and/or seminary. Although there are four basic models of the organizational framework of parish nursing described, there are already variations from these frameworks, such as the team model of parish nursing (Conrad, 1995), which is derived from the congregational unpaid organizational framework. In the team model, each nurse puts in small amounts of time in her specialized area of interest. Most important for this model is a well-developed infrastructure to support and ensure the stability of the program. It is anticipated that as communities of faith design parish nurse programs, other variations may surface. One of the strengths of parish nursing is the flexibility in the design. As different faith communities begin to integrate parish nursing into the life of their congregations, different kinds of organizing frameworks emerge.

No matter how a parish nurse program is organized, there are certain issues that need to be addressed, such as: Will there be partners involved, such as multiple churches and a health care institution? Who will they be? What resources will each partner contribute to the partnership? What will the primary accountability for the parish nurse be? What process will be used for the selection of the nurse? How will basic preparation in parish nursing be provided for the nurse? Who will supervise the orientation of the nurse? How will physician consultation be provided for this parish nurse? Will the nurse be reimbursed for travel when visiting homebound members of the church? Where will the office space for the nurse be located in the church? How will the parish nurse's phone be managed in her absence? How will this ministry interface with other ministries already functioning in the congregation? It is clear that no matter what the framework, sufficient planning must take place to ensure long-term success of the program. A matrix of issues to be considered in the planning and development of a parish nurse program is included in Appendix C for use by those implementing and in the process of developing parish nurse programs.

Pros and Cons of
Different Organizational Frameworks

Which organizational framework is the best? Some would say that, of course, the paid model is the best—and there is merit in that position. Others would be quite offended at that response, as the unpaid model is already providing a much needed service to their congregation members. The answer to the question lies not so much in the particulars of the model as in how each model is managed, integrated, and monitored. The following are important considerations in choosing an organizational framework for the administration of a parish nurse program:

1. The mind-set of the pastor and leadership of the health institution. Is the pastor and/or the chief executive officer of the institution able to provide the necessary leadership to foster the integration of the parish nurse ministry into the life of the faith community as well as the health care institution, or do the pastor and/or chief executive officer think it is a good idea and if you as a nurse would like to do this, it is OK? In the latter case, endorsement will be received but not necessarily sponsorship. The mind-set and position of the pastor and institutional leader(s) can provide limitless opportunity or can ultimately contribute to the demise of the program.

2. The willingness of the congregation and health care institution to embrace change. The parish nurse is a catalyst for change within the faith community as well as within the health care institution. This role provides the congregation and health care institution with a constant reminder of the health and healing mission of the congregation and each member's need to be a good steward of personal health resources. As health and health care changes, the parish nurse as catalyst calls the faith community and health care institution to be dynamic and to embrace the possibilities that are present in transformation.

3. The ability of the congregation and health care institution to dedicate resources to the mission of health and healing over the long term. This can range from dedication of funds to paying the full salary to, in an unpaid model, providing operating funds for the program. This relates to how well the mission of health and healing can be integrated into the life of the faith community and health care institution. If the development of the parish nurse program has to be reviewed by the finance committee of the congregation and is included in the operational budget of the health care institution, with specific funds dedicated, there will have to be an understanding of what this program will contribute to the life of the congregation.

4. The selection process that is available to choose the parish nurse. Selection of the parish nurse can be one of the most important ingredients in assuring the overall success of a parish nurse program. Congregations are not used to interviewing health care professionals, much less ones that are intended to provide whole person care. Consultation from those who have expertise in this area will be important. Just because a congregation has a nurse who worships regularly does not mean that this nurse has the spiritual maturity, competence, or skills to manage a parish nurse role.

5. Development of the necessary infrastructure to support the long-term integration of the parish nurse program. This applies to both the congregation and health care institution. Both agencies need to identify program placement and what the reporting relationships will be for the parish nurse. This necessitates clarity regarding regular evaluation of the nurse and the program, the management of market and merit increases for the nurse if paid, and provision of nursing and pastoral supervision, as well as ongoing continuing education.

6. Integration of the parish nurse program into the strategic plan of the health care institution and the goals and objectives of the faith community. If the parish nurse program is included in the organizational plans of the health care institution and/or the congregation, it will be difficult for the program to be eliminated if personnel changes. At least, if alterations are considered in the program, they are less likely to be at the discretion of one or two individuals or be the result of having the nurse or pastor leave and thus having the program cease.

These few points are but a beginning in determining which framework of parish nursing would serve best in the faith community under discussion. Others will surface as the faith community engages in the planning and study of this ministry. The more thorough the study and preparation up front, the more a successful outcome is assured.

Issues Related to the Planning and Development
of a Parish Nurse Program

Educate! Educate! Educate!

The first step in initiating the planning for a parish nurse program in a congregation is to discuss this interest with the pastor of the congregation. This may require educating the pastor on the concept of parish nursing and the congregation as a health place in the community (Solari-Twadell, 1997). It is important that the pastor not only endorse the exploration of this ministry for the congregation but take a part in the initial planning stages of the program.

The initial exploration begins with the study of health ministry. This will be an important beginning for any subcommittee or committee within the church. It will provide an opportunity for members of the group to learn what constitutes a health ministry and how health ministry supports the overall mission of the congregation and for the congregation to identify what it may already be doing that can be considered health ministry (Westberg, 1997). By engaging in this kind of study and exploration, this group will gain a better understanding of where the congregation is currently in regard to health ministry and be able to create a vision of where it would like to be in the future. It is then time for the group to begin to consider the possibilities of parish nursing. What would a parish nurse have to offer the faith community in terms of enhancing the health ministry? It is important to acknowledge that a "Minister of Health" does not have to be a nurse. Other health professionals or laypeople in the congregation who have an understanding of whole-person health, prevention, and health promotion and have skills in education and counseling may be ministers of health. However, a minister of health who is a parish nurse is a registered professional nurse. The skills, knowledge, experience, and basic preparation in parish nursing enhance the manner in which the health ministry can be developed within the life of the faith community. The capacities of the parish nurse are very well addressed in "Twelve Beatitudes for Parish Nursing" (see Appendix D).

Education is a priority throughout the life of a parish nurse program within a congregation. New members join the faith community, lay leaders rotate in and out of positions, and pastors come and go. This kind of dynamic congregational life calls for ongoing education. It can never be assumed by a parish nurse that the faith community no longer needs to have ongoing education about the parish nurse ministry within the faith community. The parish nurse ministry will grow and change with the dynamic nature of the congregation. Ongoing education about the nature of those changes is important to members' understanding of what resources are available through the parish nurse ministry.

When an institution plans to be a partner with a congregation in initiating a parish nurse program, there is also quite a bit of educating that needs to be done within the institution. Certainly sponsorship by the chief executive officer of the institution is needed, and this may require some education as to the advantages of developing partnerships with congregations in the community. The following identify a few of the positive outcomes for an institution to consider as it moves ahead in establishing these relationships with congregations:

1. A congregation's mission, no matter what the denomination, is that of health and salvation. The congregation is in the business of helping people to live their lives better. If the institution is interested in maintaining and sustaining the health and well-being of the community, partnering with a faith community with this mutual goal in mind makes sense.

2. Parish nursing is a concrete way for an institution to be socially accountable to the community it serves. Through supporting the development of a parish nurse program, the institution is able to funnel its resources in a practical way to members of the faith community and members of the community at large.

3. Supporting the initiation of a parish nurse program in a faith community allows the health care institution to be involved with people in their episodes of wellness as well as their episodes of illness. The institution has the ability to develop relationships with people in the community through the congregation before they ever need acute care services.

4. Congregations are voluntary organizations. People who are members of faith communities are often looking for ways to be of service to their neighbors. Parish nurses, through the expansion of health ministry in a congregation, identify skills and talents of members of the church and match these skills and talents with the needs exhibited by others in the congregation. In this day of shortened hospital stays and employment of both spouses, having volunteers who can provide respite care, meals, and visitation can be important to successful recovery for some. Institutions such as hospitals or health care systems are fortunate when they have a network of parish nurses that their discharge planners can work with in facilitating return-home arrangements for a patient.

5. Institutions struggle to supporting consumers in becoming more responsible for their own health. Congregations as agencies of personal transformation can assist their members to gain the mind-set of being better stewards of their personal health resources. Through education and personal health counseling, the parish nurse can assist members in preparing advance directives. A parish nurse can help members of the faith community to make important decisions about the use of health resources in the hospitals and clinics in the community, thus referring people to the most appropriate resource.

6. Parish nurses increase access to care earlier in the disease process. Thus, by reaching people earlier in their illness, often a less costly intervention or level of care can be used. This can be important for institutions interested in cost savings or managing an illness pattern in the most cost-effective way.

7. Through supporting the development of parish nursing services in partnership with congregations, institutions have a direct link to assessing the needs as well as the assets of the community. Through documentation of parish nurses' assessments and interventions, institutions have more direct information about the members they are to serve in the community. If the institution is a school of nursing, development of a parish nurse program can provide unique clinical sites for students in learning about an innovative way to provide health promotion and disease prevention services to members of the community. As with the congregation, continuing education is needed for the institution so that employees are aware of what relationships are being formed with faith

communities and how these partnerships are affecting the members of the faith community and community at large.

Organizational Approval

Once health ministry has been explored in the congregation and parish nursing has been recommended by the initial investigating group, discussion and endorsement by the pastor is essential. In addition, there needs to be approval from the congregation's lay leadership group, whether that is the church council, board of elders, or ministerial board. This is another opportunity to educate the church leadership and begin the discussion of what resources will be needed for this ministry, as well as how it will enhance the present health ministry within the congregation. This step also begins the creation of the infrastructure for the parish nurse program. Discussion will need to take place about how this program will interface with existing organizational structures and committees within the congregation. Without this kind of discussion and endorsement, the parish nurse program has the potential to become a person- or group-owned ministry rather than a congregation-supported and -endorsed ministry. Similarly, for the institution that may be partnering with a church in the development of a parish nurse program, it is necessary to have organizational approval and resources allocated for the development of the parish nurse program. This organizational approval at the highest level is key to the integration of the parish nurse program into the strategic planning of the institution.

Creation of an Infrastructure

The establishment of infrastructure supports the functional integration and the longevity of a parish nurse program within the faith community. The essence of functional integration is functional processes of a program situated so that they provide for the servicing of all members of the faith community in a coordinated manner. Functional integration is the extent to which key support functions and activities are coordinated across an organization, adding greater overall value to the system (Shortell, Gillies, Anderson, Erickson, & Mitchell, 1996, p. 57). When thoughtful consideration is given by a group educated about parish nursing to the best placement and reporting relationship of a parish nurse program, there is a commitment being made by the faith community. This commitment communicates to the members of the congregation that the faith community is the place that will help people live their lives better, make better decisions about their health on a daily basis, and become better stewards of health resources from a communal perspective. This happens when there is an infrastructure that supports the message regarding the stewardship of health being integrated into all that the congregation does.

It is the same for the institution partnering with congregations in the community to develop parish nurse programs: An adequate infrastructure needs to be in place within the institution so that resourcing of the parish nurses and enhancement of these congregational relationships can occur. Holst (1987) recommends the development of a steering committee and faculty to assist the organization in adequately supervising and educating the nurses as well as contributing to the ongoing planning for the development of the parish nurse program. The purpose of a steering committee is to function in an advisory capacity. The membership of this committee or work group may vary; however, significant managers who will be instrumental to the work of developing a parish nurse program are usually appointed or asked to participate. The members of a steering committee may include managers from human resources, public relations, legal, nursing, pastoral care, finance, community outreach, marketing, the philanthropic foundation, and the medical staff. In addition, one or two pastors from the community may be asked to participate. Initially, the work of this group is more internally focused, dealing with the development of contracts, position descriptions, policies, and procedures. After the first few years, the steering committee may meet only quarterly or twice a year and advise on the progress of the program. There may also be a decision to disband this group once the parish nurse program is well integrated into the strategic plan of the institution.

A second addition to the infrastructure of a parish nurse program in an institution is a faculty. The faculty assists in planning the continuing education programming for the parish nurse and may also assist in the interviewing of parish nurse candidates. The membership of this group is small, with participation from nursing, medicine, and pastoral care. Members of the faculty may also be members of the steering committee. The members of the faculty are available to the parish nurses on a regular basis.

Establishment of Ongoing Financial Support

Early in the development of a parish nurse program, both from the congregational and institutional perspective, there must be clarification of what financial resources are going to be dedicated to the parish nurse program. For the congregation, this means that there will need to be serious dialogue regarding the ongoing financing of the parish nurse program. At the very least, it means the creation of a line item named "parish nurse program" in the congregation budget.

From the beginning of the institution's discussion of the parish nurse program, the development of ongoing financial support has to be integral to the dialogue and planning. For those institutions that have a philanthropic foundation, personnel from the foundation should be included in the planning.

Advertising for the Parish Nurse

Regardless of the organizational model that is developed, there should be a conscious effort to seek out the best nurse for the parish nurse position. Many times a pastor learning of the parish nurse concept may know of a nurse in the congregation. This person may, with little thought of qualifications, be asked to be the parish nurse. In another scenario, a nurse in the congregation becomes excited about this concept for her church and pursues not only the initiation and development of the parish nurse ministry for the faith community but a role for herself. This method of selection may eliminate the possibility of finding the best nurse for the parish nurse position.

Most often, the best place to advertise for parish nurse positions is in church bulletins or local nursing publications. Nurses are usually present in churches and often already volunteering in many different capacities within their congregations. Seeking viable candidates using church bulletins is often a very cost-effective manner in which to attract the best parish nurse candidate.

Selection of the Parish Nurse

No matter what organizational model is chosen, it is necessary to determine a process for the selection of the parish nurse. Whether the nurse is paid or unpaid should not make a difference in the parish nurse selection process. The recommended format for selection is a series of interviews. These interviews follow verification of the minimal requirements for the position: a current registered nurse license and recent nursing experience. It is preferable that the nurse have a baccalaureate preparation in nursing because of the basic educational preparation this affords in community health. The interview process should include questions that will result in information about the spiritual maturity of the candidate, the level of communication skills, flexibility, whether the candidate is a self-starter and an independent worker, as well as creativity, the ability to maintain a sense of humor, experience with health promotion and disease prevention programming, and whether there is a compatibility with the belief structure, culture, and pastor of the congregation.

Installation of the Parish Nurse

The formal installation of the nurse selected to serve as the parish nurse is an important ingredient in the recognition of this health ministry in the congregation. It is also an opportunity to introduce the new parish nurse. This installation can be part of a regular Sunday service, or a special service can be held just for the installation. Whichever is selected, it is helpful if a reception follows so that members of the congregation will have the opportunity to meet the new parish nurse. When an institution partners with the faith community, it is important that there is representation from the institution at the installation. If appropriate, a representative from the health institution may even participate formally in the event.

Basic Preparation and Orientation of the Parish Nurse

It is important that the parish nurse have basic preparation in parish nursing. Basic preparation includes at least 30 hours of continuing education as part of an endorsed parish nurse basic preparation course as described in chapter 24. In addition, the nurse will need to participate in an orientation. Orientation takes place at the site of practice. The nurse will, during orientation, have access to the history of the congregation, meet other staff members, and learn the nature of the ministries they are accountable for in the congregation. In addition, the parish nurse will meet with each of the committees and groups in the church, not only to learn who they are and what they are doing, but to introduce the parish nurse program and herself. If there is an institution that is part of the initiation and ongoing development of the parish nurse program, there needs to be an orientation for the nurse to that institution. Time should be scheduled with each of the faculty members, so the parish nurse can learn who they are and what resources they may offer the parish nurse program. Key services that the parish nurse may be interfacing with on a regular basis may also be included as part of the orientation schedule. In addition, the new parish nurse should be scheduled to meet and spend time with other parish nurses in the network supported by the institution.

Clarification and Communication of Parish Nurse Program Goals

Different people will have different understandings of what the parish nurse program is intended to provide for the faith community. For this reason, it is important that the goals and objectives of the parish nurse program be developed in conjunction with a health and wellness committee or other sponsoring group within the congregation. Once these goals and objectives are developed, they should be reviewed and endorsed by the pastor and shared with the membership of the congregation. It is only through this kind of congregational endorsement and communication that clear understanding of the intention and purpose of this health ministry will occur.

Providing for Ongoing Visibility and Integration of the Parish Nurse Program

The parish nurse ministry is intended to be intricately involved in the life of the faith community. This begins with the parish nurse being a member of the ministerial team within the congregation, which provides an opportunity for whole person health and wellness to be considered in every dimension of congregational life. Through fostering good working relationships with the pastor and members of the staff, the parish nurse often becomes a resource to them in addressing personal health and wellness issues in their lives. In addition, collegial relationships are developed in which there is comfort in referring individuals to each other rather than seeing the parish nurse as someone that is going to infringe on the "turf" of another staff member. Where clear understanding of each staff member's skills, gifts, functions, and responsibilities are continually being clarified, good working relationships are the result. These kinds of relationships encourage others to hold up the visibility of the parish nurse role; they relieve her of having to do all her own publicizing.

Regular use of the church bulletin and newsletter is another way to keep the profile of the parish nurse ministry high in the life of the congregation. Some parish nurses find the use of a bulletin board or posters with health and wellness information another avenue for drawing attention to this health ministry (Kindelsperger, 1996).

Summary

Regardless of the organizational framework chosen, there is a need for sufficient planning for the integration of this health ministry into the life of the congregation. Appendix E shows a timeline for the development of a parish nurse program, identifying the issues previously discussed. It is far better to take the necessary time to be thorough in planning than to quickly initiate a program that has little integration, financial support, or endorsement. Such a program may struggle to provide the intended outcomes, which can be a great disappointment to all. The development of a workable parish nurse program is not done quickly or in isolation. Many people can participate in the creation of this ministry, and this requires time. The most important developer is God. Appendix F, a favorite writing by an unknown author, describes how interesting a partner God can be.

References

Conrad, D. M. (1995). Team nursing in parish nurse ministry: Even Jesus had 12 apostles. In *Proceedings of the Ninth Annual Westberg Parish Nurse Symposium: "Parish nursing: Ministering through the arts."* Park Ridge, IL: International Parish Nurse Resource Center.

Djupe, A. M., Olson, H., & Ryan, J. A. (1994). *Reaching out: Parish nursing services* (2nd ed). Park Ridge, IL: Lutheran General HealthSystem.

Holst, L. E. (1987). The parish nurse. *Chronicle of Pastoral Care, 7*(1), 13-17.

Kindelsperger, M. L. (1996). Launch the spirit. In *Proceedings of the Tenth Annual Westberg Parish Nurse Symposium: "Parish nursing: A celebration of health, healing and wholeness."* Park Ridge, IL: International Parish Nurse Resource Center.

McDermott, M. A., & Burke, J. (1993). When the population is a congregation: The emerging role of the parish nurse. *Journal of Community Health Nursing, 10*(3), 179-190.

Shortell, S. M., Gillies, R. R., Anderson, D. A., Erickson, K. M., & Mitchell, J. B. (1996). *Remaking health care in America: Building organized delivery systems.* San Francisco: Jossey-Bass.

Solari-Twadell, A., McDermott, M. A., Ryan, J. A. & Djupe, A. M. (Eds). (1994). *Assuring viability for the future: Guideline development for parish nurse education programs.* Park Ridge, IL: Lutheran General HealthSystem.

Solari-Twadell, P. A. (1997). The caring congregation: A healing place. *Journal of Christian Nursing, 14*(1), 4-9.

Westberg, J. (1997). *The health cabinet* (2nd ed). Park Ridge, IL: International Parish Nurse Resource Center.

APPENDIX A
Statement of Philosophy for Parish Nursing

Parish nursing is an emerging area of specialized professional nursing practice distinguished by the following characteristics:

- Parish nursing holds the spiritual dimension to be central to the practice. It also encompasses the physical, psychological, and social dimensions of nursing practice.

- The parish nurse role balances knowledge with skill, the sciences with theology and with the humanities, service with worship, and nursing care functions with pastoral care functions. The historic roots of the role are intertwined with those of monks and nuns, deacons and deaconesses, church nurses, traditional healers, and the nursing profession itself.

- The focus of practice is the faith community and its ministry. The parish nurse, in collaboration with the pastoral staff and congregational members, participates in the ongoing transformation of the faith community into a source of health and healing. Through partnership with other community health resources, parish nursing fosters new and creative responses to health concerns.

- Parish nursing services are designed to build on and strengthen the capacities of individuals, families, and congregations to understand and care for one another in the light of their relationship to God, faith traditions, themselves, and the broader society. The practice holds that all persons are sacred and must be treated with respect and dignity. In response to this belief, the parish nurse assists and empowers individuals to become more active partners in the management of their personal health resources.

- The parish nurse understands health to be a dynamic process that embodies the spiritual, psychological, physical, and social dimensions of the person. Spiritual health is central to well-being and influences a person's entire being. Therefore, a sense of well-being and illness may occur simultaneously. Healing may exist in the absence of cure.

The providers of educational preparation for the practice of parish nursing acknowledge that

- preparation for specialized practice and research is at the graduate level.

- the professional standard for entry into professional practice is preparation at the baccalaureate level.

- they are engaged in education for professional development of parish nurses who are prepared at a variety of entry levels—both into nursing and into parish nursing practice.

To enhance parish nurses' contribution to the nursing profession, educational providers need to

- commit resources to develop and coordinate programs to sustain the growth of this specialized practice.

- recognize that life-long learning is essential for nurses to maintain and increase competence in nursing practice and to foster spiritual formation and growth.

- develop related options to meet the diverse needs of the parish nursing population.

- recognize that a variety of educational providers can offer parish nursing continuing education and staff development.

- provide ongoing evaluation to maintain and enhance the quality and cost-effectiveness of parish nursing education.

- monitor the development of the practice of parish nursing and encourage the movement of formal educational programs into academic institutions.

Parish nurses must take responsibility for their own professional development. However, the structure and content of lifelong professional development opportunities should meet both their immediate and future goals.

SOURCE: Developed by the Philosophy Work Group, which consisted of Judith Ryan, R.N., Ph.D.; Ruth Berry, R.N., M.S.N.; Janet Griffin, R.N., M.S.; and Jean Reeves, R.N., Ph.D. This statement was refined as well as endorsed by all in attendance at the First Invitational Educational Colloquium, sponsored by the International Parish Nurse Resource Center, June 16-17, 1994, held at St. Mary of the Lake Seminary, Mundelein, Illinois (Solari-Twadell et al., 1994).

APPENDIX B
Four Models of Institutional Frameworks

APPENDIX TABLE 1 Model of an Institutional Organizational Framework

The institutionally based paid model has several distinguishing features:

1. Continuing education and consultation is available from the sponsoring institution for pastors and lay leaders on the development of the parish nurse program.
2. The parish nurse receives financial compensation for providing parish nursing services (the payment can be salaried, hourly, or a stipend).
3. Advertising, interviewing, and selection of the parish nurse is done in partnership with the institution and the congregation.
4. Access to basic preparation in parish nursing and an orientation to the institution and the congregation is facilitated for the parish nurse.
5. The parish nurse receives ongoing continuing education through the congregation's relationship with the institution.
6. The parish nurse networks with other peer parish nurses through the relationship with the institution.
7. The parish nurse receives assistance from the institution in identifying referral resources.
8. The parish nurse and congregation may receive liability coverage through their relationship with the institution.
9. The parish nurse receives ongoing nursing and pastoral counseling supervision through the relationship with the institution.
10. The parish nurse may receive benefits and reimbursement for travel through either the institution or the congregation.
11. The parish nurse will be using a documentation system that results in regular reports being generated for the congregation and institution.
12. The position description for the parish nurse is endorsed by both the congregation and the institution.
13. Physician resources and consultation are available through the relationship with the institution.
14. External funding, such as that from grants, is pursued in partnership with the institution and the congregation.

APPENDIX TABLE 2 Model of an Institutional Unpaid Organizational Framework

The second organizational model is the institutional unpaid model. Even though the parish nurse is not being paid, she operates as an integral part of the pastoral team. This model has the following distinguishing characteristics:

1. The parish nurse receives no financial compensation for providing parish nursing services. The only nursing role that may be salaried by the institution in this model is "Coordinator of Parish Nursing," who is responsible for supporting those parish nurses providing services in the congregation. In some instances, the coordinator of parish nursing may also be providing parish nursing services part-time in one or more congregations.

2. Ongoing continuing education from the institution or consultation from the partnering institution may be available for pastors and lay leaders of the congregation.

3. Assistance in the selection of the parish nurse may be provided by the institution, with the final decision made by the pastor and congregation.

4. Access to basic preparation in parish nursing and an orientation to the institution and the congregation may be facilitated for the parish nurse.

5. The parish nurse receives ongoing continuing education through the institution.

6. The parish nurse networks with other parish nurses through the congregation's relationship with the institution.

7. The parish nurse receives assistance from the institution in identifying referral resources.

8. Liability coverage for the parish nurse and the congregation will need to be secured independently through insurance vendors.

9. The parish nurse receives ongoing nursing supervision and pastoral counseling supervision through the relationship with the institution.

10. The benefits and expense reimbursement for the parish nurse will need to be negotiated by the nurse if either will be provided.

11. The parish nurse may use a documentation system that results in a regular report being generated for the congregation and the institution.

12. The parish nurse position description is endorsed by the congregation and the institution.

13. Physician consultation for the parish nurse may be available through the institution.

14. The acquisition of external grants and, therefore, grant funding for the parish nurse program is usually taken care of by the institution.

APPENDIX TABLE 3 Model of a Congregationally Paid Organizational Framework

The third organizational model is the congregationally paid model. In this model, there is no contract or covenant with any institution. The nurse is considered an integral member of the pastoral team of the congregation. The congregation supports the development of this ministry on its own. This model has the following list of distinguishing features:

1. The parish nurse receives financial compensation for providing parish nursing services. This compensation may be through a salary, hourly pay, or a stipend.

2. A position description is developed and endorsed by the governing body of the congregation.

3. Advertising for, interviewing, and selection of the parish nurse is done by a task force of the church or the health and wellness committee in conjunction with the pastor.

4. Access to basic preparation in parish nursing and an orientation to the congregation as a workplace will need to be negotiated and provided for by the pastor, health cabinet, or other designated church leadership structure.

5. The parish nurse, pastor, or health cabinet identify sources of continuing education for the parish nurse.

6. The parish nurse seeks out peers for networking.

7. The parish nurse identifies referral resources in the community.

8. The parish nurse and the congregation seek out and purchase liability coverage for the nurse and the congregation.

9. Nursing supervision and pastoral counseling supervision arrangements are made either within the congregation or through external consultation arrangements.

10. Benefits and reimbursement for travel are negotiated by the parish nurse as part of being hired by the congregation.

11. Documentation requirements are established with the pastor, health cabinet, or lay leadership of the congregation, taking into consideration the professional accountability of the nurse.

12. Physician resources and consultation are sought through the congregation or the external community.

APPENDIX TABLE 4 Model of a Congregationally Unpaid Organizational Framework

---

The fourth organizational model is the congregationally unpaid model. The nurse is still considered part of the staff of the congregation, but she operates in an unpaid status. There is no contract or covenant relationship with an institution. The defining characteristics of this model are the following:

1. The parish nurse receives no financial compensation for providing parish nursing services;
2. The job description of the parish nurse is developed and endorsed by the pastor, health and wellness cabinet, and/or lay leadership of the congregation.
3. The process for interviewing and selection of the parish nurse is determined by the pastor, health committee, or lay leadership of the congregation.
4. Access to basic preparation in parish nursing and an orientation to the congregation as a workplace is negotiated with the pastor, health cabinet, or lay leadership of the church.
5. The parish nurse, pastor, and/or health cabinet identify sources of continuing education for the parish nurse.
6. The parish nurse seeks out peers and opportunities for networking.
7. The parish nurse identifies referral resources in the community.
8. The parish nurse and the congregation seek out and purchase liability coverage for the parish nurse and the congregation.
9. Nursing supervision and pastoral counseling supervision arrangements are made either within the congregation or through external consultation arrangements.
10. Benefits and reimbursement for travel are negotiated with the pastor, health committee, or lay leadership of the congregation.
11. Documentation requirements are established with the pastor, health cabinet, or lay leadership of the congregation, taking into consideration the professional accountability of the nurse.
12. Physician resources and consultation are sought through the congregation or the external community.

APPENDIX C
Matrix Planning Tool for Use in
Developing Parish Nurse Programs

	Institutional Paid	Institutional Unpaid	Congregational Paid	Congregational Paid
Education and consultation				
Paid or unpaid				
Advertising interviewing selection				
Basic preparation and orientation				
Continuing education				
Networking				
Referral sources				
Liability insurance				
Supervision of nursing and pastoral counseling				
Benefits				
Documentation system				
Position description				
Physician consultation				
Grants				

APPENDIX D
Twelve Beatitudes for Parish Nurses

Nurses are blessed with a variety of gifts that make them uniquely attractive to faith communities striving toward whole-person health. However, these blessings, not unlike other talents, have their "dark" or "shadow" side. The following beatitudes should be understood as acknowledging that caveat.

1. Blessed be the parish nurse, for she is caring!
2. Blessed be the parish nurse, for she is available and accessible to most faith communities!
3. Blessed be the parish nurse, for she is knowledgeable about community resources and the process of referral!
4. Blessed be the parish nurse, for she is cost-effective!
5. Blessed be the parish nurse, for she has a high tolerance for ambiguity!
6. Blessed be the parish nurse, for she has had a generalist education and previous employment that have resulted in a broad variety of skills!
7. Blessed be the parish nurse, for she is process oriented!
8. Blessed be the parish nurse, for she is possessed with a generosity of spirit, both of time and of talent!
9. Blessed be the parish nurse, for she focuses on priorities!
10. Blessed be the parish nurse, for she is committed, dependable, and persevering!
11. Blessed be the parish nurse, for she has a heritage and tradition of pioneering!
12. Blessed be the parish nurse, for she is a believer in God, clients, nursing, herself, and in a better world here and hereafter!

SOURCE: Developed by Mary Ann McDermott, R.N., M.S.N., Ed.D.

APPENDIX E
Planning for and Development of a Parish Nurse Program

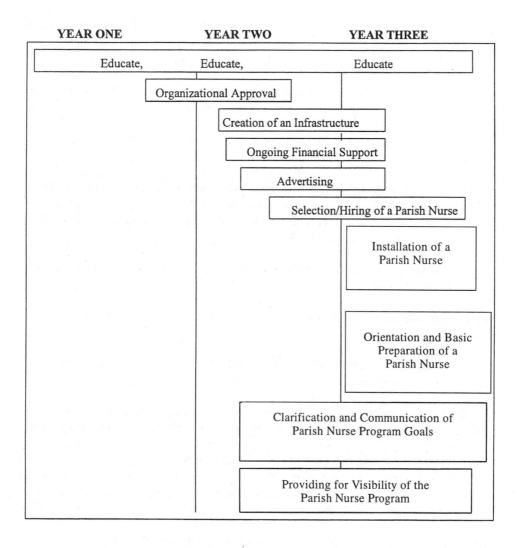

YEAR ONE	YEAR TWO	YEAR THREE

Educate,   Educate,   Educate

Organizational Approval

Creation of an Infrastructure

Ongoing Financial Support

Advertising

Selection/Hiring of a Parish Nurse

Installation of a
Parish Nurse

Orientation and Basic
Preparation of a
Parish Nurse

Clarification and Communication of
Parish Nurse Program Goals

Providing for Visibility of the
Parish Nurse Program

APPENDIX F
The Road to Life

At first I saw God as my observer, my judge keeping track of the things I did wrong, so as to know whether I merited heaven or hell when I die. He was out there, sort of like a president; I recognized His picture when I saw it, but I really didn't know Him.

But later when I met Christ, it seemed as though life was rather like a bike ride, but it was a tandem bike, and I noticed that Christ was in the back helping me pedal.

I don't know just when it was that He suggested we change places, but life has not been the same since.

When I had control, I knew the way. It was rather boring, but predictable . . . it was the shortest distance between two points. But when He took the lead, He knew delightful long cuts, up mountains and through rocky places at breakneck speeds. It was all I could do to hang on! Even though it looked like madness, He said, "Pedal!"

I worried and was anxious and asked, "Where are you taking me?" He laughed and didn't answer, and then I started to trust.

I forgot my boring life and entered into the adventure, and when I'd say, "I'm scared," He'd lean back and touch my hand.

He took me to people with gifts that I needed, gifts of healing, acceptance and joy. They gave me their gifts to take on my journey, my Lord's and mine.

And we were off again. He said, "Give the gifts away; they're extra baggage, too much weight." So I did, to the people we met, and I found that in giving I received, and still our burden was light.

I did not trust Him, at first, in control of my life. I thought He'd wreck it; but He knows bike secrets, knows how to make it bend to take sharp corners, jump to clear high rocks, fly to shorten scary passages. And I am learning to shut up and pedal in the strangest places, and I'm beginning to enjoy the view and the cool breeze on my face with my delightful, constant companion, Christ.

And when I'm sure I just can't do any more, He just smiles and says, "PEDAL."

SOURCE: Church newsletter (anonymous author).

2

Health and the Congregation

L. James Wylie
Phyllis Ann Solari-Twadell

Health is central to the congregation. Stated another way, the congregation's central mission is that of health and salvation. The Christian Church, indeed the entire community of faith globally, has no more important mission than health and healing. This chapter will focus on theological foundations for the health and healing mission in the congregation, a historical overview of the congregation as a health and healing place, and current changes along with the prospects for the future.

Theological Reflections

Not a single faith fails to address the issues of illness and wellness, of disease and healing, of caring and curing. People turn to their faiths to interpret their misfortunes, to summon the strength to fight illness, to rally their communities and a larger public to promote well-being (Marty, 1990).

One could assert from the beginning that God is about the healing or transformation of His creation. As illustrated in the Genesis narrative, God's intentions for His creation were abridged by the willfulness of humankind in various activities that are generally categorized with the simple everyday word "sin." It is the view of faith that the problems of the world in one way or another are traceable to the collective determination of human beings throughout history to willfully rebel and/or deviate from the purposes of God.

The actions of human beings can facilitate health and healing. God, however, is the source of all health and healing. In Hebrew scriptures, health is portrayed as one of God's great gifts, and responsibility is placed on people to lead lives that cherish and protect this treasure. God, however, is the source of all health and healing. One cannot be healthy if one does not simultaneously care for the body, human relationships, nature, and relationship with God. To be healthy, one has to be a responsible steward of God's many gifts (Wind & Lewis, 1994).

Both the Old and New Testaments reflect health and healing as a central ministry of the faith community (Carroll, 1995). From the perspective of faith, the Kingdom of God is in the process of being revealed and experienced as God's creation is being healed. In the Christian community, for example, the work of Jesus Christ and the ministry that He initiated is intended as a model and an example of the way in which the faithful are to proceed as the agents of God in bringing transformation to a fallen creation. It is recognized that this Kingdom will not fully come and this transformation will not fully occur during our lifetime, and, in fact, it will not fully occur until the end of time.

It is important to understand some basic terminology. The Hebrew term "shalom" encompasses the perspective of wholeness that is "the desired intent of creation." It implies the activities and behaviors that best maintain and promote the development of a peaceful, that is, *balanced,* understanding of existence. Further, it suggests the relational nature of all things—the balanced, symbiotic dimensions of the created order (Richardson, 1956, p. 165).

Historical Perspectives

The ancient Greeks and Romans perceived healing and religion as identical. Temples were used as the site of sacrifice to soothe the anger of a god or seek favor so that health could be restored. Temples were known as places of healing. The Greeks' domination by the Romans brought their knowledge of healing into the Roman culture.

Healing is prevalent in the gospels. Jesus was very focused on the restoration of health. This is known to be true because he performed more miracles of healing than of any other category (Carroll, 1995). Jesus acknowledged the scientific information available during his time; however, he did not stop there. He put great emphasis on the importance of psychological and spiritual factors in sickness and health. He stressed the interrelationship between all the factors of a total person. In some instances, psychological or spiritual factors were noted as the cause of the physical disorder (Luke 5:18-36).

Most acknowledge and accept the fact that the mission of the Christian faith community is shaped by the ministry that Christ initiated. We refer back to Christ's dusty trips with his band of 12 as the beginning of the Christian community. Paul, Peter, and their associates set about establishing congregations, or more accurately in many cases, seeking to bring the messianic understanding to existing Hebrew communities of faith.

If those early congregations had a mission statement, it would have included three elements: (a) to teach, preach, and heal; (b) to conduct worship and promote fellowship; and (c) to perform service—direct service such as healing the sick, feeding the hungry, and providing comfort and protection to widows and orphans.

One element that is of significance is that of the diaconate. Deacons and deaconesses carried the church into people's homes. It is important to note that the nursing profession traces its beginnings to these early Christian orders. It was the deaconess Fabiola who founded the first charity hospital in Rome about 300 A.D.

During the medieval age, the Church was the primary vehicle through which the healing arts were promulgated. Through this entire period, monks and some nuns were engaged in the work of healing. It was not uncommon for monasteries and convents to have rooms for the sick. Hospitals were then built in connection with some churches (Scherzer, 1984).

The Crusades, although not accomplishing their primary purpose of regaining the Holy Land, did have an influence on the Church and health. Leprosy was an illness brought back to Europe from the Orient. As it spread, the Church tried to respond. Hospitals were built and called "lazarettos" after Lazarus the Leper in the New Testament. During one period, there were 2,000 lazarettos in France and 200 in England (Scherzer, 1984).

Two events appear to have influenced the estrangement of the Church and formalized medicine. Emperor Constantine not only legitimatized Christianity, he went on to take the "service" component of the congregation's life and assign it directly to the bishops for their development and supervision. Therein, the direct ministries of health and restoration were essentially removed from the congregation (Wietzke, 1987). The purpose of this change was to bring sustaining stewardship to the service components lest they go astray at the changing whims of a congregation. About that time, the Church organization under the bishops became directly involved in supervising the service component of the congregation's activity as a function of the bishop's office. This changed the role of a specific congregation and began the institutionalization of these services. In later centuries in Europe and, to a lesser degree, in America, Protestant groups and congregations moved out on their own through what were called "mission societies," doing "service" at home and abroad as an expression of their personal faith, independent from the work of bishops and formal church structures.

A second major influence, not directly associated with the Church, fueled the separation of the Church further from its mission of health and healing. The influence of the philosopher Descartes in the mid-1600s emphasized the dualism of spirit and body. This construct had been brewing in the culture, including the faith community, for a number of years. This view of man came to be pervasive, if not characteristic, of Western civilization. This division has persisted until modern times.

Starr (1982), in *The Social Transformation of American Medicine,* gives a compelling and revealing perspective in the subtitle of the book, "A Rise of a Sovereign Profession and the Building of a Vast Industry." This book describes the impact of economic and conceptual forces that edged the Church even further from needing to focus on health and healing. The development of the medical health establishment over the past 75 to 80 years, with its interest in specialization, identifies the clergy and their associates as pursuing the matters of the spirit, certain physicians and their associates in medicine dealing with the matters of the body, and other emotional specialists dedicated to disturbances of the mind.

After World War II, a reconciliation between clergy and physicians and those two worlds of spirit and body began to occur. The midcentury contribution of physicists moved us from a Newtonian understanding of the universe to a whole person cosmology—an understanding of all elements of the universe as having a basic synergy and interrelationship. This ushered in the beginnings of an era of renewed emphasis and acceptance of whole person health.

A Definition of Health

Health is a word that has different meanings to different people. For some, the term health has a strong physical connotation. Others who are more whole person oriented will understand health to include not only physical applications but also those that are emotional, spiritual, intellectual, and environmental. An interesting exercise is to ask a convened group of people to break up into small groups and discuss their understanding of health. The ultimate task of each small group is to come to consensus on one definition of health. This exercise often illustrates not only the diverse understandings of health but the difficulty of agreeing on one definition. The following is a sampling of definitions of health:

- The World Council of Churches (1990) envisions health to be most often "an issue of justice, of peace, of integrity of creation and of spirituality" (pp. 1-4).
- Paul Tillich's definition of health is another often-quoted understanding: "Health is not the lack of divergent trends in our bodily or mental or spiritual life, but the power to keep them together. And healing is the act of reuniting them after the disruption of their unity" (quoted in Mays, 1978, pp. 3-4).
- The Institutes of Religion and Health (1981) define health as being "found in a man or woman whose living reflects a sound and liberated mind, body and spirit, freed in a healing community to have integrity, to love and to work for good."
- Another definition of health comes from David Jenkins (1981), who states, "Health is what we enjoy on our way to that which God is preparing for us to enjoy. It is a value and a vision word. Practically speaking, health is never reached. From a faith point of view, health is an eschatological idea. We seek health even as we enjoy it . . . it is a vision beyond the range of possibilities or failures of medicine" (pp. 12-13).
- J. C. McGilvrey (1981), a pioneer in the work of the Christian Medical Commission of the World Council of Churches, lays out the dilemma in his definition: "The first task in the quest for health is to recognize the confusions which obscure our understanding of it. More medicine will not give us more health. Health is not something that someone else can give to someone. Health is not a human right when in fact it is largely a matter of personal and social responsibility" (pp. 81-82).

What is clear in each of these definitions is that health is broader than physical and that the majority of individuals in this country have been misled about the relevance and meaning of health in their lives. The congregation can play an important role in assisting people to an understanding of health and their role in maintaining their own health and the health of others in their community.

The importance of this understanding for us is that it gives the rationale and foundation for efforts to reestablish the congregation, not medicine or treatment, as the primary focus for health. This becomes a key element in a social strategy to bring about a new way of thinking and behaving.

It is also important to have firmly in mind the "birthright" that we have, one to which parish nursing brings primary instrumentation. Our birthright declares the congregation as the chief and primary focus for health and salvation. When one uses these words together, they are fairly digestible. But when one drops the word "salvation" and then says, as is the title of this chapter, that the primary ministry of the congregation is a *health* ministry, that often catches in the throat. It is important for any congregation that is considering the parish nurse ministry to carefully check their mindset, or understanding, of how they see their congregation as a "health place" in the community.

Nurses, as well as others, need to be well grounded in this understanding theologically and historically. One of the reasons to be knowledgeable on this subject is that there will be a need to interpret it to a congregation that has been raised in an understanding that health is the property of the medical community. This thinking needs to be changed. Health is the property, or, better, the responsibility, of each person. When the congregation and the community of faith understands its role as a "health place" in the community, the role of the hospital is clarified as an acute care facility, with the physicians and other service providers as partners in the health enterprise. It then is easier to understand the need for active engagement with our Creator in the process of reclaiming and healing His creation. For most faith communities, retrieving their mission of health calls for a change in thinking. In other words, all need to develop a proper mindset, particularly the members of the community of faith (Wylie, 1987).

Without embracing a renewed understanding of the congregation's role in health and healing, introduction of the parish nurse may be received with much confusion and resistance on the part of the members of the faith community.

The Congregation as a Partner

Congregations work with many different agencies in the community, depending on the interest and need of the faith community. The following issues are pertinent to agencies considering approaching a faith community about being a partner in a parish nurse ministry.

1. All churches may not understand what it is to have a mission in health, or a health ministry. For a congregation to see the value in being a partner with a hospital, home care agency, or department of public health, this understanding may be an important item to assess; otherwise, resistance from the congregation may be an issue of concern for the health agency seeking the partnership.

2. Congregations are volunteer organizations. This translates into the fact that meeting times will be predominantly in the evenings and weekends. In addition, it may take longer to schedule time with a church council or particular committee, as the members are usually all volunteers meeting on a once-a-month basis. Approval on pending issues may take more time than business-oriented organizations are used to.

3. Congregations, particularly if they are small, may not see themselves as having the resources to be a viable partner with larger agencies in the community. This may be true. However, through development of ecumenical congregational coalitions, small churches can combine resources and often serve well as a partnering group. This is most evident when the congregations are geographically close to each other.

4. Denominations differ as to their organizational structure and decision-making processes. Even some congregations of the same denomination differ as to how they are organized and how decisions are made. This can be a challenge for an agency that has little understanding of church policy. It is important to become educated. Most clergy or lay leaders can be very helpful in responding to questions about their own congregations.

5. Congregations have a very active life. Usually they have goals, a mission statement, and plans for what the focus for their liturgical year will be. It is important to be considerate and knowledgeable about these plans. For example, if the major emphasis within a congregation is a building project, there may be little time or energy for developing new partnerships with other community agencies.

6. Every congregation has a history. Some congregations have a profile of being risk takers, others assume a more sedate historical pattern. When getting to know a congregation, history is important. Often ghosts of past conflicts plague congregations and keep them from moving into new and different styles of leadership. No agency wants to get caught up in nonproductive partnerships. Knowing a congregation's history can often provide insight into current functioning and leadership.

Considering the previously listed thoughts, the next set of suggestions relates to actions that can be taken by institutions and agencies interested in engaging a congregation as a partner.

- Contact your clergy friends. Usually each health agency has a few clergy in the community that they have come to know better than others. Start with those you know, and inquire. Ask what their understanding is about the congregation's mission in health. Inquire as to their interest in being a partner. Present questions that investigate what the congregation's goals and plans are for the year. See if the strengths and deficits of the congregation can be identified through early conversations.

- Contact the regional ecumenical clergy council. Usually there is such an organization present in the community. Inquire as to the nature of their meetings or gatherings. Perhaps a natural entry into meeting more members of this group is to offer to speak to the group on some aspect of the healthier community or another topic that may be of interest to the group. Again, this is an excellent place to learn about congregations and their leadership.

- Meet the clergy in their setting. Go to the congregation. Just by being in the congregation, you can gather information. What is the actual physical capacity of the building? Is it accessible to persons with handicaps? Are the grounds and building well maintained? By going to the congregation, you will be sending another message: that there is interest in doing just what is being done—getting to know the congregation and its leadership by visiting them in their location.

- Focus the conversation with clergy and lay leadership around the term *health*. Using the term *health care* tends to narrow the conversation to more of an illness and/or physical understanding. By framing the conversation with the term *health,* you will allow a broader exploration of the physical as well as the emotional, spiritual, and intellectual aspects of the person.

- Clarify the terminology being used. The word *healing* can mean different things to different people. When you define what is meant in using a term, all listeners will be clear about what is being addressed.

- Plan to move slowly into this partnership. This gives the congregation the necessary time to educate members and communicate information about future partnership opportunities fully to decision makers within the congregation. Some of the most effective ways to begin may be the simplest. Complexity can often produce unnecessary stumbling blocks in the development of the relationship.

- Be clear about what resources the agency or institution has available to contribute to the partnership. When the gifts and limitations of the agency seeking the partnership with the congregation are known up front, there is less likelihood that unavailable resources will be committed. In addition, this kind of clarification gives the congregation the sense that the agency seeking the partnership has really given this some thought. It will demonstrate a seriousness about the intention to work together.

- Identify one person who will be a consistent liaison with the congregation. There is nothing more frustrating than for clergy or lay leaders of a congregation to have multiple people with whom they will be expected to communicate about a partnership issue. It is much more considerate to have one contact person from the agency seeking the partnership and allow that person to dedicate time to nurture the relationship with the faith community.

Leadership for the Journey

Pastoral leadership is a key factor in the successful transition of the congregation to a health place and a community of healing. In a study that was done in 1994 on 635 black churches in the northern United States, a key finding was that the minister's level of education was strongly associated with church outreach activities. Of those churches whose ministers had graduate degrees, 83% offered community outreach programs. In the responses from the ministers, health issues were central to the mission of their churches (Thomas, Quinn, Billingsley, & Caldwell, 1994, p. 576).

The pastoral leader interested in fostering a healthy faith community will not just teach and preach biblical concepts but will also teach and model how to use power with responsibility, how to communicate effectively, how to respect each person in the congregation, and how to organize the congregation so that it is fulfilling its goals (Ailabouni, 1988, p. 9). Most important is the organization of the congregation to allow for maximum lay involvement in the mission of the church.

This is a tall order for anyone. It calls for a whole-person understanding of health and a dedication to one's personal responsibility to one's own health and wellness. It goes back to the saying, "You can't help someone to the top of the mountain without getting there yourself." If there is a sincere dedication to the congregation's being a place that can assist people to live healthier lives, the leadership must have the capacity to model and teach this concept. This is quite a "call" for the already busy pastor—but it is one that cannot be ignored if there is a seriousness to the mission of health within the congregation. Of equal importance is the ability of the pastor to exercise good steward-ship of personal health resources. Clergy often are encouraged to ignore good health practices because of the demands of their position. Yet the single factor that can cripple any pastor's ability to be available in ministry is ill health. Disciplined health practices need to be fostered to provide energy for the call to be of service to others.

Conclusion

The fact is that in spite of America's success, it is in the throes of a health policy struggle. Driven by concerns about cost, questions are raised as to quality and appropriateness of care, along with concerns about access and distribution. The high-tech forces are not in phase with high touch. The corporate restructuring of provider organizations characteristic of the 1980s has wound down, and the words heard more than any other across the realm are *quality—total quality management—continuous quality improvement,* and this in an industry that for years has prided itself on quality. The Joint Commission on Accreditation of Healthcare Organizations (JCAHO) and other prestigious medical leadership in this country join in the observation that quality is not documented nor reliably available in America. It is in this arena that churches seek to make entry.

The church ponders what to do, and in some cases it seeks to get involved through political advocacy. At the same time, the medical community is beginning to refocus on the spiritual dimension of caring and curing. It is a time of immense change and rethinking. In the final analysis, churches need to be there out of their own need, as well as for the good of society. The faith community needs to play a more dominant role in this new beginning. A congregation that has a clear perspective and program with regard to its health ministry, totally integrated with its activities of worship, fellowship, teaching, and preaching, is a very ready component for the social transformation that is needed in health care (Solari-Twadell, 1997).

Financially, there is a need to address more of the needs of people in the community; further, there is a need to properly allocate our technical capabilities. The opportunity at the congregational level is to form partnerships with health professionals and health care agencies, as well as getting a firm grip on the opportunities that churches have to participate in this transformation. Unique opportunities exist for the faith community that go beyond diagnosis and curing.

In summary, the central mission of the congregation is health and salvation, and in so saying, one thing has been said, not two.

References

Ailabouni, S. R. (1988). *The congregation: A healing community in need of healing.* Unpublished doctoral dissertation, Lutheran School of Theology at Chicago.

Carroll, J. T. (1995). Sickness and healing in the New Testament gospels. *Interpretation, 49,* 130-142.

Institutes of Religion and Health. (1981). *Basic mission, policies and goals.* (Working draft).

Jenkins, D. E. (1981). Foreword. In J. C. McGilvray, *The quest for health and wholeness.* Tübingen: German Institute for Medical Mission.

Marty, M. (1990). Health, medicine, and the faith traditions. In *Healthy People 2000: A role for America's religious communities.* Chicago: Carter Center of Emory University and Park Ridge Center for the Study of Health, Faith and Ethics.

Mays, L. H. (1978). Theological perspectives on health care. *Viewpoints* (pp. 3-4). Minneapolis: Augsburg.

McGilvrey, J. C. (1981). *The quest for health and wholeness*. Tübingen: German Institute for Medical Mission.

Richardson, A. (Ed.). (1956). *A theological workbook of the Bible*. New York: Macmillan.

Scherzer, C. (1984). *The church and healing*. Unpublished manuscript, Deaconess Hospital, Evansville, IN.

Solari-Twadell, P. A. (1997). The caring congregation: A healing place. *Journal of Christian Nursing, 14*(1), 4-9.

Starr, P. (1982). *The social transformation of American medicine*. New York: Basic Books.

Thomas, S. B., Quinn, S. C., Billingsley, A., & Caldwell, C. (1994). The characteristics of northern black churches with community health outreach programs. *American Journal of Public Health, 84*(4), 575-579.

Wietzke, W. A. (1987). *A precise congregational health partnership*. Unpublished manuscript. Congregational Health Partnership.

Wind, J. P., & Lewis, J. W. (Eds.). (1994). *American congregations* (Vol. 1). Chicago: University of Chicago Press.

World Council of Churches. (1990). *Healing and wholeness: The churches' role in health* (Christian Medical Commission). Geneva, Switzerland: Author.

Wylie, L. J. (1987). Primacy franchise for health: The parish. *Chronicle of Pastoral Care, 7*(1), 3-6.

3

A Personal Historical Perspective of Whole Person Health and the Congregation

Granger Westberg

It all happened quite spontaneously. A group of us had been experimenting since the late 1960s with "wholistic" health centers that were family doctors' offices in churches. Our aim was to see if we could bring about whole person health care in a church setting by having spiritually oriented family doctors, nurses, and clergy working together.

It was a project enthusiastically sponsored by the W. K. Kellogg Foundation and the Department of Preventive Medicine and Community Health of the University of Illinois College of Medicine. More than a dozen of these medical clinics were begun in neighborhood churches in upper-, middle-, and lower-income areas in cities around the country (Tubesing, 1977; *The Wholistic Health Centers: A New Direction in Health Care,* 1977; *Wholistic Health Centers: Survey Research Report,* 1976).

The evaluations of these doctors' offices in churches over a period of 10 years indicated that the quality of care offered when these three professions worked together under the same roof was measurably more whole person oriented than the average doctor's office. Further, it was clear that the nurses in each of these centers were the glue that bound these three professions together in a common appreciation of the healing talents of each.

The evaluators, who were disinterested scholars from nonreligious backgrounds, began with a bias against the possibility of scientific medicine and religion actually collaborating in a joint approach to the problems of individual patients. Over the years, they saw that it was working very well. As they tried to ascertain why it worked, they gradually came to the conclusion that most of the nurses employed in these clinics could speak two languages: the language of science and the language of religion. The nurses

35

were acting as translators. They helped the doctor and the minister communicate in ways that were helpful to a whole person approach to health care.

As inflation swept America and it became more and more expensive to start new wholistic health centers in churches, someone said, "If the nurses in these clinics have proved so valuable, why not try placing a nurse on the staff of a congregation and see what happens?" When we asked individual nurses about this idea, the response was immediately favorable. We decided to try it.

I went to Lutheran General Hospital (LGH) in 1984 because I have had a long-standing relationship with several of the founding leaders of that hospital. Lutheran General Hospital, located in Park Ridge, Illinois (a northwest suburb of Chicago), is a 608-bed hospital founded in 1959. This hospital had long been a leader in pastoral care for its patients, and it showed immediate interest in participating in a pilot project. LGH describes its philosophy of *human ecology* as "the understanding and care of human beings as whole persons in light of their relationships to God, themselves, their families, and the society in which they live" (LGH mission statement). Currently, some 25 chaplains work closely with physicians, nurses, social workers, and many other health professionals in an unusually effective team approach.

An administrative team from LGH was organized to plan and implement the first institutionally based program. I was asked to go out and meet with pastors and congregational members. We were seeking to have six churches initially participate in the program. We also decided to go to large churches of various denominations that might be able to afford hiring a nurse. Initially, we were asking the church to pay the full half-time salary of about $10,000.

As I met with the pastors and described the concept, about 75% showed great interest and 25% some interest. They readily recognized that the nurse would be a person to assist them in their ministry to people who were hurting and many whom they felt they could not adequately serve by themselves.

I then asked each pastor if there was a group of people that I could talk to some evening and describe the concept. In many cases, this group consisted of nurses and other health professionals from the congregation. The response was immediately positive. The next group I was invited to speak to was a decision-making board such as the church council. I described the overall picture of health and the role of a nurse in the church. Again, the response was very positive.

All responses were positive until I met with the finance committee. They immediately began to express concerns about their budget and finding the resources to support another position. Many felt they could not fit the position into their current budget. Each of the churches I talked to had good reason for its financial concerns. Many were involved in building or renovation projects. It was then that I realized something very important. None of these large churches had a line in their budget with funds appropriated for "risk taking." Consequently, I had to go elsewhere to find funds. I went back to the hospital and explained that none of the churches, regardless of size, were willing to risk a salary of $10,000. This was 1984.

With the help of LGH administrators, who were eager to respond to the churches' willingness to participate in such a program, a plan was developed. LGH agreed to pay 75% of the salary the first year while the church paid 25%. It was decided that in the second year, the church would increase its contribution to 50%, the third year 75%, and by the fourth year the church would be making the full payment. The hospital would continue to pay for the nurse's benefits and liability insurance.

With the new proposal that they would contribute 25% of the salary the first year, six churches were willing to participate and agree to a 3-year trial period. Four of these churches were Protestant and two were Roman Catholic. They were located as close as six blocks away from the hospital and as far as 30 miles away.

In early 1985, the hiring process began. An advertisement in a local paper brought some 30 applications for these half-time parish nurse positions. Interviewers from both the hospital and the churches discovered hidden talents in these nurses, and the quality of the candidates was deemed to be amazingly high. By and large, they were women (no male nurses applied) in their 30s and 40s whose smaller children were now in school. They all showed genuine interest in a type of nursing that would allow the kind of creativity they had always longed for.

All of the candidates were stimulated by the potential of a whole person approach to their work with people. The fact that they would be working within the context of a congregation and actually serving on the pastoral staff of that church was of great interest to them. Most of the candidates indicated that their original motivation for going into nursing was strongly influenced by a desire to incorporate the spiritual dimension into their work.

After choosing six nurses to participate in the program, we decided not to superimpose upon them a course of instruction because we were not at all sure what direction such a course should take. Instead, we invited them to spend a half day each week at the hospital in an informal discussion group where, in the presence of a teaching chaplain, a nurse educator, and a family practice physician, they could describe what they felt they needed in an ongoing educational process. The salary of the staff supporting these sessions was part of the contribution from the hospital.

Once a week, the nurses came to LGH for 3 hours; this was part of their salaried work week. We began each day by going around the circle of these six nurses and asking them to tell of their experiences in the parish during the preceding week. In the early weeks, it took anywhere from 1 to $1\frac{1}{2}$ hours for these women to tell the stories of their ministry. The telling of these stories brought about all sorts of questions, spontaneous role-playing of situations, even tears and laughter, as everybody took part. At the end of every session, we were all exhausted but also exhilarated to think that these unusual happenings were taking place simply because a nurse had been added to the staff of a church.

The parish nurses told us of their many opportunities to talk with people informally between services, at coffee hours, at meetings of church organizations, at potluck suppers, and in home visits with the sick or shut-ins. It was in the informality of it all that we saw the nurse having the unusual opportunity to talk with people in the early stages of illness. Before these people ever thought of going to see a doctor about their very minor problems, the nurse, with her unique sensitivity to early cries for help, was already responding to it.

It gradually dawned on us that churches are actually the one organization in our society most suited to give leadership to the field of preventive medicine. Scientific medicine has not been known for its contributions to preventive medicine. Jeff Goldsmith, national health care advisor, says that the nation's health care system still acts as if most diseases strike "like a fire in your house" rather than "like a fire in a pile of leaves." And as a result, he says, health care is preoccupied with climbing ladders and chopping holes in roofs instead of keeping a bucket of water and a rake nearby.

The history of the parish nurse movement is closely tied up with an understanding that churches, when they are functioning at their best, are dedicated to keeping people well. This means tending the little fires in piles of leaves. But most people do not see churches and synagogues as an integral part of our present health system (Westberg, 1988). If a pollster asks the question, "What are the health agencies in your community?" the usual reply mentions local hospitals and perhaps a well-known medical clinic.

When we speak of health care, we usually mean "sickness care." And that's where hospitals and doctors' clinics do such a good job. So we still have to raise the question, "What are the institutions of our culture that keep us well?" There are at least five: home, school, church, the workplace, and the public health department. We are well aware of the sickness that follows when any of these five is not contributing to a quality of life that builds up immunity to disease.

The churches and synagogues of America are becoming conscious of their role in keeping people healthy. They have never really seen themselves as part of the nation's health system because health was believed to deal with a complex thing called "medical technology" that was becoming more technical every day. Almost with the same suddenness, society is now realizing that many illnesses are preventable.

Most illnesses come on slowly. It is as if our bodies are trying to tell us something— something about how our way of looking at life, or our way of handling life's many problems, is making us sick. At least these things are making us more vulnerable to the germs attacking us. If a great deal of illness is related to our way of looking at life—our outlook on life, our philosophy of life—then, of course, religious institutions must be integrated into the health care system.

It is precisely at this point that parish nurses are seen to be natural organizers of congregations as community-based health centers. Almost two thirds of the people in the United States have some tangible relationship to congregations. Churches of all sizes and shapes are to be found in all corners of America—and in almost every church there is a registered nurse.

Many large churches have 25 or more nurses in their membership. Most of these churches, however, have never even thought to use these nurses in any creative manner, until recently.

During the first year or two of the parish nurse project, it became clear that there were seven areas of ministry in which the nurses were engaged. These will be described later in this book, but let me just mention them here:

1. The parish nurse is a health educator.
2. The parish nurse is a personal health counselor.
3. The parish nurse is a referral agent.
4. The parish nurse is a coordinator of volunteers.
5. The parish nurse is a developer of support groups.
6. The parish nurse assists people to integrate faith and health.
7. The parish nurse is a health advocate.

Actually, what these seven areas describe is what the parish nurses attempt to do by engaging the entire congregation in seminars, workshops, Sunday forums, and so on, where all can grapple with the concept that true health includes the spirit, that it is not all physical or nutritional.

Sixty years ago, a best-selling book by the famous missionary to India E. Stanley Jones (1930) titled *The Way* contained the following quotations that help us understand that the Christian Way provides an excellent foundation for healthful living.

> When we live the Christian Way, we are living the way we were made to live . . . made in the inner structure of our being.
>
> Evil is a turning of the natural into the unnatural—it is a living against life.
>
> Self-love, the natural, can become selfishness, the unnatural.
>
> Self-respect, the natural, may be lured into pride, the unnatural.
>
> Love, the natural, can be beguiled into lust, the unnatural.
>
> Sex desire, the natural, can be lured away from its God-intended creative function and become an end in itself.

These simple, natural functions, dedicated to God and controlled by God, bring life—life to the whole person. But if they *become* god, become ends in themselves, there is one result: death—death to development, to happiness, to the whole person (Jones, 1930).

E. Stanley Jones and many other Christian divines through the centuries were remarkably aware of the wholeness concept that many of us are coming to see as a sensible approach to health. It gives validity to the entrance of churches into the health field.

Many active, dedicated church members of all branches of Christendom are searching for ways to make the message of Christian faith more relevant to our age. They are fascinated by the way Jesus in his healing ministry always dealt with people as whole persons. They are disturbed that our present highly technical health care system tends to neglect the spiritual dimensions of illness. Just as the ecological movement has captured the imagination of youth throughout the world, so now it is just possible that the whole person emphasis in health care will be included in those splendid concerns.

Many churches want to make a more meaningful contribution to society. They feel that they are stagnating because they spend so much of their time just talking. They want to become involved in action that leads to a healthier society. It is time to bring religiously oriented people into the discussion of what is meant by high-level wellness. If we can agree on a number of major religious concepts—stated clearly and succinctly—concerning what we believe *health* to be all about, then our chances of getting church people and health care people to work together on joint projects will increase greatly.

Let me suggest nine statements that could possibly be accepted by a wide variety of religious people:

1. Health is intimately related to how a person "thinketh in one's heart."
2. Physical health is not to be "our chief end in this life"—only a possible by-product of loving God and one's neighbor as oneself.

3. Health is closely tied up with goals, meaning, and purposeful living: It is a religious quest, whereas illness may be related to a life that is empty, bored, without purpose or aim.

4. Our present disease-oriented medical care system must be revised to include a strong accent on modeling and teaching prevention and wellness.

5. Our present separation of body and spirit must go, and an integrated, whole-person approach put in its place.

6. There is a difference between merely existing and a life lived under God, responsive to the prompting of God's spirit.

7. The body functions at its best when a person, who is the body, exhibits attitudes of hope, faith, love, and gratitude.

8. True health is closely associated with creativity by which we as people of God participate with God in the ongoing process of creation.

9. The self-preservation instincts of the human can be happily blended with the innate longing to love and to help others. (Westberg, 1982)

We who have been engaged in the parish nurse movement have found much meaning and challenge in the widespread determination to understand the meaning of the word *health* as much broader and deeper than ever before. It is a natural part of the vocabulary of the Bible and of Christian theology. "And thy health shall spring forth" is a famous quotation from Isaiah. *Health* and *salvation* are words used interchangeably throughout the scriptures. Parish nurses are engaged in doing the Lord's work when they assist in encouraging people to move toward the whole-person goals of the highest scriptural injunctions.

Parish nurses are now serving in hundreds of churches throughout the country, united in their desire to bring salvation to people, understanding that the basic meaning of the word *salvation* is *being made whole.* The Great Physician knows that not everyone wants to be made whole. Churches are in the motivation business. They understand how important it is to motivate people to want to live healthier lives. Christ himself asked that question of the man at the pool of Bethesda: "Do you want to be made whole?"

The whole person movement takes a person's belief system seriously. If one's belief system is faulty, it affects the way the body functions. If whole person concepts can be integrated with one's religious beliefs, then each will provide motivation for the other.

This is a time in history when the Church is sorely needed to help motivate people to put body, mind, and spirit together and to convince them that the integration of these three can lead to truth, health, and wholeness.

Let us sum up some of our reasons for believing that churches provide a natural setting where parish nurses can do their most effective work as health educators, health counselors, coordinators of volunteers, agents of referral into our complex medical system, and integrators of faith and health.

1. Churches are to be found everywhere, out in neighborhoods where people live—urban, suburban, rural—and their buildings are largely unused during the weekdays.

2. Churches have a long history of serving their communities through social activities and continuing education programs.

3. Churches symbolize our need to take seriously the problems of the human spirit that are so often related to the causes of illness.

4. Churches provide a remarkable reservoir of dedicated people who are willing to volunteer their services to assist in humanitarian endeavors.

5. Church members have a growing appreciation for the opportunity to model, in their own church buildings, the need for cooperation between scientific medicine and religious faith.

The role of parish nurses is basically a reaching out for more whole person ways of ministering to people who are hurting. There is a slowly growing desire among many health care professionals to integrate human caring with the achievements of high-tech medical care. Most of these professionals are under such restraints of time and bottom-line concerns that they cannot practice what they know would be better health care.

Parish nurses have the unique opportunity to demonstrate effective ways of combining the strengths of such collaboration between the humanities and the sciences.

References

Jones, E. S. (1930). *The way.* New York: Asssociation Press.

The wholistic health centers: A new direction in health care (Experience report). (1977). Battle Creek, MI: W. K. Kellogg Foundation.

Tubesing, D. (1977). An idea in evolution. In *History of the wholistic health centers project.* Hinsdale, IL: Society for Wholistic Medicine.

Westberg, G. (1982). The church as health place. *Dialog, 27*(3), 189-191.

Westberg, G. (1988, November/December). Parishes, nurses and health care. *Lutheran Partners,* pp. 26-29.

Wholistic health centers: Survey research report. (1976). Hinsdale, IL: Society for Wholistic Medicine.

4

Spiritual Caregiving

A Key Component
of Parish Nursing

Marcia Schnorr

Nurses claim to be concerned about the whole person, but their emphasis often lies in the physical dimension of care. Nurses generally identify the psychological, social, and spiritual dimensions as they describe humankind, but there is often a psychosocial and spiritual maze that may lead anywhere—or nowhere.

Many nurses hesitate to include spiritual care because they "don't want to push religion," "religion is the job of the minister," or "religion is too personal." Some nurses are uncomfortable discussing religion. Other nurses believe that they have considered the spiritual needs of their patients by inquiring about their religious preference upon admission. Parish nurses, by their very nature, may be more attuned to the religious needs of their "patients." Religious affiliation may be identified, and religious needs may be addressed, but what about spiritual care? Unlike other nurses, parish nurses not only *can* provide spiritual care, they *should* be spiritual caregivers.

This chapter describes, in part, the research for my doctoral dissertation, "Spiritual Nursing Care: Theory and Curriculum Development" (Schnorr, 1988). Although it seems that there has been increased interest in the topic of spiritual nursing care, there continues to be some general hesitation on the part of some nurses to include spiritual care in their nursing care. Some nurses continue to confuse spiritual care with psychosocial care. Some nurses advocate spiritual care, choosing alternative therapies. Other nurses are determined to provide spiritual care that is consistent with Christianity or other faith traditions.

Definitions

Spirituality and *religion* are words that are often used interchangeably, but they are not synonymous. Several writers have provided insights concerning the similarities and differences in these two concepts. For the purposes of this chapter, the following collective definitions will be used.

Spirituality is that life principle that pervades the entire being, integrating and transcending all other dimensions of life. It gives meaning to life and death. It offers love and relatedness. It includes the need for forgiveness. It includes hope, trust, and faith. It involves a belief in a supernatural or higher power (Bell, 1985; Carpenito, 1993; Carson, 1997; Conrad, 1985; Dettmore, 1985; Gordon, 1992; Granstrom, 1985; Mayer, 1992; McFarland & Wasli, 1986; Sumner, 1998).

Religion, on the other hand, is an organized system of beliefs and practices. It is the spiritual application of the relationship between people and their God (Carson, 1997; Granstrom, 1985; Kennedy, 1984).

Spirituality and religion are *related,* but they are not identical. Religious and spiritual care are also related, but they are also not identical.

Review of the Literature

This brief literature review will consider two major themes. First, indications for spiritual nursing care will be considered. Second, research related to spiritual nursing care will be presented.

Indications for Spiritual Nursing Care

Steiger and Lipson (1985) stated that many nurses are troubled regarding the extent to which they should intervene in the spiritual needs of patients. They warn that the nurse should, however, assess and support the spiritual dimension of the patient (see also Fish, 1995; Price, Stevens, & LaBarre, 1995).

Piles (1990) continues to report that many nurses are reluctant to provide spiritual nursing care. Hamner (1990) reports that some nursing schools provide minimal content in spiritual health and distress. Boutell and Bozett (1990) surveyed 238 practicing nurses and found that the majority did not assess spiritual needs. Taylor, Highfield, and Amenta (1995) studied the practice of oncology nurses and found that the majority did not feel comfortable providing spiritual care.

The American Nurses' Association Congress for Nursing Practice (1980) developed the *Social Policy Statement,* which says that nurses must concern themselves with anything that has the potential to affect the health of an individual. Soeken and Carson (1986) stated that the *Code of Ethics* of the International Council of Nurses requires that nurses be responsible for spiritual care and not just for the more familiar concerns of nursing.

The *Standards of Practice for Parish Nurses* developed by the Health Ministries Association (1997) states, "Parish nursing . . . focuses on the promotion of health within the context of a faith community. . . ." Standards of Practice for Parish Nursing within the Lutheran Church Missouri Synod (1994) identifies Spiritual care as a component of each of the roles of the parish nurse.

Research Related to Spiritual Nursing Care

Highfield and Cason (1983) completed a study to determine the awareness by nurses of spiritual concerns of patients. The results indicated that most of the nurses believed the spiritual to be part of psychosocial health.

Haase, Britt, Coward, Leidy, and Penn (1992) studied the relationship between spirituality, hope, acceptance, and self-transcendence in health. Their findings suggest that each of these concepts provides a connectedness that seems to be a positive factor in attaining a higher level of wellness.

Stiles (1990) reports that providing spiritual care gives meaning and spiritual growth to the patient and nurse. Mickley, Soeken, and Belcher (1992) found a positive relationship between spiritual well-being, religiousness, and hope among women with breast cancer.

Stepnick and Perry (1992) provided helpful guidelines for preventing spiritual distress in the dying client. The authors incorporated the phases of spiritual development described by Peck (1987) in developing a framework to preserve the spiritual integrity of dying clients.

Corrine, Bailey, Valentin, Morantus, and Shirley (1992) provided insights regarding the provision of spiritual care to women experiencing spiritual distress related to the death of an infant or child, sudden infant death syndrome, miscarriage, or infertility. Spiritual interventions were identified as important in minimizing spiritual distress and enhancing spiritual health.

Research to Develop a Theory of Spiritual Nursing Care

In the past, most research related to spiritual nursing care was conducted in hospital settings. Most of these studies identified perceived spiritual needs and the inadequacy of nurses in recognizing and responding to these needs.

I completed research to develop a substantive theory in spiritual nursing care that may be helpful to nurses in any setting (Schnorr, 1988). This study used the principles of grounded theory methodology, a method that is especially appropriate for applied professional fields such as nursing.

For this study, the unstructured interview was used to collect data. Although there was no structured interview schedule, a guideline was used that included demographic questions and questions related to the research questions.

Health care providers and health care recipients were asked to recommend registered nurses who (a) were involved in direct patient care, (b) included spirituality in their nursing care, and (c) did not equate spiritual care with proselytizing. Nurses who were recommended to this researcher were invited to participate in voluntary, confidential interviews, and interviewing continued until theoretical saturation was reached (until no new information was being discovered).

The final research sample included 46 registered nurses, representing 12 states, 1 territory, and 2 foreign countries. The sample included nurses with varied sources of paid or voluntary practice and diverse areas of practice and specialty areas. The sample included nurses from each of the three basic educational programs that qualify one to take the licensure examination for a registered nurse. The nurses in the sample had from 1 to 42 years of nursing experience. Although the nurses were not asked about their religious affiliation, 44 of them identified themselves as Christian; the other two nurses described themselves as "nontraditional."

Overview of the *CIRCLE* Model of Spiritual Care

As a result of the data collection in my study (Schnorr, 1988), the CIRCLE Model of Spiritual Nursing Care was developed (see Figure 4.1).

Setting

The nurses in this research sample had different professional backgrounds, and they identified settings for spiritual nursing care that were just as varied. One of the interviews could be summarized as "Any situation can elicit a spiritual need." Spiritual care can, and should, be a part of nursing care in any setting.

Recipient of Spiritual Nursing Care

The "identified patient" is the most obvious recipient of spiritual nursing care, but the care could and should extend to the families, friends, other personnel, and nurses themselves. Everyone who is playing a significant role in the life and care of the "patient" has a potential need for spiritual care.

Provider of Spiritual Nursing Care

The provider of spiritual nursing care can be any nurse who has the interest, knowledge, skills, and commitment necessary to care for the whole person. This nurse is not limited to a particular setting or by a specific educational program. She is limited only by her personal philosophy of nursing care.

Nursing Process

Assessment. The three main "tools" identified for assessing spiritual needs are (a) religious cues, (b) emotional cues, and (c) assessment guides.

Religious cues may be direct statements regarding a religious need, the use of religious jargon, religious comments, and/or a specific request. Religious cues may, however, be indirect—references to "the man upstairs," asking the "why me" question, or hiding the request in humor. The nurse may also pick up on religious cues from items in the environment (e.g., religious literature, religious works of art, jewelry, or artifacts).

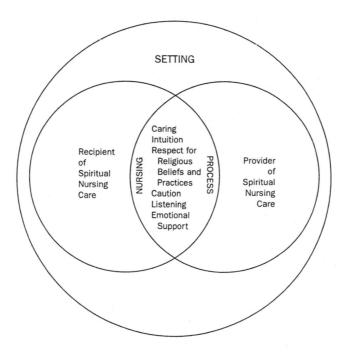

Figure 4.1. CIRCLE Model of Spiritual Care

Assessment guides are helpful in specifically addressing the spiritual dimension. Unfortunately, few nursing assessment guides provide more than a cursory glance at the spiritual dimension. Stoll (1979) developed an assessment guide that is specific to the spiritual dimension of humankind. This guide continues to be a useful tool for nurses. A "Family/Individualized Health Survey" is available from the Health Ministries of the Lutheran Church Missouri Synod (Board for Human Care, 1989) and addresses the whole person, including spiritual health issues. A "Parish Nurse Whole Person Inventory," which is available from the International Parish Nurse Resource Center (1989), also includes a section specific to the spiritual dimension of health.

Planning and intervention. The six specific concepts included in spiritual nursing are (a) caring, (b) intuition, (c) respect for religious beliefs and practices, (d) caution, (e) listening, and (f) emotional support. The first letter of each of these concepts form the acronym *CIRCLE.*

Caring is the foundation for any nursing care, and spiritual care is no exception. Caring includes (a) demonstrating care and compassion, (b) possessing a caring attitude, and (c) caring enough to take or use the available time.

Nurses must demonstrate care and compassion—not just *say* that they care. Nurses have consistently referred to "tender loving care" as an important part of nursing care. What the nurse does speaks much louder than the words that the nurse uses. Nurses need to *show* that they care.

Nurses also have to have a genuinely caring attitude. It is the caring attitude that gives meaning to the caring behaviors.

Nurses need to take or use the available time. It is not so much the amount of time that is available; nurses are always busy. It is taking advantage of the time that you have, rather than wasting it on empty words and hurried routines. Spiritual care can be incorporated into the time spent taking care of other basic needs.

Intuition, as simple as it may seem, may be valuable in spiritual nursing care. Intuition includes (a) possessing instinctive feelings, (b) acting on instinct, and (c) sensing the unspoken message.

Nurses who give spiritual care often describe a "feeling," an "instinct," a "gut feeling," and/or a "hunch" that there is a spiritual need. These feelings are, of course, grounded in an awareness of the spiritual dimension, practical experience, and an openness to respond to the spiritual needs of people. These nurses stated that they "follow their hunches" and are generally right. Many times it is the unspoken message of the individual that reveals the spiritual need; nurses must learn to "read between the lines."

Respect for religious beliefs and practices includes (a) making appropriate referrals, (b) praying, (c) encouraging devotional activities, (d) providing for specific rites and sacraments, and (e) offering religious conversation.

Referral can be an important part of spiritual nursing care. Referral, however, should not be done for the sole convenience of the nurse. Referral should be made at the proper time and to the proper person—as determined by the needs of the individual. Some persons prefer to talk to nurses because they are perceived to be less threatening than the clergyperson who "represents God" and, therefore, is more intimidating. Some persons may prefer to talk to the clergyperson because their concerns can only be relieved by "the authority." Other persons may find their spiritual needs met best by a specific family member, friend, or an individual who has had a similar experience.

The need for prayer must be recognized and respected. Nurses may pray for patients, nurses may pray with patients, and nurses may allow patients to pray for themselves. The decision about how to pray, when to pray, and what to pray for should not be made before some basic assessments have been made. Prayer, whether for, with, or by the patient, must take into account the patient's needs to be meaningful.

Nurses can encourage devotional activities such as reading, listening to inspirational music, and attending worship services. Some individuals find private devotions meaningful; other individuals prefer to participate in group devotions. Nurses can encourage the person to participate in personal or group devotions; nurses can also offer to share a devotion with the individual (patient, family member, etc.).

Nurses should know the religious belief of their patients and the rites and sacraments practiced by that religion. It is important that the nurse be prepared to perform or make arrangements for appropriate sacraments or rites in case of emergency (e.g., baptism). Nurses also need to be aware of dietary regulations, significant artifacts (e.g., medals or beads), and other religious practices that may be meaningful to the patient. When the caregiver has the same religious affiliation as the recipient of care, this happens almost automatically. However, when the caregiver and the recipient of care do not share the same religious beliefs, the nurse must address the religious needs of the recipient of care and not those of the caregiver.

Religious conversations can be quite informal and nonthreatening. These simple conversations can, however, be meaningful approaches to allowing the individual to sort out spiritual concerns.

Caution is an important concept in spiritual nursing care. Caution includes (a) declining to proselytize, (b) avoiding judgments, and (c) giving choices.

Nurses should never push, manipulate, or force religion onto their patients. Patients will "choke" if nurses try to "cram religion down their throats." Nurses need to be natural and live their beliefs, not preach them.

Nurses should not judge their patients; judging will only result in antagonizing them, and the nursing care will be less effective. It is the responsibility of the nurses to minister to the whole person needs of the patients.

On the other hand, nurses should not hesitate to *offer* the patient spiritual care, including religious ministration. When nurses do not offer, patients are not given the choice, and spiritual needs are not met. If, however, the offer meets with resistance, it is the patient's right to have other needs met without being forced to participate in spiritual and/or religious care.

Listening includes (a) making an effort to hear what the person feels and (b) encouraging the person to express feelings. Listening is the most important skill the nurse can use.

Listening includes more than hearing the words that are spoken. Listening includes catching feelings expressed and understanding the meaning these feelings have for the individual. Listening involves getting to know people, their interests, their supports, and their aspirations.

Nurses must not only listen, nurses must encourage their patients to express their feelings. Nurses need to support and encourage people to express their feelings; nurses also need to *accept* both the feeling expressed and the person who expressed them.

Emotional support provides the vital link between psychosocial and spiritual dimensions of care. Emotional support includes (a) working through feelings, (b) showing love, and (c) touching.

Feelings that are repressed will reemerge later, often presenting a greater threat. Feelings, including those related to spiritual distress, must be worked through.

Love and respect can and should be shown to all persons. At times, nurses need to be firm; this firmness, however, must not be devoid of love. Empathy, not sympathy, is an important component of nursing care. It is difficult, however, if not impossible, to demonstrate empathy without feeling love.

A hug, a pat on the back, quietly being present, holding hands all convey a message that often evokes emotional and spiritual healing. The nurses must also respect the individual who indicates discomfort in being physically touched and discover alternative ways to "touch" that person.

Evaluation. Sometimes the result of spiritual nursing care may not be immediately known. At other times, however, a positive change can be identified. These changes may be relational, physical, emotional, intellectual, and/or religious.

The following are examples of implementation of the CIRCLE model of spiritual care used by the parish nurse. The examples are genuine, but the names have been changed for confidentiality.

Mr. Smith came to the blood pressure screening that is held after each worship service one Sunday a month. His initial blood pressure reading was 182/110. Mr. Smith returned three times that Sunday to have his blood pressure rechecked; each time it was essentially the same.

Although the "reason" for his visit was to have his blood pressure checked, the parish nurse was also able to assess his emotional distress. Mr. Smith was worried. He expressed that his father had died of a stroke some years ago. It was clear that Mr. Smith worked hard in his job as well as with several church and community organizations. Lately he had been subjected to a number of stressors. Mr. Smith's blood pressure was not his only problem.

The parish nurse *cared* about Mr. Smith and demonstrated this through her attitude, presence, and time. *Intuition* told the parish nurse that Mr. Smith was worried and fearful that he might have a stroke like his dad. The parish nurse also suspected that he had some questions about the future. Through Mr. Smith's behavior and conversation, the parish nurse knew how important his religion and spiritual life were to him. *Respect for his religious beliefs and practices* was exhibited by the parish nurse through sharing religious conversation, referring to scripture, and encouraging him to continue in the sacraments and religious practices that he found meaningful. *Caution* was used by the parish nurse; she did not judge him in any way or assume that she really knew him and his spiritual resources. The parish nurse *listened* to what he said and didn't say. She tuned in to the meaning and the feeling of his communications, verbal and nonverbal. *Emotional support* was offered by the parish nurse by words, caring, and the use of touch.

Don't think for a moment that the 182/110 blood pressure was ignored. The parish nurse referred him to his physician for medical management. His pressure is now 132/84. By making herself available to the needs of Mr. Smith's whole person, care was made available through using the CIRCLE model.

The parish nurse received a telephone call informing her that Tommy (a child not quite 2 years old) had been taken to the local hospital following a fall. The parish nurse was told that he was under "routine" observation and that it was not necessary to visit until the next day. Before the next day, however, the parish nurse received another call. Tommy had "taken a turn for the worse" and had been transported by helicopter to a pediatric intensive care unit in a nearby city.

The parish nurse immediately went to visit Tommy and to let the family know that she *cared.* She learned that Tommy had been diagnosed with bacterial meningitis and the prognosis was guarded.

The parish nurse observed that the family was close, and her *intuition* told her that there would be many people there and an outpouring of different emotions. She was right. She instinctively knew they would appreciate her visit. They did. Most of the family (parents, grandparents, aunts, and uncles) are members of the parish nurse's congregation. Many of them are active participants. The grandmother and one aunt are involved in the music program. *Respect for their religious beliefs and practices* was demonstrated. The parish nurse prayed together with the family. The parish nurse and the family spoke of God's love. During one of the times that Grandma was at Tommy's bedside, the parish nurse suggested that they all sing "I Am Jesus' Little Lamb" for the unconscious child. Singing, they wept prayerful tears.

The family had many questions. The doctors had few sure answers. The parish nurse used *caution* when attempting to respond to their questions. They wanted at least *some* answers. They needed reassurance. The parish nurse wanted to provided some answers—but no false hope.

The next 2 weeks were a roller coaster. The situation seemed better, then worse. The doctors did not always agree. Tommy was transferred from the pediatric intensive care unit. This, however, did not mean that the news was all good. Doctors warned that Tommy might be blind, deaf, retarded, and/or physically challenged. The parish nurse *listened* as the family members shared their hopes, their fears, their anxiety, their grief, their searching. *Emotional support* was provided through shared hugs, tears, and caring.

Tommy was finally discharged and began a long, carefully planned comprehensive therapy plan. The parish nurse continued to show concern and support. Tommy was in the congregation's prayers. Tommy was finally fitted with hearing aids and glasses, and he continues to regain coordination through physical therapy.

Summary

The relationship between the patient and the nurse is often closer when a nursing response includes spiritual interventions. Relationships between family members often improve when spiritual issues have been recognized and addressed. Spiritual care can result in mending relationships that have been weakened by conflict and strain between individuals.

Some nurses reported, in the data collection for the research that culminated in the CIRCLE model, that they had patients who required less sedation or less analgesic after they received spiritual care. Other nurses reported that patients "seemed sicker" before their spiritual needs were recognized and included in the nursing care.

Spiritual care can have a calming effect and reduce patient anxiety. Patients, families, and other recipients of care seem more relaxed when their spiritual needs are met. Spiritual care "takes the edge off"; people are less afraid. Patients get a sense of peace and are better able to deal with things when their spiritual needs are met. They are better able to accept the situation and make "healthier" decisions. They are more settled—not plagued by so many questions that have no answers.

Individuals may maintain or regain meaning from their religion as a result of spiritual nursing care. There may be a sense of renewal, reaffirmation, and reconciliation with their God, their church, and their inner self.

A parish nurse is not just a nurse in the parish. Parish nursing was founded with spiritual care as the core of the practice. Parish nurses must never hesitate to provide spiritual care. Parish nurses should be comfortable with psychosocial nursing skills but not confuse them with spiritual nursing care.

Parish nurses, like other nurses, may have varying degrees of comfort in providing spiritual care. Unlike other nurses, parish nurses are in a setting that makes spiritual care an accepted (even essential) component of their ministry. Practice in assessing spiritual needs and assets, suggesting or implementing spiritual intervention will improve the parish nurse's comfort and skill level in ministering spiritually to others who can be considered more advanced.

To be proficient, parish nurses must take advantage of opportunities to develop their spiritual caregiving expertise. Attending educational programs, which should include spiritual caregiving, is important for parish nurses. Some programs provide instruction specific to new parish nurses. Other programs offer more eclectic, alternative modes for spiritual caregiving. Parish nurses need to take advantage of spiritual growth opportunities that are available within the community of faith. Nurses who work in congregations but do not have spiritual care as the core of their practice may be nurses in the parish, but they are not parish nurses.

References

American Nurses Association and Health Ministries Association. (1998). *Standards of practice for parish nurses.* Washington, DC: American Nurses Publishing.

American Nurses Association Congress for Nursing Practice. (1980). *Nursing: A social policy statement.* Kansas City, MO: American Nurses' Association.

Bell, H. K. (1985). The spiritual care component of palliative care. *Seminar Oncology, 12*(4), 482-485.

Board for Human Care, Lutheran Church Missouri Synod. (1989). *Family/individualized health survey* (mimeograph). St. Louis, MO: Author.

Boutell, K. A., & Bozett, F. W. (1990). Nurses' assessment of patients' spirituality: Continuing education implications. *Journal of Continuing Education in Nursing, 21,* 172-176.

Carpenito, L. J. (1993). *Nursing diagnosis: Application to clinical practice* (5th ed.). Philadelphia: J. B. Lippincott.

Carson, V. B. (1997). Spirituality and patient care. In A. W. Burgess (Ed.), *Psychiatric nursing: Promoting mental health* (pp. 143-149). Stanford, CT: Appleton & Lange.

Conrad, N. L. (1985). Spiritual support for the dying. *Nursing Clinics of North America, 20,* 515-526.

Corrine, L., Bailey, V., Valentin, M., Morantus, E., & Shirley, L. (1992). The unheard voices of women: Spiritual interventions in maternal-child health. *Maternal Child Nursing, 17,* 141-145.

Dettmore, D. (1985). *Nurses' conceptions and practices in the spiritual dimension of nursing.* Unpublished doctoral dissertation, Columbia University, New York.

Fish, S. (1995). Can research prove that God answers prayers? *Journal of Christian Nursing, 12*(1), 24-27.

Gordon, M. (1992). *Manual of nursing diagnosis.* St. Louis, MO: Mosby Year Book.

Granstrom, S. L. (1985). Spiritual nursing care for oncology patients. *Topics in Clinical Nursing, 10,* 39-45.

Haase, J. E., Britt, T., Coward, D. D., Leidy, N. K., & Penn, P. E. (1992). Simultaneous concept analysis of spiritual perspective, hope, acceptance and transcendence. *IMAGE: Journal of Nursing Scholarship, 24*(2), 141-147.

Hamner, M. L. (1990). Spiritual needs: A forgotten dimension of care? *Journal of Gerontological Nursing, 16*(12), 3-4.

Highfield, M., & Cason, C. (1983). Spiritual needs of patients: Are they recognized? *Cancer Nursing, 6,* 187-192.

International Parish Nurse Resource Center. (1989). *Parish nurse whole person inventory* (mimeograph). Park Ridge, IL: Author.

Kennedy, R. (1984). *The international dictionary of religion.* New York: Crossroads.

Lutheran Church Missouri Synod. (1994). *Standards of practice for parish nurses in the Lutheran Church Missouri Synod* (mimeograph). St. Louis, MO: Author.

Mayer, J. (1992). Wholly responsible for a part, or partly responsible for a whole? *Second Opinion, 17*(3), 26-55.

McFarland, G., & Wasli, E. (1986). *Nursing diagnosis and process in psychiatric mental health nursing.* Philadelphia: J. B. Lippincott.

Mickley, J. R., Soeken, K., & Belcher, A. (1992). Spiritual well-being, religiousness and hope among women with breast cancer. *IMAGE: Journal of Nursing Scholarship, 24*(4), 267-272.

Peck, M. (1987). *The different drum: Community making and peace.* New York: Simon & Schuster.

Piles, C. (1990). Providing spiritual care. *Nurse Educator, 15*(1), 36-41.

Price, J. L., Stevens, H. O., & LaBarre, M. C. (1995). Spiritual caregiving in nursing practice. *Journal of Psychosocial Nursing, 33*(12), 5-9.

Schnorr, M. A. (1988). *Spiritual nursing care: Theory and curriculum development* (Doctoral dissertation, Northern Illinois University). *Dissertation Abstracts International, 50,* 601-A DA8912525.

Soeken, K. L., & Carson, V. T. (1986). Study measures nurses' attitudes about providing spiritual care. *Health Progress, 67,* 52-55.

Steiger, N. J., & Lipson, T. G. (1985). *Self-care nursing theory and practice.* Bowie, MD: Brady Communication.

Stepnick, A., & Perry, T. (1992). Preventing spiritual distress in the dying client. *Journal of Psychosocial Nursing, 30*(1), 17-24.

Stiles, M. K. (1990). The shining stranger: Nurse-family spiritual relationship. *Cancer Nursing, 13,* 235-245.

Stoll, R. (1979). Guidelines for spiritual assessment. *American Journal of Nursing, 79*(9), 1574-1577.

Sumner, C. H. (1998). Recognizing and responding to spiritual distress. *American Journal of Nursing, 98*(1), 26-31.

Taylor, E. J., Highfield, M., & Amenta, M. (1995). Spiritual care practices of oncology nurses. *Oncology Nurses Forum, 22,* 31-39.

5

Parish Nursing Practice With Underorganized, Underserved, and Marginalized Clients

JoAnn Gragnani Boss

The exclusion of the weak and insignificant, the seemingly useless people from a Christian community may actually mean the exclusion of Christ. In the poor, Christ is knocking at the door. We must, therefore, be very careful at this point.

—Dietrick Bonhoeffer

Overview

The unique manner in which the seven functions of the parish nurse are made manifest with underorganized, underserved, and marginalized populations will be explored in terms of "being present" in complex relationships. Guidelines within the parish nursing practice for healing broken social structures are examined. Strategies for support and renewal for nurses working in this setting are identified throughout.

To illustrate the above points, material has been gathered from 10 parish nurses who collectively have over 60 years of experience in urban parish nurse ministry. Several have a decade of practice in this specialty, and 3 years was the shortest time spent as a parish nurse. The average length of service is about 6 years. This empirical approach

AUTHOR'S NOTE: The author wishes to extend the deepest gratitude to the parish nurses and staff at Advocate Health Care, Park Ridge, Ilinois, for the important part they have played in contributing to this chapter and to her ongoing spiritual formation.

captures the qualitative human interactions that best represent the heart of inner-city parish nursing.

Impoverishment: The Context for an Inner-City Parish Nurse Practice

"Inner city" brings to mind a number of images. A portrait of poverty is accompanied by a collage of related problems and deficits: unemployment, crime, gang activity, homelessness, mental illness, alcohol and drug abuse, abuse of all varieties, and limited access to all types of services, including health care. Ethnic diversity, which might be perceived as an asset in another community's landscape, is here a limiting characteristic, as it is most often complicated by language barriers and sometimes uncertain legal status. Safety issues may result in isolation. A sense of perpetual crisis pervades the environment.

Inner-city parish nurses talk about the economics of those in poverty. Sheer multiplication of financial, social, mental or emotional, and spiritual deficits compound the destitution of this population. Some individuals have been isolated for years. They overtly show their underorganization by transferring attachments from others to objects: They may carry their "precious" belongings with them everywhere. Because they overaccumulate, narrow pathways are the only passages through their rooms. Many do not access health care services located within blocks of their dwelling. Their wallets may contain "treasured" pieces of torn paper or stained business cards with phone numbers once tried or never used.

Inner-city parish nurses talk about their practice among people surviving on the edges of poverty who have various family configurations and are from different cultures that challenge the nurses' worldview. Many of the urban parish nurses' parishioners and community members are "unchurched" but have very strong preconceived ideas about religious matters. Being present with those whose orientation is dramatically different can be both refreshing and challenging.

Psychospiritual approaches educate and refresh the parish nurses from getting overwhelmed by the daily oppression and deprivations in their ministries. Important to the parish nurses is regular attendance at parish nurse meetings sponsored by the employing health care institution where meaningful time is spent in prayer, sharing, and theological reflection. Through these means, the parish nurses stay connected and open rather than remaining aloof or sure of their worldviews. Insights are discovered that affect their relationships, problem-solving abilities, and program strategies.

Mutuality: A Framework for Promoting and Sustaining Urban Parish Nursing Services

For parish nurses to care for their clients, it is important to know and understand the clients' values, beliefs, attitudes, and feelings about the situations that confront them. Before a parish nurse can advocate effectively for another's right or assist others who have different assumptions, the nurse needs to become aware of the client's positive and negative responses to the situation. When parish nurses acknowledge their own personal perspectives, new ways of relating to others begin to emerge.

> My professional struggles continue to lead me on a search for a fuller understanding of how to companion persons whose lives are crisis managed. I'm a little slower to react, less inquisitive in my asking, more willing to listen, more likely to focus on what the other wants now. (Boss, Parish Nurse Program, 1992, p. 4)[1]

The traditional whole-person assessment tools give way to building relationships through sharing one's story. The parish nurse's concern can translate into quality time with the person or family. It means listening and responding to their stories. Through the city dweller's stories are insights into their psychospiritual world. Sometimes, faith is their lifeline; sometimes, lack of religious or spiritual involvement parallels lack of interpersonal attachments.

The parish nurse uses the stories evoked by needs, wants, problems, feelings, or strengths in developing a relationship with the unorganized, underserved, and marginalized. These stories are entry points into their lives. Both the parish nurses' and the community members' worldviews become clearer; the richness of meaning is revealed.

In "An Emerging Theory of Human Relatedness" (Hagerty, Lynch-Sauer, Patusky, & Bouwsema, 1993), mutuality is described as "the experience of real or symbolic shared commonalties of visions, goals, sentiments or characteristics, including shared acceptance of differences that validate the person's world-view" (p. 294). A sense of belonging, reciprocity, synchrony, and mutuality are the four social processes that create movement towards involvement with others, report Hagerty et al. They state that disconnectedness occurs when one experiences low levels of these four processes. Furthermore, "disruption in client's relatedness contributes to biological, psychological, and social disturbances" (p. 291).

The direction and approach to inner-city parish nursing practice evolves around this spoken or unspoken standard of mutuality. The brokenness of the impoverished inner-city dwellers has penetrated deep within their bodies, minds, hearts, and souls. Mutuality is the context in which brokenness can be healed.

Mutuality can be bonded with a faith development process. Elements of sharing acceptance of commonalties or differences can be woven into building faith communities. These conditions are "praying together, studying together, ministering together (or at least sharing together about our ministry), dialoguing together and socializing together" (Fonck, 1983, p. 23).

A link between the psychospiritual realm and mutuality is found in the BeFriender's Model (*BeFriender Ministry Coordinator Manual,* 1995) for developing mutual relating skills. This model divides mutuality into four behavioral building blocks: "telling our story appropriately, understanding another's story accurately, giving feedback respectfully, and receiving feedback with a measure of openness" (Section II.5).

Tanner, Benner, Chesla, and Gordon (1993) state that getting to know a family or community member is "primary caring practice" (p. 275). They asserted,

> Knowing the patient is central to skilled clinical judgment and is broader than what is captured in formal assessments of physical systems. Knowing the patient is a practical nursing discourse that points to specific nursing skills of seeing and involvement.

Knowing the patient creates the possibility of advocacy. Knowing individual patients
sets up learning about patient populations. (p. 277)

Leininger (1991) described the activities of presence (spending time and listening)
as "signs of respect for patients as human beings . . . 'good care' by being attentive,
compassionate, and empathic to their needs" (p. 8).

This fundamental value and spiritual practice of mutuality, therefore, also extends
to the ministerial team, as often the needs of church members are not addressed by one
staff member alone. Some parish nurses can feel they are "team players" with the parish
staff, church councils, and volunteers. However, some nurses can feel like outsiders or
lone workers functioning independent of staff and volunteers. Quality time and attention
is needed to develop mutuality in ministry among all members of the parish staff and
lay volunteers. The areas of team building and shared ministry are critical for the mission
of a healthy, healing church community.

The parish nurse's interventions can be instrumental in influencing health standards
in individuals and communities. Health policy monitoring as a defined intervention of
the Nursing Interventions Classification (NIC) taxonomy (McCloskey & Bulechek,
1996, p. 310) is very appropriate for urban parish nurses. For example, across the street
from one inner-city parish is a single-room-occupancy hotel (SRO) that serves as a
residence for the chronically mentally ill. Many of the SRO residents come to the church
for clothes, food, and companionship. Usually at this time the parish nurse hears
descriptions of "life inside the walls" from some of the SRO residents. When the parish
nurse, along with another staff member of the church, requested a meeting with the
building owner, they found that the complaints were all true: The building was in terrible
disrepair, the food was minimal, and violence occurred due to lack of rules and trained
supervision. But this particular matter needed a higher degree of attention.

Sitting in a court room and feeling alone, the parish nurse faced the city housing
inspectors and the current owner of the SRO. As an advocate for the residents of the
SRO, the nurse brought up questions to the court about the owner's alleged goodwill.
This was possible because of validation provided by the parish staff. Sometimes follow-
through requires more organization than the urban poor can or care to provide. If this
inadequate system of care had continued without some attempt to stop it, the parish nurse
and ministerial staff, too, would be culpable (Corbett, Parish Nurse Program, 1992, pp. 6-7).

The parish nurse nurtures healthier one-to-one relationships. Through this effort, a
supportive faith community grows. The inner-city church can become a haven, a
stabilizing place. Community members can stop in for coffee, talk, get warm, and state
their latest problems.

The Expanding Role of Inner-City Parish Nurses:
Presence in Complex Relationships

Inner-city work takes tenacious determination because of the comprehensive life
problems of the people. Being deprived, depleted, and drained psychologically, emotionally, physically, culturally, and spiritually plunges the urban poor into frozen development processes as their bodies grow older and weaken. The accumulation of violence
and oppression takes its toll.

Ethnic language restraints and cultural diversity prevail. As one parish nurse so poignantly described,

> Whether it be language barrier or cultural norms—as parish nurse, I often find energy and time being consumed in establishing a communicable relationship. This relationship establishment can be so involved that any actual health intervention or teaching often is an unreached goal. (Cox, 1995, p. 3)

Parish nurses guard against becoming the indispensable comforter in whatever form that may look like: taking on family role responsibilities, performing community health nursing activities like changing dressings or giving injections, or being their own best volunteer. Enabling the recycling of unhealthy behaviors occurs if parish nurses are too attached to *doing* nursing.

> A couple of very important points [that] I've learned from these reluctant friends are: (1) preventive health is important, but still they will wait until they are "real" sick before seeking medical attention. (2) I must be patient and non-judgmental in accepting their decision as to when it is the right time for them to make changes. (Galvan, Parish Nurse Program, 1990, p. 10)

The second point is critical. In postponing medical attention, clients must also be ready to accept consequences. Ironically, many times they are surprised by the severity of their disability. One person comes to mind: Because of her refusal to follow medical orders, she developed renal failure. This life-threatening state forced the choice for her. Finally, she was ready for the doctor's care. Now she receives dialysis treatments three times a week. Still, some clients seem never to come to terms due to a state of ongoing denial.

There have been times when voluntary cooperation on the part of the individual was overridden by the parish nurse. Respectful "Tough Love," limit setting, abuse protection from self-harm or harm to others, petitioning, and legal guardianship have been discussed. These interactions take a concerted effort on the part of all members of the ministerial and/or health team. They are difficult experiences for all of the interacting parties. The consolation is that basic human needs are being met, even though the intervention is perceived as inflicting pain.

"Perpetual crisis" is a way of life for many in parish communities of need. There seems to be only the narrowest window of betterment between the crises. The alcoholic man's congested heart failure improves, but he soon goes back to daily drinking. The battered wife is provided with temporary shelter one day, but she is back with the offender the next day. For months, a teen group plans for an outing, but on the day of the event, no one is able to attend.

The hardiness, resilience, audacity, and even stubbornness of the people encountered is remarkable. One thinks they are invincible and may survive beyond all possible odds. In "Nursing as Informed Caring for the Well-Being of Others" (Swanson, 1993), the author reported on one of the five interrelated processes of the theory, stating, "It is sustaining faith in the capacity of others to get through events or transitions and face a future with meaning that initiates and sustains nursing care" (p. 345).

It is no accident that some of the clientele in the inner city call the parish nurse "Mom" or "Sister." Parish nurses may see the relationship in a different light, but what counts is how the parishioner interprets it. Many deprived of healthy attachments long for these "imagined" relationships to bring healing to the present moment.

Parish nurses are called to be *in the moment* and "choose life" when confronted with life-threatening situations. The following story is valued as a critical element of how a parish nurse can be present and relate in the most healing way:

> Sophie refused to go to a hospital even though it was clear she had pneumonia, a fever, was emaciated and could hardly move. I did not insist. We talked and prayed together and before I left, I said I would return early the next day. Sophie had the courage to refuse medical and hospital help, which would only prolong her loneliness. Even in her utterly miserable living situation, she refused.
>
> She created an internal conflict in me: I was the nurse and knew what would make her feel better. That was my job. She knew what was hers. She did not want to put off death any longer. She had seen her sister in a dream the night before and she believed in God. (Five weeks earlier her sister and lifetime companion [had] died.) The way I could "help" her was not to insist on doing it in a particular way or in a cleaner place. In her apartment she was among her neighbors and in a setting in which she [had] lived for 30 years. She died alone on the couch.
>
> When I arrived the next day, I found her dead on the couch. Her eyes were still open, her left arm held in a position to ward off death, or perhaps to link arms to welcome the new dance she was now starting. She used to plead with me to not leave her alone, to be "sure to come back." Her faith was nourished by first Friday holy communion, visits by the parish staff. Holy cards, religious medals and rosary beads surrounded her room. She and others remind me again that to make this final crossing one needs familiar religious symbols and supportive people rather than life-support machines. (Corbett, Parish Nurse Program, 1993, p. 5-7)

Sophie and other members of the church families confirm the importance of parish nursing's fundamental concept of human relatedness: Clients receive visits and attention even if they do not "go along with the program." The inner-city parish nurse continues to visit because it is requested.

Inner-city parish nurses can be pulled into a centripetal force. The nurses' comforting and healing presence merges into this force, which leads them to the Life Source. Seeded deep in all aspects of presence is prayer: prayer for, prayer with, and prayer offered up by the congregation, volunteer ministries, and staff.

Inner-city parish nurses are unknowingly led down mazes, dead ends, and blind cul-de-sacs. However, mutual relating and presence transform the road to labyrinths with open and center-directed paths.

"Poverty" Nursing:
Guidelines for Healing Broken Social Structures

David Hilfiker (1995) states, "The absence of clear guidelines is virtually the hallmark of medical practice among the poor. It is not diseases that are different . . . it's the science that is different" (p. 8). New standards are needed that are appropriate to the environment of poverty.

> We who practice in poor communities are in the process of creating new "medical" approaches to dilemmas the profession has too long ignored and mishandled. Most of my patients have already, after all, fared badly in the traditional medical system and are often disinclined to submit to standard procedures like interviews and examinations, not to speak of expensive tests for vague or minor complaints . . . or even for serious ones. A new art of caring is needed for the poor. (p. 12)

Inner-city parish nursing is interconnected with "poverty nursing." It is not a "lowering" of nursing standards that is intended. Metropolitan parish nursing can develop standards of practice appropriate for impoverished communities of need whose members and environmental conditions are calling out to be made whole.

Sharing struggles, coping strategies, feelings, and progress with our neighbors in our churches is an intervention many nurses were told was not professionally appropriate. Breaking a professional "tradition" of nondisclosure only comes after one shifts professional loyalties and engages in new ways of relating to the poor (Voss, 1993, p. 105). The following guidelines for inner-city parish nursing are offered:

1. "Creativity" in applying the nursing process to at-risk populations is essential: (a) Trust is gained more through listening than questioning. (b) A 15-minute home visit provides more helpful, accurate data than a 1-hour office interview. (c) First impressions of the parish nurse and the parish community member are often inaccurate. (d) Don't assume that you know the problem—or the solution. (e) Time and experience confirm that few situations are crises.

2. Parish nurses continue to provide transportation, companionship, and share over coffee or tea on a selected basis. "Nontherapeutic services" can be very therapeutic (Voss, 1993, p. 106).

3. "You may find you are doing more work than the client. Therefore, choose with love what you want to do. Don't expect results, yet always hope" (Boss, 1994, p. 13).

4. "De-institutionalization is a journey all must make some effort to take" (Corbett, Parish Nurse Program, 1991, p. 6).

5. The intensity, the frequency, and the duration of interacting and networking are as variable as the people we serve. People drop in and out of the relationship, but they seldom leave completely.

Some other lessons inner-city parish nurses learned from tenacious "co-journers" have been these:

1. People value affirming relationships over advice-giving ones. Give the health care speeches between affirmations.

2. Health problems may be the entry point into people's lives, but love keeps you interested and intersecting even after death.

3. Loving your neighbors, while not easy, is less difficult than detaching from your own will.

4. The Spirit utters words to us in unexpected ways. Listening takes all the senses to comprehend! Practice! Practice! Pray!

5. Stop to smell the flowers. When I come across those hard-to-tolerate smells, I remember the helpful hint I was taught in public health class—mouth breathe.

6. Ministry to the poor is both communal and one-on-one. When both come at you at once, this is when a coffee or tea break helps, though it never seems appropriate. Pray for quick wit.

7. Sometimes our souls say yes before it registers with our minds or intellect. The "Incarnate Word" is more about our yes to the "big picture" than about informed consent for every minute detail. (Boss, 1996, pp. 3-4)

The incredible ethnic and socioeconomic diversity present in the city affects the role of the parish nurse in health promotion. Parish nurses keep a more global view of health and accountability to others when in touch with such diversity (Cox, 1995, p. 2).

In one urban parish, workshops have been presented according to needs determined by a church questionnaire and general health assessment of the community. In an attempt to further reach out to the people and provide a health component not previously available, one workshop obtained certification for the state to administer vision and hearing screening. Another parish nurse's blood pressure clinic, held after church once a month, provides one step to teach persons health responsibility (Ruch, 1995, p. 2).

Education in the inner city for at-risk populations may be determined by the statistics given by the local department of health. Residents of a local family shelter were taught about HIV/AIDS. A Latino parish was targeted for an American Cancer Society mammography project. Back-to-school health fairs were held to facilitate children getting their physicals and required immunizations before classes began. Frequent health talks on various topics are scheduled to help both a homeless shelter and a seniors' lunch program (Cox, 1995, p. 2).

Parish nurses need to consider how they are delivering parish nursing services. Do we empower or hinder the person and the community by our practice? The recommendations listed below can be helpful in discerning the level of healthy people and community making in our practice. This religious and spiritual view of health promotion offers a perspective of empowerment.

C. Parks (1995), a health behavior and health education instructor, examined community health promotion and prevention from this point of view. Listed (p. 4) are five strategies for empowerment:

1. Adopt a philosophy that more and better health services do not translate into better health—focus on how do services get utilized and what do the people need.

2. Develop a new vision of poor communities and communities of color.

3. Employ methods, services, and activities that help communities address the root causes of their problems and not just their symptoms.

4. Take Nehemiah's approach; look for the Nehemiahs in your neighborhood—people have a mind to work so advocate for, not do for.

5. Approach the community in the same manner that Jesus did—ask the right questions: Do you want to be made whole? What do you have to give?

In one multicultural neighborhood, the parish nurse and the health educator from the city's department of health organized lay health promoters and volunteer personnel groups. If "neighbor helping neighbor" programs have worked in Third World countries, why would it be different here? Urban parish nurses often struggle with finding qualified volunteers and people who will commit on a regular basis. After a series of introductory classes, ongoing education classes were scheduled biweekly. Prayer, discussion, role play, and potluck luncheons were essential parts of the curriculum.

To further develop ties and skills, one-to-one personal training sessions were held by the project's coordinator under the guidance of the parish nurse. Funding for this coordinator's position was available through an organization experienced in peer education movements in foreign countries.

The lay health promoters' modest successes include two small health fairs, blood-pressure screenings once a month at a food pantry, a series of grief support groups, and exercise classes. Participation in these events by the lay health promoters has increased their attendance at worship services.

Parish nurses assist in identifying the possible physical, emotional, and spiritual needs of all age groups. They have worked with children and youth through the Sunday school, summer programs, and vacation church school. As coordinators of volunteers and small groups, the nurses work with mothers of children, members experiencing the loss of a loved one, volunteers with the homebound, and children of aging parents (Knapp, 1995, p. 2).

Quality takes precedence over quantity. Participating in developing support groups has been an enlightening experience for all inner-city nurses. Generations of addicted family systems and dysfunctional social structures are not healed with brief encounters. Learning to trust and support each other's within-group process is an acquired skill for the community members. Rallying like-minded and committed volunteers seems to be the key to success. The support groups tend to be small in number, and the parish nurses find that projects done on a smaller scale build support (Galvan, Parish Nurse Program, 1993, p. 8).

Community networking will also validate the reasons for staying in the struggle as an inner-city parish nurse (Gillis, Parish Nurse Program, 1993, p. 11).

> I find it positive that a good majority of individuals I work with live within a few block radius of the church. That makes a true sense of neighborhood ministry possible. I have been grateful for a rather extensive network of social service agencies which service the homeless and low income in the city. (Cox, 1995, p. 2)

Even with the best networking system, there are no quick fixes in the city. Connelly, Keele, Kleinbeck, Schneider, and Cobb (1993), through their research on empowerment, describe four levels of empowerment: participating, choosing, supporting, and negotiating. "Each level subsumes the previous level; therefore if someone is at the supporting level they also will be participating and choosing" (p. 300). For inner-city parish nurses, the practice has less to do with physical health care than with healing relationships through the greater use of presence and mending broken interpersonal relationships and social structures through the empowerment process. Parish nurses in the urban ministry are learning how to do all three (Corbett, Parish Nurse Program, 1993, pp. 6-7).

Inner-city parish nursing programs can improve the quality of life for underorganized, underserved, and marginalized people—one person at a time, one faith community at a time.

> No one organization can fill in all the service gaps—affordable housing, employment, transportation, accessing the health system (even with nearby neighborhood hospitals). . . . My [the parish nurse's] mission is to model how other Christians can help . . . as we live the belief that the church is a place of healing. (Squier, 1995, p. 2)

Parish nursing in the city is a team effort. Coordinating financial and human resources takes creativity and adherence to building relationships and networks. Parish nurses can make their way into institutional systems to provide better care for individuals and the community.

With managed care, parish nursing can work itself into the providers' market as a member of the interdisciplinary team. Engaging actively with case managers in discharge planning is an avenue to explore further. Networking with other parish nurses and within the nursing profession is vital for the maturation of the practice of parish nursing.

Note

1. The *Parish Nurse Report* was an annual compilation of reports from parish nurses associated with the Columbus-Cabrini Medical Center, Chicago. Each time the *Parish Nurse Report* is cited in this chapter, the name of the nurse whose report is being quoted is provided first.

References

BeFriender ministry coordinator manual (Rev. ed.). (1995). St. Paul, MN: University of St. Thomas.

Boss, J. (1994). Being a professional caretaker can be dangerous to your health. *Health & Development, 4,* 10-14.

Boss, J. (1996). Lessons learned over time: Great teachers—St. Francis, St. Clare, and Eleanor. *Health & Development, 2,* 17-19.

Connelly, L. M., Keele, B. C., Kleinbeck, S. V. M., Schneider, J. K., & Cobb, A. K. (1993). A place to be yourself: Empowerment from the client's perspective. *IMAGE: Journal of Nursing Scholarship, 25*(4), 297-303.

Cox, S. (1995). *Interpretation of the roles of a parish nurse in an inner-city practice.* Unpublished manuscript, Advocate Health Care, Oak Brook, IL.

Fonck, B. A. (1983). *Fully mature with the fullness of Christ* (Rev. ed.). (Available from Resource Center: HC 06 Box 339C, Park Rapids, MN, 56470)

Hagerty, B. M. K., Lynch-Sauer, J., Patusky, K. L., & Bouwsema, M. (1993). An emerging theory of human relatedness. *IMAGE: Journal of Nursing Scholarship, 25*(4), 291-296.

Hilfiker, D. (1995). Poverty medicine. *Health & Development, 1,* 8-17.

Knapp, M. (1995). *Interpretation of the roles of a parish nurse in an inner-city practice.* Unpublished manuscript, Advocate Health Care, Oak Brook, IL.

Leininger, M. M. (Ed.). (1991). *Culture care diversity & universality: A theory of nursing* (Pub. No. 15-2402). New York: National League for Nursing Press.

McCloskey, J. C., & Bulechek, G. M. (Eds.). (1996). *Iowa intervention project, nursing interventions classification (NIC)* (2nd ed.). St. Louis, MO: Mosby-Year Book.

Parish Nurse Program. (1990). *Annual report: Parish nurse program.* Chicago: Columbus-Cabrini Medical Center.

Parish Nurse Program. (1991). *Annual report: Parish nurse program.* Chicago: Columbus-Cabrini Medical Center.

Parish Nurse Program. (1992). *Annual report: Parish nurse program.* Chicago: Columbus-Cabrini Medical Center.

Parish Nurse Program. (1993). *Annual report: Parish nurse program.* Chicago: Columbus-Cabrini Medical Center.

Parks, C. P. (1995, November). *Empowerment vs. encumbrance.* Paper presented at the 7th Annual Conference of the Christian Community Development Association, Denver, CO.

Ruch, J. (1995). *Interpretation of the roles of an inner-city parish nursing practice.* Unpublished manuscript, Advocate Health Care, Oak Brook, IL.

Squier, C. (1995). *Interpretation of the roles of an inner-city parish nursing practice.* Unpublished manuscript, Advocate Health Care, Oak Brook, IL.

Swanson, K. M. (1993, Winter). Nursing as informed caring for the well-being of others. *IMAGE: Journal of Nursing Scholarship, 25*(4), 352-357.

Tanner, C. A., Benner, P., Chesla, C., & Gordon, D. R. (1993, Winter). The phenomenology of knowing the patient. *IMAGE: Journal of Nursing Scholarship, 25*(4), 273-280.

Voss, R. W. (1993, Summer). Pastoral social ministry in the ecosystem of the poor: Breaking through the illusions. *Journal of Pastoral Care, 47,* 100-108.

6

Perspectives on a Suburban Parish Nursing Practice

Saralea Holstrom

The congregation where I serve as parish nurse is one of the fastest-growing faith communities in the Chicago suburban area. It started as a mission congregation in 1956. This is the congregation my family and I have worshipped in since 1976. The parish nurse program was initiated in May 1985 as a result of Granger Westberg's work with Lutheran General HealthSystem. When the parish nurse program began, the congregation had a membership of approximately 2,600 members. Today the membership is more than 4,000. I have a clear memory of my first week as a parish nurse. The focus was learning about what I would "do" as a nurse on a church staff. When I met with the senior pastor, one of the first things we talked about was my attending regular pastoral staff meetings.

Participating in multidisciplinary "staffings" was not new; it had been part of my experience in a hospital setting. I was eager to learn how to integrate my role of parish nurse with other staff members in the congregation as they planned programs and worship services, solved problems, shared goals for the future, and cared for the members of the congregation.

At the same time, however, feelings of uncertainty were part of my transition from being a member of the congregation to also being a staff member. I knew that some of the congregation and probably some of the staff were not quite sure if we actually needed a *nurse* on staff in a paid position. They wondered just what I would be doing to earn my salary. In addition, there was the personal struggle, as some women in the parish had previously done some of the things in my job description as volunteers.

During my first 6 months, I did a lot of careful listening, observing, and learning at our staff meetings and slowly, cautiously at first, developed relationships with the other staff members. I gained a great deal of respect for each one of them as individuals as well as for the skills they have in their specific areas. During that learning process, I also began interacting with our parishioners to assess their needs, using the nurse's keen sense of observation and, especially, listening skills. Time passed, and I became more knowledgeable about my role and experienced the wide dimension of challenges that were included. I began to more fully understand what I heard Granger Westberg say when he spoke about his belief that the church is a place for the care of the whole person, mind, body, and spirit, and that a nurse on the church staff could direct an assertive approach to wellness management, prevention of disease, and whole person caring.

Pastoral Leadership That Fosters Collaboration

The mind-set of the senior pastor and how that is lived out in the management of the staff of the congregation is extremely important. I was most fortunate that the pastor of the congregation embraced Granger Westberg's vision of the church as a place for health and healing and took pride in that heritage. The pastor's basic understanding and commitment to the parish nurse program has been of great value as I have served as parish nurse. I know there is strong pastoral endorsement of the program, but also on a personal level, I know he respects me as an individual.

Framework for Working Together

When I worked with the pastors in responding to parishioners' specific needs, it became clear that we needed a more deliberate way to coordinate the responses to concerns that arose. A pastoral care team was formed that consisted of pastors, a seminary intern (when there was one), a counselor, and the parish nurse. Each week we met at a set time and reviewed the needs of the congregation members to coordinate which staff members would respond. Many times staff brought concerns about which the other staff members did not know. Always, the staff member involved first requested the parishioner's permission to share the concerns with the pastoral care team, and of course this meeting was conducted in a confidential manner. The pastors, intern, and parish nurse would take hospital call on a rotating basis, a week at a time. Discussions held at the pastoral care team meetings provided me with an opportunity to ask questions, to seek the pastor's and counselor's advice, and to learn from their experience and input. This contributed to my continuing growth and development as a parish nurse. Between meetings, pastoral care notes were distributed to all team members to keep everyone informed on situations. The staff person on call would write an update at the end of the week that was put in each pastoral care team member's communications box. The addition of seminary interns provided an opportunity to share the parish nurse concept. This sharing gave the interns a basic understanding of the parish nurse's role on the church staff.

Once I had adopted the parish nurse role, it did not take me long to gain respect for the support staff. Patiently they oriented me to the office routines and equipment and put me at ease. I learned to be sensitive to their stressful days, especially around Christmas, Easter, and annual report time, and to plan ahead for my mailings, bulletin inserts, and articles in our newsletter. The church receptionist gently reminded me to notify her of my schedule when I was going to be out of the office so she could relay messages to me. She also helped me with names of volunteers and parishioners so I could greet them by name. Regularly, I remind myself to show the support staff my genuine appreciation. Their partnership is invaluable to operating as a team in ministry.

Serving on a church staff, I have learned that nothing "just happens" by chance. Behind each vibrant and relevant worship service and each program are the staff members who together prayerfully organize and plan it—seriously, carefully, and devotedly. The parish nurse embraces the church staff's goal to help create an atmosphere that is healthy and vital for ministry. The goal is to create a hospitable place where anyone who enters is met with a smile and a genuine caring response.

Seven Functions of the Parish Nurse

During the past 12 years, my role as parish nurse has included the seven functions of the parish nurse role. These functions are health educator, personal health counselor, referral agent, trainer of volunteers, developer of support groups, integrator of faith and health, and health advocate.

Health Educator

The health committee chairman and members have been a constant support. They assist in the development of goals to promote an atmosphere within the faith community that supports the healing mission of the church. This committee strives to instill in the members of the congregation the desire to be responsible stewards of their own mental, physical, and spiritual health. The identification of health education programs was done in cooperation with this group. Blood drives organized by the parish nurse and health committee are held twice a year to provide blood products for the community. A member conducts low-impact exercise classes, and community-sponsored weight- and stress-management programs are held regularly in the church building.

Over the years, attendance at the scheduled educational programs was low. It was determined that there were so many health promotion education programs offered throughout the local hospitals and other community agencies that the efforts to offer health promotion education programs within the church were redundant. Today the work is to maintain up-to-date lists of current health promotion programs offered in the community. My work is to see that the congregation members are aware of these offerings. In addition, if I know that a certain congregation member is struggling with a particular health-related issue, I will know where in the community I can refer him or her for pertinent education.

Personal Health Counselor

The parish nurse role encourages personal health counseling to take place in the church, home, and long-term care facility, to name just a few locations. Relationships develop over time with those who have received care. This work has provided a fulfillment of a personal vision, which includes adapting my nursing skills beyond the realm of medical technology. A close relationship with clients develops, particularly those seen regularly due to chronic illness or those "filled with years" who are growing frail and fragile. One 89-year-old lady, who had been a faithful church worker for many years but was now "shut in" due to multiple medical problems, felt her mission in the church now was to care for our pastors, intern, and myself during our time with her. We knew we had to set aside a block of time (sometimes a challenge) when we visited her to allow time for quiet prayer, discussion of church matters, family sharing time, and a cup of tea. She saw this as a time we could relax and be away from the busyness of our office. I saw her weekly to check her blood pressure and go over her medications. As her physical condition declined, her family was referred to home health care for someone to help with her personal health needs. I lost a dear friend when she died.

People in our community have become familiar with the presence of the parish nurse. One afternoon I received a call from a hospice nurse with whom I had worked in referrals for care for several of the families in this faith community. She asked if I would talk with someone she knew who was going through a very difficult time. The staff policy has always been to respond to those in need. I made an appointment for this lady to come into my office. Her 23-year-old son was dying of AIDS, and one of her main concerns was that she felt she "couldn't" tell her elderly mother about this, "It would kill her." She shared that she belonged to another Lutheran church in our town but felt she could not bother her pastor with this. She had not shared this with any of her friends; "What would they think?" She and her spouse were trying to manage this sorrow all on their own. We talked about trusting and giving her pastor and friends the opportunity to share her sorrow and care for her. I drew from my experience in geriatric nursing, and she was reassured that the elderly are many times stronger than we realize. It was suggested that she confide in her mother about what was going on in her life. She called me a week later and said she had talked to her pastor and friends. They were very loving, compassionate, and offered her support. I asked about her mother, and she said, "Yes, she accepted this quite well." Her mother told her she knew her grandson was gay from the time he was in high school. She was relieved that now they could all be honest with each other and show him how much they loved him.

Referral Agent and Liaison With
Congregational and Community Resources

The pastor of Visitation Ministries and the parish nurse work closely together with those who are ill or shut in. Many times we make visits together, particularly for an initial assessment to plan how the client can best be supported. The pastor brings communion, and the parish nurse observes the client's clinical status, safety in the home environment, personal care needs, nutritional needs, and so on. Does the client need home health care? Would a Stephen Minister be appropriate? (The Stephen Ministry is an interdenominational, nationwide lay ministry for people in crisis situations.) Does the client need help with transportation to therapy or doctor's appointments? Is this a situation for hospice care? Appropriate referrals are provided, and in some instances help is given to make phone calls. Joint efforts are an example of accomplishing whole-person care of body, mind, and spirit.

The pastoral care team continues to help make connections between the parish nurse and parishioners by coming to the parish nurse with a need of which the team is aware. For example, the director of outreach told the parish nurse about two elderly sisters she met one Sunday when they visited us for worship. On Monday the parish nurse took them a bouquet from the altar flowers, which is done frequently for someone who is in the hospital, had a birth, death, or accident in the family, or perhaps to welcome visitors; they were then invited to the next senior lunch. As we talked, I learned that they needed a physician referral and were planning to walk to church next time they attended (they were 90 and 97 years old). When I returned to my office, I called a few of the volunteers from the congregation and set up a rotating schedule to drive them to worship on a regular basis. These volunteers have become friends of the two ladies, who were alone and new in the area.

There have been opportunities for the parish nurse to join the staff in participating in developing and maintaining a relationship with the community that perceives the church as a place for health. Recently a call was received from one of the county health department nurses. She was looking for a site to hold a wellness clinic with an infant and child immunization program in the geographic area of the congregation. She had heard that our church had a parish nurse on staff and so felt the congregation might be open to providing building space for this program. I was excited about a new use for the church building as part of a wellness program and immediately checked it out with the pastor. He asked me, "Do you feel this is a good use of our building?" My answer was a quick yes. He did not hesitate for a moment to OK this project. I notified the rest of the staff about this program because I knew there would be new people in the building asking directions to the room. People of many different ethnic backgrounds, as well as parishioners, are now coming to the church for this preventive health clinic.

About a year ago, the church receptionist told me about a call she had received from a man who was obviously distressed. It turned out he had been hospitalized for an addictive disease, had been discharged, and was in the process of continuing his after-care program. The problem was that the facility where he had received care was closing, and he did not know where his group would be able to meet. I reassured him that they would be welcome to use one of the rooms in this church building for their weekly 12-step Cocaine Anonymous meeting. The congregation also hosts a weekly Alcoholics Anonymous group that has been meeting here for many years.

Developer of Support Groups

As numerous as the needs are in this congregation, there is opportunity for the development of support groups. The constant stress of being a caregiver can have an impact on all aspects of a person's health. Physical, emotional, social, and spiritual well-being are affected (Campanale, 1996). The parish nurse facilitated the development of a caregivers' support group for members and people from the external community at different times. The parish nurse gets quite a few calls from parishioners dealing with aging parents, who sometimes are in this geographic area and other times in another part of the country. Counseling is provided about options for housing, personal care, safety and nutrition, and the adult children's role and limitations in this concern—the sandwich generation concept is a reality.

For some reason, DuPage County has the highest incidence of breast cancer in the state of Illinois, and some of our parishioners are now cancer survivors. After viewing a television series on the Mind/Body Connection on the Public Broadcasting System, two women parishioners spoke to me about having a cancer survivors support group in their church, rather than them attending a community-based program. This group has been meeting twice a month for almost 2 years; they pray together, do some guided imagery and meditation, laugh and cry together, and share stories.

Trainer of Volunteers

The parish nurse collaborates with congregational volunteer structures such as Ministers of Care, Stephens Ministry, and BeFrienders. In addition, the parish nurse serves as a clinical resource and support to volunteers, who broaden and extend sources of assistance within the congregation (Djupe, Olson, & Ryan, 1994). There are many talents and gifts present in a congregation, and they may all be seen as opportunities to be in service to our neighbors. With *service* as the basis of a spiritual life, the congregation offers to others opportunities for personal spiritual growth through volunteering to serve others. To ensure that volunteers are informed and knowledgeable in serving others, however, it is helpful if there can be opportunities for them to come together and learn with others.

The pastor supports the parish nurse in attending community information meetings on issues such as senior housing, family shelter services for domestic violence situations, and employment training and education opportunities for single mothers. This facilitates keeping the parish nurse informed about the resources available in this area. One of the parishioners, a family practice physician, approached the parish nurse about organizing nurses from the congregation to assist with a medical clinic at Hesed House, a local facility for the homeless. A schedule was developed by the parish nurse for a group of nurses who assist the physician, volunteering their time. Clients are seen there two evenings a month, October through May.

Integrator of Faith and Health

Every contact made by a parish nurse is an opportunity to assist the client in identifying more deeply the relationship of the client's faith with his or her health. Parish nurses have chosen this specialized work because of the unique opportunity to be with individuals, families, and the congregational community, discovering the deeper beliefs and values that affect their health. The sacraments, liturgy, and symbols used in the faith community enhance not only worship but also a deeper understanding of a faith tradition (Djupe et al., 1994).

Health Advocate

More and more, as the present-day health delivery system becomes more complex, people in the community are in need of advocacy. This function is woven into all of what a parish nurse does. Whether it is advocating for an adjustment in medication or better living arrangements for an older adult, the parish nurse works with the client, faith community, and primary health care resources to provide whatever is in the best interest of the client from a whole-person perspective. The function of health advocate is based on knowing the client, being able to listen carefully, supporting the client to do what it is he or she can do, and being the client's voice when he or she has none.

Change

Change weaves experiences into the fabric of our lives. With change we are invited to stretch ourselves beyond what was thought possible. (Solari-Twadell, 1994, p. 3)

Change is certainly a part of all our lives, and the church staff has become somewhat expert in adapting to the many changes that the staff experience together. Thank goodness the Good Lord has made us adaptable creatures. Building additions, with the construction noise, dust, relocation of offices, and so on, required patience, adjustments, and good humor. At one point, the pastor gathered us in his office, which was about to be demolished, for a brief "Closing of the Office" service adapted from the Lutheran Book of Worship Occasional Service Book.

Of course, the staff undergoes personnel changes. There is a sharing of the sadness that goes with saying good-bye, along with celebrating new positions as staff relocate. It is very difficult to say farewell to beloved pastors and staff. Tears have been shed together and with the congregation in this process. This is indeed a true loss and grieving process that the staff try to aid each other in experiencing. Some of these emotions are deliberately focused on a "bang-up farewell" celebration to lighten the feelings of loss. The staff's skits and shenanigans are enjoyed by the congregation, as well by as the one who is leaving.

It is therapeutic and healing for each staff member to bring out special remembrances with which to good-heartedly tease each other as we say good-bye. Staff members work closely and share part of themselves with each other as each goes through personal family crises, illnesses, weddings, and even deaths of loved ones together as part of a faith family that does the ministry of the church together.

Renewal comes from staff retreats, birthday luncheons, and holiday celebrations at our senior pastor's home, with his wife's wonderful hospitality as a gift to us all. Time away from the office together is restoring and strengthening.

Welcoming new pastors and staff members is carefully planned by staff and includes the congregation. The parish nurse aids in their orientation process by helping them become acquainted with the people to whom she is ministering so they can quickly feel at ease with these parishioners. All staff try to help each other remember names because it is a challenge, yet so important, to know everyone by name. New pastors and staff members bring many gifts that help energize and sustain the staff and congregation. The congregation hosts seminary interns, who are welcomed. Staff members share with the interns the work each does in the parish. The eagerness and gifts of the interns are put to good work.

The changes keep coming! Collaboration with church staff is neverending; the parish nurse program continues evolving as God's grace permits us to serve together, moving into the future, listening for God's spirit to guide and direct.

References

Campanale, R. (1996). Respite care and parish nurse programs: Healing ministries made for each other. In *Proceeding Book, Tenth Annual Westberg Symposium: "Parish Nursing: A Celebration of Health, Healing and Wholeness."* Park Ridge, IL: International Parish Nurse Resource Center.

Djupe, A. M., Olson, H., & Ryan, J. A. (1994). *Reaching out: Parish nursing services.* Park Ridge, IL: Lutheran General HealthSystem.

Solari-Twadell, A. (1994). *Perspectives in parish nursing.* Park Ridge, IL: International Parish Nurse Resource Center.

7

Parish Nursing
in Rural Communities

Janet Griffin

In the United States, the nursing profession has long been concerned about health in rural communities. "Ellen M. Wood established a pioneer rural nursing program in 1896 serving Westchester County, New York . . . [and] in 1911, Lydia Homan established an independent nursing service in the Appalachian mountains" (Bullough & Bullough, 1990, p. 542). Expansion of rural nursing across the country came in 1912, when the Red Cross began the Rural Nursing Service that was later known as Town and Country Nursing Services. Qualities attributed to the early rural nurses included cheerfulness, enthusiasm, patience, love of work, a sense of humor, knowledge of local traditions, and the ability to teach (Clement, 1914). The same traits are evident in today's parish nurses. Through the Rural Nursing Service, nurses provided bedside care for the sick and offered health promotion services such as prenatal care and education related to hygiene and sanitation (Bullough & Bullough, 1990; Kalisch & Kalisch, 1995).

Before taking a closer look at parish nursing in rural settings, it is important to understand characteristics of rural communities, distinctive aspects of rural family life, rural attitudes toward health, and the special health care needs of rural residents. These characteristics present both opportunities and challenges for rural churches.

A Profile of Rural Communities

Approximately 55 million Americans live in rural areas (Hearn, 1996). Although there is great diversity in rural environments, some general characteristics exist among

AUTHOR'S NOTE: I would like to thank Harriet Olson, Coordinator of Special Projects for Trinity Regional Health System's Parish Nurse Program, for her help in writing this chapter. Her rural "roots" provided valuable insight into the special needs of rural communities.

rural communities. Rural villages have a high percentage of elderly, greater levels of unemployment, fewer children, and a higher ratio of females to males than urban communities. Moreover, rural households tend to be large, with several generations sharing the home (Bushy, 1993).

Traditionally, rural villages have had small, intergenerational, family-owned businesses such as grocery stores, service stations, banks, restaurants, farm implement dealerships, and farm supply stores. A recent trend, however, is for large corporations to replace family-owned businesses. The poor farm economy also contributed to the closing of small businesses that had been supported by local residents. As a result, unemployment rates are high in rural communities, and salaries are low for those who are employed.

Over the past several decades, many rural schools have consolidated. Schools were once a focal point of activity for rural communities, but families must now travel to neighboring towns for school functions, and children have long bus rides. Both family time and community cohesiveness have been negatively affected by school consolidations. For elderly rural residents with failing health, housing options are often limited. For some, the county nursing home has been stigmatized as the "poor farm" that is to be avoided at all costs. On the other hand, premature placement in nursing homes may be necessitated by a shortage of assisted living facilities or handicap-accessible apartments that could be an intermediate step. Additional challenges are imposed by the environment. Individuals sometimes feel isolated due to distances between homes, the absence of public transportation, or travel limitations related to weather conditions that cause country roads to be hazardous.

Rural people tend to be independent and self-reliant; perhaps this is due to the distance between homes. They work well alone and have good problem-solving skills. Rural residents also tend to have conservative views morally and politically, and they value dignity and privacy. Many rural residents have lived in the same locale all their lives. In some cases, earlier generations homesteaded the area. Due to a shared history, a strong sense of belonging and loyalty among residents has developed in rural communities. People are quick to offer help when neighbors experience illness or accidents. Family life is unique in rural areas because people live in their work settings. Occupations are related to the land, and there is a strong work ethic. Furthermore, both work and recreational activities are cyclic, based on seasonal changes.

Historically, among rural residents, there has been strong emphasis on traditional gender roles. Women focused on family nurturing and coordination of activities; men took responsibility for earning a living. Under such circumstances, when husbands die or couples are divorced, women are at risk for living in poverty because their homemaker roles have not produced an income, social security, insurance coverage, or retirement benefits. In recent years, due to the poor farm economy, more women have taken jobs outside the home to supplement the family's income. Economic problems have also forced many farmers to seek other jobs and do their farming at night. Some have given up hired help and are now depending on assistance from their wives or children, who may have limited knowledge about farm equipment.

Another trend in rural communities is for fewer young people to enter farming as a profession. The cost of land and equipment makes it difficult to get started. In families where the younger generation does continue the farming tradition, however, the young farmers are often college educated. They approach their work with a business orientation, using computerized record keeping, high-tech farm machinery, and research-based production strategies. Although these advancements are a source of pride for many rural residents, they can be threatening to those who resist change.

Access to Health Care

Out of all medically underserved areas in the United States, 70% are rural (Johnson, 1994). Over the past 2 decades, many rural hospitals have closed, and there is a scarcity of physicians. Not only are basic services lacking, the shortage of specialty services is even more critical. Inadequacy of rural medical services can be attributed to declining rural populations, economic stagnation, and the urban orientation of health care professionals (Bushy, 1994; Johnson, 1994; Rost, 1994). Distance to medical services, therefore, becomes a barrier to accessing needed care. Because of the time and transportation necessary to reach health care providers, rural residents are inclined to delay interventions and may seek help only in emergencies. These problems are easily overlooked by policy makers because rural areas have low population density.

Another common barrier to appropriate medical care is the lack of health insurance. Self-employed rural residents often cannot afford insurance, and when families do have insurance, the policies may be inadequate or have excessive deductible payments. Lack of adequate insurance is a significant deterrent to preventive medicine as well as early intervention for problems that are considered minor.

Attitudes toward health may also interfere with timely medical interventions. Although there is not a singular concept of health that is common to all rural residents, some attitudes do seem to be more prevalent. Rural residents tend to define health as the ability to work. This attitude, coupled with a strong work ethic and land-based occupations that do not allow for "sick days," can lead to delays in seeking care. Furthermore, the preference for contact with "insiders" results in reliance on family, friends, and neighbors for advice related to health concerns. This informal care network is both available and affordable (Long, 1993).

Health-Related Needs

Because rural residents are often self-employed, unsafe work habits can easily go unnoticed. Common problems include failure to use protective clothing or devices, inadequate sleep, delayed meals, and use of outdated equipment. Rural residents continue to work later in life than their urban counterparts. Older workers experience changes related to aging and side effects from medications that may impair coordination, reaction time, and mental alertness. The National Safety Council reports that "agricultural work accidents resulted in 1300 deaths and 120,000 disabling injuries in 1990. The accidental death rate in agriculture was 42 per 100,000 workers, as compared with 9 per 100,000 worker in all other industries" (Wright, 1993, p. 253).

Rural health hazards are not limited to accidents. Weather conditions, such as extreme temperatures, wind, and precipitation, can also affect safety. Sun exposure increases the risk for skin cancer, chemical exposures contribute to respiratory problems, and in some areas environmental pollutants have contaminated well water. Seasonal farm workers experience additional challenges because they are often poorly housed, if at all, and have poor access to bathing and toilet facilities.

Rural residents also face the same health problems as urban residents—substance abuse, AIDS, domestic violence, teen pregnancy, depression, cancer, cardiovascular disease, and so on. Yet, although education can be an important tool for preventing such problems, access to education is frequently limited by distance to services.

The Church as a Partner in Health Care

Although shops, schools, and hospitals have closed in many rural communities, local churches have usually survived. Rural churches provide both social and religious functions and reach people of all ages. Church buildings serve as gathering places for ice cream socials, bazaars, recreational activities, weddings, funerals, and receptions—events that bring together the entire community, not just members of the congregation. In short, churches are ideal partners for meeting the health care needs of rural communities.

Rural churches are trusted by community residents because the churches have a long history in the community and reflect the local culture. Pastors are generally involved in community activities and have established relationships with agencies serving the region; pastors are therefore commonly consulted when help is needed. Unfortunately, the number of clergy ministering in rural churches has declined, and, consequently, some pastors are serving two or more churches, which limits their availability to each congregation. Rural congregations have good informal networks of caregivers. Concerns travel quickly along the "grapevine," and members reach out to one another to offer support and practical assistance.

Another striking feature of rural congregations is the strong sense of spirituality evident among those who depend on the land for their livelihood. Rural residents generally feel a deep connection to creation, along with a reverence for the Creator. An old Italian proverb affirms, "The man who helps things to grow is never too far from the smile of God" (Buscaglia, quoted in Halversen, 1996, p. 95). This connection between land-based occupations and spirituality should not be surprising. Both the Old and New Testaments of the Bible contain frequent references to rural occupations and care of the land. The following scripture passages illustrate such biblical teachings:

> Now the Lord God had planted a garden in the east, in Eden; and there he put the man he had formed. And the Lord God made all kinds of trees grow out of the ground—trees that were pleasing to the eye and good for food. In the middle of the garden were the tree of life and the tree of the knowledge of good and evil. (Genesis 2:8-9)[1]

> The kingdom of heaven is like a mustard seed, which a man took and planted in his field. Though it is the smallest of all your seeds, yet when it grows, it is the largest of garden plants and becomes a tree, so that the birds of the air come and perch in its branches. (Matthew 13:31-32)

A farmer went out to sow his seed. As he was scattering the seed, some fell along the path, and the birds came and ate it up. Some fell on rocky places, where it did not have much soil. It sprang up quickly, because the soil was shallow. But when the sun came up, the plants were scorched, and they withered because they had no root. Other seed fell among thorns, which grew up and choked the plants. Still other seed fell on good soil, where it produced a crop—a hundred, sixty or thirty times what was sown. (Matthew 13:3-8)

Let my teaching fall like rain and my words descend like dew, like showers on new grass, like abundant rain on tender plants. (Deuteronomy 32:2)

I planted the seed, Apollo watered it, but God made it grow. So neither he who plants nor he who waters is anything, but only God, who makes things grow. The man who plants and the man who waters have one purpose, and each will be rewarded according to his own labor. For we are God's fellow workers; you are God's field, God's building. (I Corinthians 3:6-9)

The cyclic nature of land-based occupations also reinforces a sense of hope. Just as spring always follows winter, times of drought or disease are followed by times of abundance. The message is clear: "The Lord is good, a refuge in times of trouble. He cares for those who trust in him" (Nahum 1:7).

Parish Nurses Working in Rural Communities

Within the context of rural communities, there are many opportunities for parish nurses. Rural residents usually have a strong commitment to stewardship of natural resources, and parish nurses can help individuals expand this commitment to care for their own bodies. The Bible provides a foundation for this focus: "Don't you know that you yourselves are God's temple and that God's Spirit lives in you? If anyone destroys God's temple, God will destroy him; for God's temple is sacred, and you are that temple" (I Corinthians 3:16-17).

As noted earlier, rural residents prefer to receive health care from people they know. In most cases, parish nurses are working in their own congregations. Consequently, church members already know and trust the nurse, and her services are provided in familiar surroundings. Awareness of cultural ties also helps the parish nurse be sensitive to the congregation's preferences. Parish nurses focus on health promotion, and this focus is often missing in rural communities. In a church setting, people of all ages are reached, and there are no financial barriers to participation. Familiarity with the congregation helps the nurse tailor health promotion activities to the group's needs and preferred methods of obtaining information. A potential challenge for rural parish nurses is maintaining confidentiality. Because area residents are well acquainted with each other, information travels quickly throughout the community. There is, however, a strong preference for privacy among many rural individuals, and therefore, to preserve the element of trust with clients, parish nurses must use care in what they disclose.

Many rural churches have a high percentage of elderly members. As members become frail and isolated, the parish nurse monitors for changes in health status. Through home visits, the parish nurse is able to accurately assess the health of the client as well as the safety of the environment. Elderly members may be reluctant to access services to which they are entitled, but the parish nurse can explain available options and help them through the application process.

The informal network of caregivers in rural communities is an important resource for parish nurses. As needs are identified for respite care, transportation, meal preparation, or friendly visits, friends and neighbors usually come forward to lend a helping hand.

In addition to church responsibilities, parish nurses typically participate in a variety of community activities. This facilitates interaction with community members and increases the visibility of the nurse. An amazing number of contacts made by parish nurses occur at school or community functions, the grocery store, the village restaurant, or other local sites. Because rural women are usually seen as responsible for the family's health, it is important for parish nurses to include them in health promotion activities. This is done through bulletin board displays, one-to-one teaching, distribution of resource materials, health fairs, or group classes.

As time and distance are barriers to participation, health promotion events will be better attended if they can be combined with other events. For example, the parish nurse may add a summer safety component to vacation Bible school, include a substance abuse awareness presentation at a youth meeting, show a video on farm safety for the church's men's group, or organize a heart-healthy luncheon for the women's group. Health promotion activities are also done in cooperation with existing community groups such as 4-H, scouts, parent-teacher associations, home extension, county fairs, or community festivals.

The amount of time a parish nurse devotes to her role varies greatly from church to church. In some churches, the parish nurse position is a paid staff position; in other churches, the parish nurse is volunteering for the role and may also be employed elsewhere. For many small rural churches, the option of having an unpaid parish nurse allows the congregation to enhance its health ministry without further straining the church budget. However, a nurse who is unpaid may have very limited time to dedicate to the role. Her time can be used to best advantage by establishing a wellness committee and a lay caregiving group so the parish nurse program is implemented through a team approach.

The value of having parish nurses in rural communities is illustrated by the following examples:

Parish nurses from churches in a cluster of rural communities coordinated a prostate cancer screening clinic. Staff for the screening was provided by medical personnel from a regional hospital. In just one evening, 70 men participated in the clinic.

To increase access to children's preventive care, a parish nurse works collaboratively with the Visiting Nurse and Homemaker Association from a community about 15 miles away. Immunization and lead-screening clinics are offered quarterly at the church. The local school helps publicize the clinics by printing the schedule on the back of the monthly lunch menu that is distributed to students.

Rural churches have unique opportunities to integrate spirituality into members' life experiences. For example, worship services incorporate blessing of the seeds in the spring and celebration of harvest in the fall, and pastors and parish nurses serve on crisis intervention teams that respond to farm accidents.

Rural parish nurses reach out to elders from the community in a variety of ways—a monthly prayer service at a nursing home located near the church, blood-pressure screening at senior meal sites, and educational programs at the county senior center.

Residents of rural communities are being encouraged by parish nurses to make healthy lifestyle choices. Using age-specific assessment tools, parish nurses are meeting with existing church groups (e.g., youth groups, Sunday school classes, and fellowship groups) to identify personal health risks. Participants are then encouraged to set goals for improving personal habits, and parish nurses provide education and emotional support.

A parish nurse invited elderly ladies from her church to a tea party. The party, which was held under a tree on the lawn of the nurse's farmhouse, provided a time for old friends to get together, enjoy a garden setting, and reminisce about past experiences.

Colo-rectal kits are being distributed by many parish nurses as part of a regional health coalition's efforts. The free screening is promoted through bulletin board displays and notices in the churches' newsletters and bulletins. Individuals are able to pick up the test kits at the churches and mail them back for processing. Results are mailed to participants, and the parish nurse receives an aggregated report indicating number of participants and number of positive tests.

Several rural churches jointly offer confirmation classes, and they have added a human sexuality component to the classes. A pastor and parish nurse teach the sessions collaboratively, emphasizing Christian values.

As the troubled farm economy has resulted in the loss of family farms, parish nurses have responded by referring families to supportive services. One parish nurse commented that, in such cases, it is especially important to anticipate the family's needs because individuals who previously were self-sufficient have difficulty asking for help.

When surveyed following hospitalization, a woman from a rural church commented, "I appreciated [my parish nurse's] reassurance and care during and following my recent surgery. If I had to vote between heat in the church or a parish nurse, I would pick the parish nurse because I can always put on more clothes."

It is clear that parish nurses have an important role within the context of rural communities. As the face of rural America changes, parish nurses are able to assess the needs of the congregations they serve and develop strategies to meet those unique needs.

The result is a better quality of life—in body, mind, and spirit—for people who live in rural America.

Note

1. All biblical quotations in this chapter are taken from the New International Version.

References

Bullough, B., & Bullough, V. (1990). *Nursing in the community.* St. Louis, MO: C. V. Mosby.

Bushy, A. (1993, March). Rural women: Lifestyle and health status. *Nursing Clinics of North America, 28*(1), 187-197.

Bushy, A. (1994, July). Women in rural environments: Considerations for holistic nurses. *Holistic Nursing Practice, 8*(4), 67-73.

Clement, F. (1914). American Red Cross Town and Country Nursing Service. *American Journal of Nursing, 14,* 1074.

Halverson, C. (1996). Health ministry in the agricultural community. In *Westberg symposium proceedings book* (pp. 205-213). Park Ridge, IL: International Parish Nurse Resource Center, Advocate Health Care.

Hearn, W. (1996, July). Health on the outskirts. *American Medical News, 39*(25), 20-23.

Johnson, S. (1994, May). Rural poor denied work, health care and respect. *Insight on the News, 10*(20), 9-11.

Kalisch, P., & Kalisch, B. (1995). *The advance of American nursing* (3rd ed.). Philadelphia: J. B. Lippincott.

Long, K. (1993, March). The concept of health: Rural perspectives. *Nursing Clinics of North America, 28*(1), 123-130.

Rost, K. (1994, July). Physician management preferences and barriers to care for rural patients with depression (Abstract). *Journal of the American Medical Association, 272*(3), 178E.

Wright, K. (1993, March). Management of agricultural injuries and illness. *Nursing Clinics of North America, 28*(1), 253-266.

Additional Reading

Anderson, J., & Yuhos, R. (1993, March). Health promotion in rural settings: A nursing challenge. *Nursing Clinics of North America, 28*(1), 145-155.

Bigbee, J. (1993, March). The uniqueness of rural nursing. *Nursing Clinics of North America, 28*(1), 131-144.

Johnson, J. (1996, May). Social support and physical health in the rural elderly. *Applied Nursing Research, 9*(2), 61-66.

Lee, H. (1993, March). Rural elderly individuals: Strategies for delivery of nursing care. *Nursing Clinics of North America, 28*(1), 219-230.

Weisgrau, S. (1995, Fall). Issues in rural health: Access, hospitals, and reform. *Health Care Financing Review, 17*(1), 1-13.

Whitener, L. (1995, Summer). Families and family life in rural areas. *Journal of Rural Health, 11*(3), 217-223.

8

The Community as Client

Assessment of Assets and Needs of the Faith Community and the Parish Nurse

Phyllis Ann Solari-Twadell

The Parable of the Dangerous Cliff

'Twas a dangerous cliff, as they freely confessed.
Though to walk near its crest was so pleasant;
But over its terrible edge there had slipped
A duke and full many a peasant.
The people said something would have to be done,
But their projects did not at all tally.
Some said, "Put a fence 'round the edge of the cliff,"
Some, "An ambulance down in the valley."
Said one, to his plea, "It's a marvel to me
That you'd give so much greater attention
To repairing results than to curing the cause
You had much better aim at prevention.

For the mischief, of course, should be stopped at its source,
Come, neighbors and friends, let us rally.
It is far better sense to rely on a fence
Than an ambulance down in the valley."
"He is wrong in his head," the majority said:
"He would end all our earnest endeavor.
He's a man that would shirk this responsible work,

AUTHOR'S NOTE: I acknowledge Anne Marie Djupe for her early work and contributions to this chapter.

But we will support it forever.
Aren't we picking up all, just as fast as they fall,
And giving them care liberally?
A superfluous fence is of no consequence,
If the ambulance works in the valley."

The lament of the crowd was profound and was loud,
As their hearts overflowed with their pity;
But the cry for the ambulance carried the day
As it spread through the neighboring city.
A collection was made, to accumulate aid,
And the dwellers in highway and alley
Gave dollars or cents—not to furnish a fence—
But an ambulance down in the valley.

"For the cliff is all right if you're careful," they said;
"And if folks ever slip and are dropping,
It isn't the slipping that hurts them so much
As the shock down below—when they're stopping."
So for years (we have heard), as the mishaps occurred
Quick forth would the rescuers sally,
To pick up the victims who fell from the cliff
With the ambulance down in the valley.

The story looks queer as we've written it here,
But things do occur that are stranger.
More humane, we assert, than to succor the hurt,
Is the plan of removing the danger.
The best possible course
Is to safeguard the source;
Attend to things rationally.
Yes, build up the fence, and let us dispense
With the ambulance down in the valley.

—Author Unknown

This parable has several themes that are pertinent to these times and parish nursing. The first is the focus of prevention as the initial response. The second is the importance of community assessment. The third is the point that the solution that was funded was the more costly one and the one that does not address the risk. This scenario plays out over and over again in our communities. A risk is identified, it goes unaddressed, and the result is an intervention that is expensive and often required over a long period of time. Parish nurses have the opportunity to change this through working with the faith community to encourage strategies that will reinforce modification of present health risks, which will result in an improvement in health status.

The Faith Community as a Client

The faith community, also referred to here as a congregation, is an assembly of people whose beliefs about God combine with a common identify, a shared history, regular worship, and common values to effect personal and social transformation (Anderson, 1990). Congregations are often the most stable and respected associations in the community. Health leaders are realizing that future improvements in health will come about only as people assume greater responsibility for their own health and for the health of the community at large. This is a spiritual problem calling for changes in behavior, not a medical problem calling for a medical breakthrough. Faith communities promote health through community building, enhancing the meaning of life, nurturing care, spiritual values, and sponsoring health-related programs (Droege, 1995, p. 188). As a community association, a faith community identifies with the following characteristics:

- Communities are interdependent—to weaken one part of the community is to weaken all;
- The community environment is constructed around the recognition of fallibility rather than the ideal, thus there is room for many leaders;
- Such associations have the capacity to respond quickly because they do not have to move issues through an institutional, corporate structure before taking action;
- The development of community associations allows for the flowering of creative solutions;
- Community associations are usually small, face-to-face groups, so the relationship is very individualized, which results in "hand-tailored" responses;
- Communities can provide care that represents consent versus control; and
- Community is the forum in which citizenship can be expressed. (McKnight, 1987, p. 56)

The philosophy of parish nursing identifies the client as the faith community. The parish nurse, then, is called to

1. Assist members of the faith community to identify factors of the faith community that are pertinent to health;
2. Work with members of the faith community to identify strategies to address the identified factors;
3. Identify at-risk groups within the faith community;
4. Work with others within the faith community to establish priorities in addressing identified health problems; and
5. Identify essential health services that can be used as referral sources for members of the faith community and that are accessible, acceptable, and affordable.

Faith community as client refers to the concept of a faith community of people as the focus of nursing service. The scope of this service includes individuals, families, groups, subpopulations, populations, and the faith community itself (Spradley & Allender, 1996). In coming to know this faith community, it is important to assess the assets of the congregation as well as the needs. The assets of the congregation will be most important as the parish nurse looks to develop needed groups of volunteers to be involved in this health ministry. Only through identification of the assets will the parish nurse be effective in "multiplying the ministers." Through identification of individual assets of the members of the faith community, the nurse encourages the congregation to see the parish nurse not as "the Health Minister" but as a facilitator of the growth and development of the health ministry in the congregation. This is important for the well-being of the parish nurse as well as the faith community (see Appendix A).

In beginning to know the faith community, the parish nurse needs to study the location, population, and social system of the faith community. Study of the location includes the boundaries of the faith community (if any), the location of health services, the geographical features of the physical plant of the congregation and the surrounding external community, and the human-made environment. Review of the population of the faith community includes the size, composition, rate of growth or decline, cultural characteristics, denominational characteristics, social and/or educational level, and mobility. The nurse's awareness of the social system grows when she pays attention to the congregation's participation in worship and other events held or sponsored by the church in addition to the power and decision-making structure communication patterns (Spradley & Allender, 1996). Gathering of this information is encouraged in the early stages of the parish nurse role (see Appendix B).

Assessment of the Assets and Needs of the Faith Community

Assessment is an important function of any parish nurse. However, how this assessment of the faith community takes place is equally important. An assessment of a faith community is defined as the process of determining real or perceived needs and assets of the faith community (Spradley & Allender, 1996).

There are different types of community assessments. They are comprehensive assessment, familiarization, problem-oriented assessment, and a faith community subsystem assessment (Spradley & Allendar, 1996).

Comprehensive Assessment

A comprehensive assessment seeks to discover all the pertinent information related to health. This includes a review of existing information, such as the demographics of the faith community, past and recent studies or surveys that were done, and any historical data that may be available. This assessment also includes the interviewing of key individuals in the faith community. This type of extensive assessment is not done often, as it is time consuming and expensive.

Familiarization

This type of assessment involves a review of data that is already available. Included in this would be the "windshield survey": driving through the surrounding community to observe the environment. It could also include a visit to the local department of public health and local hospital marketing departments to review any available information of disease patterns by age, prevalence of disease, cause of death by age, and other information that could be offered to one working with a faith community. Familiarization includes assessing the corporate health of the congregation. The corporate health of the congregation has a focus on the whole. The faith community is highlighted rather than the individual member (Wietzke, 1980). It is important to note what the mission of the faith community is and how it appears to be played out in the activities and worship of the congregation. An observant walk around the physical plant can help assess this dimension. What messages are communicated through bulletin boards, banners, signs, and posted announcements? How is space allocated? Is there designated space, with flexible use of other space? Is the congregation accessible to the handicapped? When was the last renovation or construction? Is the physical plant well maintained? What accommodations are made for the older adult, such as large-print Bibles and hearing devices? Is there a reference area or library? What kind of books and information are available?

The budget of the congregation is an essential document to review early as part of an orientation to the congregation and the parish nurse role. Again, as with the demographics of the congregation, how has the budget changed over the past 5 to 10 years? How are current resources of the congregation being allocated? This is an important perspective to have when considering any proposals for expenditures related to the parish nurse program.

Most important is to familiarize yourself with the other staff members. Knowledge of their history with this congregation and other congregations they may have worked with in the past, as well as their current areas of responsibility, is invaluable in learning to know them as individuals and resources. It may be helpful to know about the history of services offered. When was the last time an assessment related to programming was done in the congregation?

Problem-Oriented Assessment

The problem-oriented assessment is the most common type of assessment done by parish nurses. It begins with a single problem, such as, What are the health education assets and needs of the faith community? The most common method of assessment is the paper-and-pencil checklist (see Appendix C). A caution with the use of this method is that although it is the cheapest and quickest, it usually results in the lowest rate of return. This is an important consideration. If the rate of return is low, a minority poll could dictate the results, and these ultimately may not determine the real assets or needs of the whole. Other methods used with problem-oriented assessment are telephone survey and personal interviews. No matter what method is used, it is extremely important to share the results with the faith community. This may encourage better participation in future surveys if the members understand that their input is important.

No matter what method or format is used, it is important that the content be pertinent to the faith community. Parish nurses interested in doing assessment may seek permission to use a survey that has been developed for another faith community. Such a practice may not get at the issues important to the faith community being surveyed, as the content was not tailored to that specific congregation. Remember, the results are only as good as the questions that are asked.

Community Subsystem Assessment

A subsystem assessment of assets and needs focuses on a single constituency of the faith community (see Appendix D). For example, perhaps there is interest in knowing what the older-adult group is wanting, as well as what they may have to offer. Development of a tailored survey can be most effective, particularly if the survey can be completed as part of a regular meeting where the majority will be gathered.

In summary, before doing an assessment, the following questions may be helpful:

1. *What information is needed or wanted?* It is important to be clear about what information is wanted and for what purpose. Clarity about this will assist in the development of the questions for a survey. Each faith community has a distinctive nature. Surveys used in other churches may be reviewed and discussed by the health committee and parish nurse. In addition, the survey tool may be piloted with a small group of parishioners. This can provide valuable input in shaping the survey.

2. *Is the information that is wanted already available?* Some of the information, such as the demographics of the congregation, is probably already available. By reviewing the predominant age groups, one can often determine the prevalence of disease patterns. If the information needed is going to be used to plan health education, it may be important to check and see what is offered in the community already, avoiding needless duplication.

3. *Are there resources in the community that can assist with the gathering of necessary information?* If there is a nearby college or university, it may have students who are in need of a community-based project. This is helpful, as the student will usually bring along the expertise of a faculty member. In this way, the congregation can link with the college and at the same time receive expertise it would otherwise not have.

4. *What is the best method for collecting the needed information?* Getting a representative number of responses is the biggest problem in doing an assessment. It is the work of the health and wellness committee and parish nurse to recommend the best method, based on the unique features and resources of the congregation.

5. *What resources are available to complete the assessment?* Each method of assessment has a cost. The cost can often be removed or partially negated if a college, hospital, or other resource in the community is willing to participate. The telephone survey is often the quickest—and most expensive—option. It is important that, if this is the option selected, an outside party that is able to insure confidentiality, consistency in telephone interviewers, and integrity in administration of the process be selected to manage the project. Use of a focus group may take longer, but it is a way of obtaining information that also fosters relationships. If the parish nurse has experience in doing

focus groups, then it is also an opportunity for members of the faith community to get to know the parish nurse and vice versa.

6. *What will the information be used for once it is collected?* Part of the determination for collecting information is clarity as to how the information will be used and how the results will be communicated to the members of the faith community.

Guidelines for the process of assessment include the following:

1. Never do for others what they can do themselves.
2. Find another's gifts, contributions, and capacities and use them. This will give them a place in the community.
3. Encourage people-reaching-out-to-people when possible rather than using purchased services.
4. Acknowledge each member of the congregation for whatever he or she can contribute— all, even the poor, disabled, and illiterate, have a contribution to make.
5. Develop a sense of hospitality. Create a sense of hospitality in administering this assessment.

Parish Nurse Self-Assessment

There are certain myths that often can be found in the parish nurse community (see Appendix E). It is important that each parish nurse can find a way through these myths to what is important. For the parish nurse, personal balance is a necessity. This calls the parish nurse to nurture the personal disciplines of "self-wisdom" in caring for her own physical, emotional, intellectual, spiritual, and social capacities. Without attention to and experience in the struggle for personal self-care, the parish nurse will struggle to find the ability to assist others to learn effective health care strategies. Each individual has personal gifts and human limitations. Self-assessment results in the parish nurse being aware of personal capacities, what needs to be changed, and what can be changed. Important to personal change is surrender. Surrender is being able to see and accept a situation while realizing that "I am powerless." This calls for help outside of oneself. Surrender is essential for change (Keller, 1991). At one time, it was thought that if people gained insight about themselves, they would change—but it takes more than insight. True change finds its way through the heart. It is important that a parish nurse be serious about attending to the personal. Individuals in the faith community tend to look to the parish nurse as a role model. This can place a demand on the nurse that can be personally challenging. This knowledge encourages the nurse to be disciplined about incorporating into her personal life pattern a time for personal reflection or prayer that seeks an intimate contact with her Higher Power and implies contact with self. This includes the ongoing process of self-emptying and openness to sharing and receiving. There is a certainty of God's providential care, which creates a trust that makes the nurse's own struggle and commitment more meaningful.

In Lane's (1987) article "The Care of the Human Spirit," she discusses not only the works of the human spirit but the activities of the human spirit. These activities are

- inward turning—the ability for introspection and reflection,
- surrendering—the experience of letting go and letting be,
- committing—the ability to attach or bond oneself to another, and
- struggling—the piecing together of a number of life's elements to find meaning, cohesion, and unity in life.

The nurse, ministering to others through the role of parish nurse, is ultimately involved with this process. The nurse can recognize these activities of the human spirit in ministering to others while experiencing the same process in ministering to self.

Reflection on the Spiritual Dimension

Thomas A. Droege (1991), in his book *The Faith Factor in Healing,* notes that the key term for making the connection between health and spirituality is faith.

Herbert Benson (1975), author of the text *Beyond the Relaxation Response,* promotes the healing effects of the relaxation response. In his research, he identified a *faith factor* that further enhances healing. Benson explains that the use of the simple relaxation response, combined with a person's deepest personal beliefs, can create other internal environments that can help the person reach enhanced states of health and well-being. The combination of these two dynamics is what Benson refers to as the "Faith Factor."

Sharon Fisk and Judith Allen Shelly (1978), in the text *Spiritual Care: The Nurse's Role,* speak of spiritual health occurring when a person is able to experience God as the source of meaning and purpose, love and relatedness, and forgiveness. These factors are the essence of spiritual health, which is that dynamic and personal relationship with God.

Donald and Nancy Tubesing (1991), in their text *Seeking Your Healthy Balance: A Do It Yourself Guide to Whole Person Well-Being,* discuss the spiritual as referring to "that core dimension of you—your innermost self—that which provides you with a profound sense of who you are, where you came from, where you are going, and how you will reach your goal" (p. 86). The Tubesings go on to state that "the spiritual dimension provides one with principles for living—commitment to God or some ultimate concern, engenders a spirit of selflessness, sensitivity to others and a willingness to sacrifice for people in need" (p. 86).

How does the work of the parish nurse incorporate faith and spirituality? The incorporation of faith and spiritual care is the foundation for parish nurses. This can occur only when the parish nurse has integrated the nurturing of her own faith and spirituality into her daily self-care. You can only effectively teach someone something that you yourself have come to learn and integrated into your own life's practices.

Journey as Metaphor

The integration of faith and spirituality is a little like going on a long journey. When preparing for this kind of trip, there are several things that people will usually do.

Those heading for unknown territories will often go to the library and find literature that will give them clear and current information about the people they will meet, the customs of the country, and the type of food that may be available. It is the same for learning about spiritual care. Read and study about it. Learn how others have provided it in caring for others, and read with the intent to learn how your own faith and spiritual life may be enhanced.

It is always exciting, when planning to travel to an unknown destination, to know and talk to others who have been there. What fun it is to find others of like mind who have a little more experience relating to where you are planning to travel. There is little difference when the focus is the spiritual. It is good to know others who are concerned about their faith life as well as their spiritual growth and development and are interested in stretching themselves. Find other individuals or a group that you can talk with, and share your spiritual journey. In reading and talking with others, one of the primary things you will be interested in is what you are going to need for this journey. What kinds of clothes should you take? How much money should you plan on for the trip? How much luggage should you take? Oftentimes, the best resource for this kind of information is those who have most recently been to your planned destination. It is not too different with a spiritual journey. It is a gift when you can identify others who have preceded you and are willing to share what made this particular spiritual journey a little easier and more joy filled. They will often graciously be glad to share their experience, strength, and hope.

It is important when planning a long journey to judge carefully what you really need to take and what can be left behind. If one packs too much in one's suitcase, there is a significant amount of energy that is lost carrying unnecessary baggage. It is similar with a spiritual journey. Often it is important to be able to unburden oneself. In the unburdening, energy is freed up for other purposes. It often is not easy to "unburden oneself" or "become empty." However, for the vessel to be filled, it must be at least partly empty.

It is much more fun to have a companion when traveling long distances to new destinations. There is security in being with another. There is someone to talk and laugh with, to share the adventure with, and to be present if something unexpected arises. Again, this is very similar to a spiritual journey. Having a spiritual director or companion can make the continuing journey into spiritual maturity a more joy-filled experience.

Valuing the Spiritual and the Theological

At times, it may be important for oneself or in working with others to reflect on what is valued from a spiritual perspective. Table 1 in Appendix F includes a tool that can be used for review and reflection to gain insight into what is important and what is spiritually dominant or more secularly dominant in one's life. Honesty is required. Only in being honest in this reflection will an individual come to know what needs to be addressed to produce a more spiritual stance in life. The second table in Appendix F can be used in a similar way. This table lists attitudes that reflect both a spiritually dominant stance and a secularly dominant stance. Review of one's current dominant attitudes can also indicate where work needs to be done to adjust attitudes to reinforce a more spiritually centered posture.

Individuals, through their involvement in their own faith communities, adopt and integrate a faith belief system to which they can refer daily. No matter what this faith belief system is, there are theological underpinnings, stories, and/or examples that relate to health. It is important in the role of parish nurse to become familiar with these health-related writings and scripture. This familiarity will be of assistance to the parish nurse in ministering to self as well as when doing personal health counseling, praying with another, or creating liturgy for the faith community. An example of this is found in Appendix G.

Each individual nurse brings different gifts to the practice of parish nursing. All come with basic human limitations, experience in various nursing positions, and unique life experiences. All of this, interwoven with the individual's faith beliefs and spiritual maturity, will assist in defining each parish nurse's distinctive pattern of providing health ministry. Daily life brings with it stress, pain, anxiety, fear, and sometimes loss, as well as love, laughter, forgiveness, compassion, and companionship. Striving for a healthy balance in our lives gives an appreciation of and sensitivity to the struggles of others as they strive for a healthy balance in their lives.

References

Anderson, H. (1990). The congregation as a healing resource. In D. S. Browning, T. Job, & I. S. Evinson (Eds.), *Religious and ethical factors in psychiatric practice* (pp. 264-287). Chicago: Nelson-Hall in association with the Park Ridge Center for the Study of Health, Faith and Ethics.

Benson, H. (1975). *Beyond the relaxation response*. New York: Avon.

Droege, T. (1991). *The faith factor in healing*. Philadelphia: Trinity.

Droege, T. A. (1995). Congregations as communities of health and healing. *Interpretation, 49*(2), 117-129.

Fisk, S., & Shelly, J. A. (1978). *Spiritual care: The nurse's role*. Downers Grove, IL: InterVarsity.

Keller, J. E. (1991). *Alcoholics and their families: A guide for clergy and congregations*. San Francisco: Harper.

Lane, J. A. (1987, November-December). The care of the human spirit. *Journal of Professional Nursing,* 332-334.

McKnight, J. L. (1987, Winter). Regenerating community. *Social Policy,* 54-58.

Spradley, B. W., & Allender, J. A. (1996). *Community health nursing: Concepts and practice*. Philadelphia: Lippincott.

Tubesing, D. A., & Tubesing, N. L. (1991). *Seeking your healthy balance: A do it yourself guide to whole person well-being*. Duluth, MN: Whole Person.

Wietzke, W. R. (1980). *In league with the future: The people of God in ministry*. Minneapolis, MN: Augsberg.

APPENDIX A
Personal Gifts Form

Each member of the faith community has personal gifts they can share with others. Please take the time to reflect on the gifts you can share with the members of this faith community.

1. If you have had experience in any health topic and would be willing to teach or share your experience, please put your name and telephone number below. Please note the topic you are familiar with.

2. I am willing to help in the following areas as a volunteer for _____

    _____ Provide meals for special situations
    _____ Provide transportation to church, doctor's office, other
    _____ Baby-sit or provide elder care
    _____ Grocery shopping for shut-ins
    _____ Bereavement
    _____ Visitation to sick or shut-ins
    _____ Setting up for an educational program
    _____ Providing refreshments at an educational program
    _____ Other

3. Name:

    Phone number (   )

If you have any questions regarding the Parish Nurse Ministry or are interested in helping to organize this committee, please contact

Thank you for taking the time to complete this survey.

APPENDIX B
Projected Stages of Parish Nurse Development

Stage 1

"Who am I, and what do I do?" This stage is characterized by questions such as

- Where do I begin?
- What is expected of me in this role?
- Who can help me?
- Where are my resources?

The primary focus is on educating the congregation and building relationships. Identifying support for self in this role is important.

Stage 2

This stage is known by questions such as

- Why did I take this job?
- What is the nature of this role as it develops?
- What strengths do I have that assist me in this role?
- How do I balance the demands of this role with other areas of my life?

The primary focus is reevaluation of the role, self, and time management.

Stage 3

Toward the end of the first year, the parish nurse usually feels comfortable in the role. However, as the end of the first year rolls around, there is again time for evaluation, and usually there is some anxiety for the nurse. This issue is particularly emphasized for salaried nurses as the church determines its budget for the coming year. If the church is taking on more of the salary of the nurse, it may be critical to question the impact of the program. Questions that arise are

- Am I effective in the role?
- How will the congregation and staff understand, as well as value, the parish nurse program?

This is usually a time to report to the congregation at an annual meeting about the ministry's activities, programs, and outcomes.

Stage 4

This stage represents a time of resolution. Even though this is a new type of a role with many questions and uncertainties, this is where the nurse wants to be. That does not mean there are no periods of discouragement and questioning, but overall, the nurse feels settled in the role. There also seems to be a shift in the nurse's implementation of the role. There is a shift from program activities and very visible actions to more one-to-one counseling and referrals. The parish nurse becomes much more involved in the concerns and needs of individuals and families. At this point, the parish nurse also tends to reach out into the community by responding to community needs. This results in even more interaction with community programs and agencies.

APPENDIX C
Parish Health Ministry Survey

To help plan for health ministry in our faith community, your assistance in answering the following questions is important. There is no need to sign your name—unless you want to. All information is confidential and will be used for planning programs in this church.

Please put an X by the correct answer.

1. Your age: ___under 20 ___20-29 ___30-39 ___40-49 ___50-59 ___60-69 ___70+

2. Sex: ___Female ___Male

3. Marital status: ___Single ___Married ___Divorced ___Widowed

4. Employment status: Employed? ___Yes ___No ___Full-time ___Part-time
   ___Retired ___Planning retirement within 5 years

5. How do you rate your health? ___Excellent ___Good ___Fair ___Poor

6. Do you engage in regular exercise? ___Yes ___No
   If yes, please explain briefly:

7. Health status: Please check if you have or have had any of the following conditions. Place a "C" by any current conditions and a "P" by those conditions you have had.

   ___Heart disease   ___Lung disease
   ___High blood pressure   ___Cancer
   ___Arthritis   ___Mental illness
   ___Diabetes   ___Physical disability
   ___Depression   ___Other

8. Support groups can be developed to meet the interests of the greatest number of people. Please indicate if you would participate in any of the following. You may mark as many as you would participate in on a regular basis.

   ___Diabetes   ___Arthritis
   ___Weight control   ___Caregiving to aged relative
   ___Parents of preschoolers   ___Parents of elementary schoolers
   ___Single parents   ___Stepparents
   ___Parents of teens   ___Unemployed/underemployed
   ___Living with chronic illness/disability   ___Caregiving to chronically ill/disabled
   ___Families of persons with mental health problems
   ___Other

9. The following are health promotion classes that may enhance your emotional, physical, and spiritual health. Classes will be developed to meet the interests of the greatest number of people. Please indicate if you would participate in any of the following. You may mark as many as you would participate in on a regular basis.

   ___Communication skills   ___Exercise
   ___Healthy eating   ___Prayer
   ___Aging process   ___Stress reduction
   ___Time management   ___Women's health issues
   ___Preretirement planning   ___Men's health issues
   ___Marriage enrichment   ___Adolescent health issues
   ___"Break a habit"   ___Sexuality:
                                       ___Teen   ___Young adult
                                       ___Middle age   ___Elderly
   ___Other

(continued)

10. What day of the week and time would you be willing to attend a class or group?
    ___Monday ___Tuesday ___Wednesday ___Thursday ___Friday ___Saturday ___Sunday
    ___Morning ___Afternoon ___Evening

11. What is(are) your major health concern(s)? This includes emotional, physical, and spiritual.

12. What is(are) your major health concern(s) for your family? This includes emotional, physical, and spiritual.

13. If you have had experience in any health topic and would be willing to teach or share your experience, please put your name and telephone number below and indicate what topic you are familiar with.

14. Name (optional)

Thank you for taking the time to complete this survey.

APPENDIX D
Health Ministries—Meeting the Needs of Seniors

In each category, check *one* only:

Age	Who Are You Living With?	This Questionnaire Was Completed By
___ 65-79	___ Spouse	___ Self
___ 80+	___ Relatives	___ Spouse
	___ Nursing home	___ Son/daughter
Sex	___ Alone	___ Friend
___ Male	___ Other (state below)	___ Other (state below)
___ Female		

Check *all* areas that apply to you:

1. With which of the following physical needs can we assist you?
   ___ Preparation or delivery of meals
   ___ Transportation to doctor or dentist's office, church, social events
   ___ Running errands (example: buying groceries)
   ___ Housework or yard work
   ___ Other
2. With which of the following social needs can we assist you?
   ___ Having someone visit you on a regular basis
   ___ Planning group meals (potlucks, picnic, dining out)
   ___ Planning more group activities for seniors
   ___ Providing ways to help you become involved with helping others
   ___ Other
3. With which of the following spiritual needs can we assist you?
   ___ Organizing small group Bible studies
   ___ Regular visits from the pastoral staff
   ___ Feelings of guilt
   ___ Spiritual doubts (example: salvation)
   ___ Other
4. With which of the following emotional and mental needs can we assist you?
   ___ Learning or teaching hobbies
   ___ Maintaining or improving self-worth, self-esteem
   ___ Marriage enrichment series
   ___ Dealing with feelings of loneliness or depression
   ___ Other
5. In which area listed below do you have the greatest need?
   ___ Physical
   ___ Social
   ___ Spiritual
   ___ Emotional and mental
6. Would you participate in all activities in which you indicated a need if these areas were provided by the church? ___ Yes ___ No
7. Please list other areas or needs we can assist with that were not included in this questionnaire.
8. What personal gifts or talents do you have to share with this faith community?

Name (optional)

Phone ( )

Thank you!

APPENDIX E
Myths About the Parish Nurse

Myth #1: The Parish Nurse Has All the Answers

"You are a nurse, certainly you have read the latest about that new test for cancer." "What do you think about flu immunization?" "Should I see a doctor for this pain? If so, which one?" The list of questions goes on and on. A parish nurse may be seen as the key medical consultant in the congregation, the person who has the latest information on all subjects and for all age groups. The reality is that each nurse comes to this role with various experiences and expertise. The new parish nurse may feel this burden. One nurse commented that she felt like she had to memorize *Tabor's Medical Dictionary*. It is important to recognize one's limitations and develop a network of clinical resources to obtain answers for the parishioners. To establish credibility, the nurse must provide sound advice and recommendations, so it is important that she learn to say to people, when she is unsure, that she will be happy to find out and get back to them.

Myth #2: The Parish Nurse Is the Perfect Model of Health

Parish nurses seem to struggle with this issue a great deal. If a parish nurse is teaching others about health and wellness, how could she personally experience physical or emotional illness? The parish nurse may feel that she needs to be the proper weight, exercise daily, and eat a well-balanced, nutritious diet. The parish nurse may also feel that she must always be able to handle stress effectively and balance all the demands in life effortlessly. Whereas these are certainly admirable goals for everyone, they must not be viewed as necessary burdens in fulfilling the role. Parish nurses have described the inner struggle and guilt when they experienced illness. The parish nurse is a role model for health to the members of the congregation. However, that does not imply perfection. Health is a process, and perfect health in the whole-person sense is not attainable here on Earth. The parish nurse must come to a place where she can accept her humanness and struggle but also recognize the opportunity and challenge to model healthy behaviors. It is an issue of maintaining balance and a realistic perspective on one's life.

Myth #3: The Parish Nurse's Family Always Behaves Properly

The parish nurse may begin to experience some of the feelings common to the clergy. One of those relates to the feeling of being "on stage" or the center of attention. This is particularly true for nurses working in their own congregation. Suddenly, the nurse and her family may be viewed in a different light. Just as the nurse may feel the need to always be healthy and whole, she may also have a new awareness of how the congregation is viewing her family. Certainly, if the parish nurse is supporting and counseling others regarding their relationships and lifestyle, there may be the feeling that her own family must be a model for others. Parishioners may become critical of the parish nurse's family, just as they often have of the clergyperson's family. The pastor often feels that his or her family is a reflection of his or her faith and trust in God. The nurse may also begin to experience this and may feel particular stress when her own family goes through periods of disruption and disharmony. The nurse may feel additional pressure, when difficulties do arise, to handle them effectively. Again, the issue of humanness arises.

Myth #4: The Parish Nurse Cannot Be Friends With Members of the Congregation

The parish nurse may feel uneasy about special friendships in the congregation. The issues seem to center around confidentiality as well as feelings about whether the parish nurse may be showing favoritism to some members in the congregation. This may be especially true for nurses who grew up in that particular congregation. The parish nurse may either feel awkward about continuing friendships in the congregation or, at the other extreme, feel she must be friends with everyone. It is analogous to a staff nurse moving up into a management role in which she must reassess friendships and relationships in light of the new role. There may be the feeling that the nurse can no longer look to congregational members as a main source of support and encouragement. This is why it is so important for parish nurses to form their own network and have support from each other as well as developing support systems with the parish and pastoral staff.

Myth #5: The Parish Nurse Helps Everyone Who Asks

The parish nurse is carving out a niche in a new role. She feels that she must respond to needs as they arise. Before long, the needs begin to exceed her time and abilities. The parish nurse then has to come to grips with personal limitations and learn when it is OK to say no and not feel guilty. This is where support is vital for the nurse. This is a common struggle for professionals in the helping professions, and parish nurses need to help each other deal effectively with this issue. It is extremely helpful when members of the pastoral staff or health cabinet can support the parish nurse in setting priorities and limits. This seems to be a critical issue that must be addressed for the nurse to be able to continue in the role for any period of time without feeling frustrated and "burned out."

The parish nurse who has become very involved in this role may begin to hear people saying that they will not call her because she is "too busy." One nurse heard a parishioner say that "the nurse always has time for me, but she doesn't have time for everyone." It may become somewhat of a status symbol for parishioners to have their "own special nurse." This can be very manipulative, and what was intended to be helpful and caring becomes unhelpful. It is important to listen to these comments and to understand their messages.

Myth #6: The Clergy Are Above Human Struggles

Over the years, parish nurses have become a source of support not only for members of the congregation and the community but for the parish staff. This role can be extremely important, as the pastoral staff may feel a lack of personal support. Clergy also struggle with many of the myths listed above. Whereas the nurse may feel very positive in this supportive role, it also may bring with it feelings of disappointment and disillusionment. The nurse may have grown up with the concept of the clergy as being "special" people who do not experience the same frustrations and struggles as others. It may be difficult to suddenly come face to face with the reality that the clergy share these same feelings and frustrations.

Myth #7: The Parish Nurse Is on Call 24 Hours a Day

Each nurse must determine her own limitations within the role of parish nurse. Just as the minister may be called at any time during the day or night, so may the parish nurse, and she must decide how she will handle the calls. She must decide her limitations and develop back-up systems, which may include the purchase of an answering machine. Otherwise, the nurse may feel unable to take vacations or personal time. Time is a very precious commodity, and the nurse must decide how hers is to be used most effectively.

When the parish nurse is a member of the congregation in which she works, she may feel that she is never off duty. When the parish nurse comes to the church to worship or participate in an activity, she is seen by the parishioners in the role of parish nurse. As with many clergy, nurses may feel they must actually be away from the parish to have time for themselves or that they have to worship elsewhere to fully participate in worship. The nurse needs to find ways to feel supported and spiritually nurtured.

Myth #8: The Parish Nurse Is Accountable to Everyone

When there is a cooperative program between a health care institution and a congregation, the parish nurse may feel accountable to the hospital, the pastoral staff, the health cabinet, and the congregation. This may feel very fragmented, particularly when the lines of communication and authority are not clearly delineated. The parish nurse may begin to feel expectations from many directions and wonder where the allegiance really belongs. This issue must be confronted and discussed as it arises and clarified whenever possible. It may be helpful to designate one person as the contact person for the parish nurse. It is also important early on in the program to determine who will be evaluating the nurse herself as well as who will be making decisions regarding the continuation of the program.

Myth #9: The Parish Nurse Is a Pseudo-Minister

As parish nurses develop their roles, they get involved in many pastoral activities, such as participating in services, bringing communion to parishioners, and visiting the sick. It is an ongoing issue to maintain a balance between pastoral and nursing activities. The foundation of nursing knowledge and practice must be an underlying theme in all activities. This is what makes the parish nurse role unique, and it must be preserved. As the role is developed, defined, and evaluated in various settings, this issue must constantly be confronted and discussed. This is a new role for the congregation and the clergy, and there are no simple answers or specific limitations to the role, so we must continue to define the role out of experience. There has to be a balance. It is critical to the parish nurse role that nursing knowledge continue to be a foundation for practice.

Myth #10: The Parish Nurse Is Always Happy

This myth again refers to the nurse feeling as though she is always on stage and always "up." This is commonly expressed by the pastoral staff as well. One of the pastors said that he could never have a "bad day." He said it was difficult to find places where he could let down and truly be himself. This again reinforces the need for ongoing support and supervision with which the parish nurse can discuss feelings and get feedback. It is also important to discuss these feelings with the pastoral staff. If this issue is not addressed, it will eventually affect the nurse's family members and other significant relationships.

Appendix F
Review of Spiritual Values and
Principles of Healthy Spiritual Living

Appendix Table 1 Review of Spiritual Values

	Secular Dominant	*Spiritual Dominant*
Value:	Things, money, power, success, sex	People
Goal:	Acquire the above	Quality of relationships
Commitment to:	Power, control, do what I want, having it my way	Faithfulness, integrity, doing God's will
Achievement:	Competition, getting	Caring for others, giving of self, behaving in ways that enhance self-esteem
Self-worth:	Being superior, being perfect, seeking to avoid vulnerability	Being me, letting others be themselves, being human, accepting limitations, affirming strengths, being productive, being responsible and accountable for attitudes, feelings, and behaviors
Internal feelings:	Pride, self-pity, self-preoccupation, insensitivity, seeking praise	Trust, humility, gratitude, awareness of others, openness, empathy

SOURCE: Carl Anderson, as modified and cited by Keller (1991). Used with permission.

APPENDIX TABLE 2 Principles of Healthy Spiritual Living

Human wholeness (completeness, fulfillment) is experienced through surrender of self-will to a relationship (partnership) with a higher power. This relationship restores balance, harmony, and self-acceptance, giving humans the freedom to be human.

Health	Illness
Surrender of ego (self-will) (yes, yes)	Compliance with reality (yes, no)
Acceptance of limits and dependence	Fighting limits: "If only I had. . . ."
Recognition of incompleteness	Self-sufficient
Realization that I am not God	Desire to be like God (control)
Honesty	Deception
Ability to enjoy humor	No laughter, sad, gloomy
Self-responsibility	Blame others
Opportunities to act	Self-pity, feel controlled
Acceptance of self	Perfectionism, achievement
Acceptance of others	Manipulate others
Success equals quality in relationships	Success equals quantity of things, money, power
Care, love, worth through relationships	Accumulate things, money, power
Cooperate	Compete
Action, choices	React, "victim" role
Free for	Free from
Acceptance of humanness	"I'm only human"
Use things, money, power for relationships	Use relationships for things, money, power
Serenity	Tension

SOURCE: Carl Anderson (from lecture notes and outlines).

APPENDIX G
The Life of Jesus as a Role Model of
Healthy Behaviors and Balance

Jesus was a human. He was a child, experienced adolescence, and grew into manhood. He had feelings and lived with human limitations. The following are a few of the characteristics that contributed to His state of wholeness.

He Didn't Do It Alone

Jesus carefully selected the 12 apostles. Once He was gone, His ministry could have ended if He had tried to do it alone. In His time on Earth, He fostered a fellowship of believers who fostered forgiveness and restoration of healthy relationships in community. That community is worldwide today.

He Prepared Others to Help Him

His work was spent in teaching all. Special time was taken in role modeling the behavior and skills needed to carry on the ministry.

He Had a Close Group of Friends Who Listened to Him and Cared About Him

Jesus developed good relationships with men and women. These relationships were ones in which He could relax, share His frustration, and be supported.

He Exercised Regularly

Jesus walked almost everywhere He went. His mission depended on Him being in good health.

He Loved

Jesus loved His Father and those He worked with and those He reached out to in His ministry. His death on the cross was an act of love for us all.

He Looked to Others for Support but Not to Take Care of Him

There were many times in the life of Jesus when He relied on those close to Him for support. However, He never expected them to do what He needed to do Himself.

He Rested and Slept Regularly

Jesus did grow weary. His human limitations were apparent, and He did what He needed to do for Himself so He would be in the best position to serve the Father.

He Ate Healthfully

Jesus did not have a McDonald's or Wendy's fast-food restaurant along his route. His diet was simple. He ate what He needed to provide the necessary fuel for His work.

He Prayed Often

Jesus prayed for courage, strength, and guidance to do His Father's will.

He Practiced Solitude

This time of solitude was the time away from the distraction of the world. Solitude gave Him time to refocus and develop clarity about His mission.

He Was Open to All People

Throughout His life, Jesus interacted with all people: the very sick, the poor, the wealthy, the farmer, and the hypocrite. All became part of His mission and work.

He Trusted

Jesus's trust in His Father was without fault. He trusted that the Father would provide for Him anything He needed to do His work.

He Did God's Will

Jesus fulfilled the prophecies. He planted seeds and role-modeled to all how they could do the same.

He Went About His Work in Spite of All Problems

Problems were acknowledged and dealt with. However, there were times when He was tempted to be distracted from His primary mission.

SOURCE: Solari-Twadell (revised 1998).

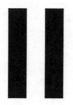

PARISH NURSING
A Collaborative Practice

9

Listening to Faith Communities

Collaboration With Those Served

Robert Lloyd
Patti Ludwig-Beymer

In this chapter, listening as a fundamental principle of continuous quality improvement (CQI) is identified and explained. The concept of collaboration and the role it plays as a means to foster listening is also explored. Finally, research designed to listen to the "Voice of the Customer" (VOC) will be described, along with a discussion of how the data have been used to enhance collaboration between parish nurses and those they serve.

Quality

Everywhere in health care, the concept of quality is gaining ground. Whether it is called quality management, continuous quality improvement, quality deployment, total quality management, or the search for excellence, the concept is ever present in health care. This new perception of quality is different from the old view of quality assurance. Rather than identifying quality deficiencies, the new perspective focuses on striving to continually improve the quality of the health care services and products delivered.

The concept of CQI is also gaining acceptance within Christian churches. As described by Kallestad and Schey (1994), implementing "Total Quality Ministry" will result in many benefits, including empowering congregations, evaluating processes rather than criticizing people, excellence in ministry, emphasizing God's mission and vision for the congregation, keeping the focus on the customer, preventing problems, and creating an open atmosphere.

CQI is basically a management philosophy that involves a never ending cycle of continuous improvements in quality (Deming, 1986). Parish nurses who experienced hospital quality assurance (QA) programs prior to the 1990s may be surprised to learn of the differences between QA and CQI. Traditionally, QA looked at quality in terms of standards. When standards were not met (or thresholds were not reached), action was taken with the individuals deemed responsible for the failures. CQI, on the other hand, looks at quality as a dynamic phenomenon. Rather than blaming individuals, CQI looks at processes to determine why a process is producing outcomes that do not meet or exceed customer expectations.

CQI is grounded in three basic principles: (a) it is customer focused, (b) it analyzes the processes that customers experience, and (c) it uses data to make decisions (Carey & Lloyd, 1995). CQI occurs when all three of these concepts come together on a daily basis. Pursuit of only one or even two of these principles will cause organizations to fall short of the true potential of CQI.

CQI begins with listening to the "Voice of the Customer" or client (VOC). In the past, health care professionals often forgot the importance of the client, believing that only they (and not the patients) could understand and appreciate the complexities of the health care industry. However, the health care industry is increasingly coming to understand that clients can and should help to define quality and set the expectations for performance. Although clients may not know the specifics of how the technical dimensions of care are delivered, they can certainly identify how they feel about the ways in which they were treated and the outcomes they experienced. This chapter concentrates on listening as a key responsibility of parish nurses.

After listening to the clients and determining what they want, need, or expect, the next step is to gain an understanding of the processes in place that will either delight or repel. One of the most frequently used tools to assist in this stage of CQI is the flowchart. By making a flowchart of the current process, parish nurses will gain a deeper appreciation of the complexity of the process and identify opportunities for improvement. Clients do not own the processes; parish nurses do. It is their responsibility, therefore, to not only understand the processes in place but to understand which components of the process are having the greatest influence.

The final CQI principle is that data are needed for making good decisions. A criticism of the health care profession has been that anecdotal rather than objective data frequently drive decision making. Organizations embracing CQI rely on current and objective data to evaluate the processes delivering products or services to customers. Using data in this way is characterized as listening to the "Voice of the Process" (VOP). When VOP data are combined with listening to the VOC, CQI can flourish and improvements may be realized.

Listening to the Voice of the Parishioner

Listening is not a new concept. The value of listening over talking is taught and reinforced in childhood. Adults, however, frequently forget some of the simple, yet profound, lessons from their youth. More specifically, health care professionals are often criticized by those served as being quick to give advice but slow to listen. This may be true in some sectors of the health care field, but parish nurses represent one group of health care professionals who build listening into all that they do.

Continuous quality improvement begins with listening to the VOC. Parishioners, whom we may think of as clients, patients, or in other terms, must be listened to. Clients are the ones who define quality and set the expectations for performance. It is not difficult to find examples of this perspective in every industry. The driver of a car does not need to know about the technical aspects of fuel injection, but he or she does expect a smooth-running engine. Similarly, the customer at a department store does not really care about the inventory replacement system, but he or she does expect to obtain products as requested. In short, listening to the VOC provides clear messages about the expectations of those served. How providers respond to these data will set the tone for the future. Clients are the reason health care providers exist!

Collaboration

One word that is synonymous with parish nursing is collaboration. The concept of collaboration is fairly straightforward. It basically means working together or jointly toward a common goal.

As initially conceived by Granger Westberg (1987), parish nursing is grounded in the idea that health and well-being are easier to maintain in collaborative arrangements than in isolation. A parish nurse strives to understand a person's wellness needs (i.e., listens to the VOC), places these needs within the context of a whole person approach to health, and then works with the individual to identify appropriate courses of action and/or referral(s) for continuous improvement. Collaboration is not only the guiding principle behind an individual parish nurse's efforts; it also serves as a fundamental approach to organizing parish nurses into an integrated team of professionals.

True collaboration, however, requires much more than merely saying that you believe in it or that you understand it as a concept. Furthermore, although it may seem to be a fairly simple concept to grasp, implementing and making collaboration an integral part of daily life may not be straightforward. This is due to the fact that collaboration may not follow a linear way of thinking and it may not always be done in the same way. Consistent and successful collaboration requires a strong sense of systems thinking, teamwork, nonlinear thinking, and a willingness to be flexible. It is as much an art as it is a management concept—and in some ways, it is a behavior that reflects a way of viewing the world and human interaction rather than a skill learned in formal education courses.

There are, basically, two levels of collaboration that occur within parish nursing: (a) collaboration at the individual level and (b) collaboration at the group or collective level. Both levels require the parish nurse to be sensitive not only to the needs of those involved but to the different tools and techniques that enhance the chances of success. Ultimately, if all of these considerations are integrated and balanced, collaboration will be optimized.

The first level of collaboration occurs when a parish nurse interacts with another individual. This may be with a parishioner who has a personal or family need, or it can be with a pastor, a lay leader of the congregation, another parish nurse, or a referral agent. This level of collaboration requires strong interpersonal skills, an ability to listen and identify specific needs, empathy, and knowledge of how to develop creative solutions.

The next level of collaboration occurs when a parish nurse works with groups of individuals. These groups vary in size and may include families, teams of health care professionals, or an entire congregation. Most of the skills used to develop collaboration with individuals can also be used within a group setting, but there are several additional skills that need to be fostered. For example, the nominal group technique (NGT), brainstorming, affinity diagramming, multivoting, rank ordering, structured discussion, sociograms, cause-and-effect diagrams, and force-field analysis are important tools and techniques that can be used to foster collaboration within a group context (see Scholtes, 1993, for additional tools and explanation of the tools and techniques listed here).

Advantages and Challenges of Collaboration

Nearly everyone would agree that collaboration makes sense. But what does it really mean to collaborate? Cheaney and Cotter (1991) offer a simple yet insightful response to this question: "Ask a kid!" Yes—just ask a child why working together (collaboration) is better than competing. In their book, Cheaney and Cotter tell the story of Adam (age 9), who was asked why he thought it was a good idea to work together in teams. He pondered briefly, then said, "Well, you can get done faster, because you are all working together." Adam continued by saying that, "You can do better, because if you're all working together, you should agree on what you're working on." When asked why it was important to agree, he responded, "Because, if you agree, there is a better chance that you are right." Rightfully so, the authors end this story by saying, "Sometimes the most powerful ideas are the simplest. Ask a kid."

The advantages of collaboration seem obvious. Yet how often is the vision of Adam missing? Kohn (1986, 1993), for example, has developed extensive arguments about the devastating effects of competition within our society. He argues that competition is inherently destructive and leads to dysfunctional relationships between individuals, within families, and even between countries. Cooperation and collaboration, for Kohn, are the building blocks for success.

The challenges faced by those who wish to develop collaborative relationships are numerous, however. These challenges become more complex when moving from individual collaboration to a group setting. Parish nurses must be skilled at both levels, but they will find their greatest challenges at the group level. For group collaboration to exist, therefore, a parish nurse must be able to *simultaneously* (a) figure out all the multiple agendas in the group, (b) detect any hidden agendas, (c) know when and how to use each of the tools and techniques listed above, (d) be part diplomat and part street cop, and (e) have the patience of Job! Knowledge of CQI tools and techniques provides a strong foundation for building these collaborative relationships.

Listening to Those Served

When students take their first health care course, one of the messages that is constantly repeated to them is that the patient is at the center of all they do. This suggests that health care providers not only listen to those served but also use the input received to make decisions about the care that will be delivered. This may sound good in theory, but in reality health care professionals have done a rather poor job of actually listening to those they serve and an even poorer job of incorporating what they hear into the delivery of care. For example, patients indicate that they do not want to travel to many different parts of the hospital to complete their preadmission testing. Yet, the lab is located on one level, the radiology department is located on another, and the blood bank is in still a third location. The reality experienced by patients does not demonstrate listening to the customer.

Health care professionals have difficulty in listening closely to those they serve. This was especially true during the early years of modern medicine (e.g., prior to 1940) when the profession was much more paternalistic and hierarchical than it is today. Many consumer groups maintain, and it is widely acknowledged, that even today, health care professionals frequently approach their jobs with a fairly closed perspective toward the customer. Despite all of the advancements in the health care field, there is still a concern that health care provider ears often seem to be deaf to the voice of the customer, which then makes it extremely difficult to incorporate what the customer wants or expects into the delivery of care.

Scherkenbach (1991) has written extensively about listening to the voice of the customer. He writes,

> The voice of the customer communicates to you the producer, the wants and needs of your customers, as you perceive them. It can also be more generally viewed as the forecast, goal, plan aim, prediction, objective, target, "druthers," or as Dr. (W. Edwards) Deming sometimes said, "facts-of-life." (p. 12)

For parish nurses, the challenge is twofold: (a) to understand, very clearly, what the voice of the customer is trying to tell them and (b) to facilitate collaborative behaviors that will meet or exceed the customer's expectations.

Listening Three Times

Ideally, we should be listening to our clients at three distinct points in time: before service is delivered, as service is delivered, and after service has been delivered. Each phase of listening is outlined below.

Preservice assessments are valued because they help define what clients want, need, or expect. Typically, this form of listening is done as organizations are designing (or redesigning) new services or facilities. For example, the parish nurses frequently survey or solicit information from congregation members before initiating the development of health education programming.

Point-of-service feedback is gathered while the clients are still receiving care. This allows for (a) rapid response to meet client expectations and (b) remedial action to keep potentially negative situations from blossoming into major trouble spots. In this case, a parish nurse will interview a client while the client is still receiving care. Because respondent bias is a major challenge, it is wise to consult with individuals skilled in conducting structured interviews or focus groups before embarking on this method of listening to the customer.

Postservice evaluations are conducted after patients leave care. The most popular approaches are mailed or telephone surveys. Sometimes, organizations attempt to do postservice evaluations on their own. This requires people knowledgeable about survey design and construction to create reliable and valid surveys. Hayes (1992) provides a very good overview of the essential steps needed to create valid and reliable surveys; Dillman (1978) highlights the pathway for effective telephone survey methods.

A comprehensive VOC measurement system should combine all three types of assessments. The challenge is to be familiar with all the different tools and techniques that can provide VOC data and then know when to use each one. Table 9.1 summarizes several of the more frequently used techniques to gather input from the VOC. For each entry, the advantages and disadvantages are presented. The most frequently used approach is to conduct a survey. Unfortunately, most surveys are developed by sincere people who have little knowledge or experience with proper survey construction techniques and methods. This is particularly true in parish nursing. Often surveys developed by parish nurses receive poor response rates, which lead to broad results.

Surveys can be a very powerful method for listening to the voice of the client, but care must be taken to ensure that they are developed and tested properly and that an integrated approach to the distribution and collection of the surveys has been agreed upon. Those interested in reading more about proper survey development should consult Dillman (1978), Hayes (1992), and Carey and Lloyd (1995).

Focus groups are another frequently used way to listen to the voice of the client. As shown in Table 9.1, the major advantage of a focus group is that it can provide a great deal of in-depth information. A skilled focus group facilitator uses structured questions to probe the members of the group about a particular subject or event. Then the facilitator will develop a summary of the session. The major disadvantage of a focus group approach (particularly if only one session is conducted) is that there is little generalizability that emerges from the session. All that can be said about the results is that on this day, at this hour, these people felt this way or that about this topic.

Less frequently used approaches to listening to the voice of the client include observation, complaint letters (or letters of praise), suggestion boxes, historical records, and customer defections. Webb, Campbell, Schwartz, and Sechrest (1969) discuss the advantages and disadvantages of many of these approaches in their book *Unobtrusive Measures: Nonreactive Research in the Social Sciences*. The leading complaint against using these approaches is that the amount of information obtained from each approach can be limited. For example, complaint letters usually provide a great deal of insight from one person, but the central question is, How pervasive is this complaint? Does it reflect one voice or many? Letters of praise or complaint may, however, be aggregated and analyzed qualitatively, as described by Ludwig-Beymer et al. (1993). Such analyses, although time consuming, are helpful in identifying issues of importance to patients and family members.

In summary, there are many ways to listen to those served. How health care providers listen is important. However, in many ways it is even more important to be clear about why providers want to listen and what they intend to do with the information once they have obtained it.

TABLE 9.1 Selected Approaches to Gathering Input From Customers

Tool/Approach	Cost	Advantages	Disadvantages
Surveys	Moderate to high cost depending on the methodology used	• Generalizability • Offers continuous monitoring • Provides comparative reference data • Versatility • Reasonably quick to implement	• Requires rigorous protocols and valid/reliable instruments • May require sampling • Not highly flexible • Unwillingness of individuals to participate • Inability of respondents to recall
Focus groups	Moderate to high cost depending on the number conducted and who conducts them	• In-depth qualitative data • Does not require large samples • High flexibility • New issues/concerns may be identified during session	• Low generalizability • Requires skilled facilitators • Not anonymous
Observation	Low cost	• Easy to do • Highly flexible	• Low generalizability • Low value for comparisons • Limited to publicly observable behavior • Requires considerable time and effort
Personal interviews	High cost	• Very detailed data • Easy to probe for additional data • Effective with all socio-economic levels	• Very labor intensive • Very time consuming • Quality of data depends on skill of interviewer • Not anonymous
Unsolicited feedback	Very low cost	• Identifies extreme dissatisfiers/satisfiers	• Virtually no opportunity to generalize findings
High-tech tools	Very high cost	• Provides real-time feedback • User-friendly • Flexibility	• May not be appealing to certain groups of respondents • No control over sample of respondents
Experiential (the "mystery shopper")	High cost	• Tremendous depth of data • Can cover all aspects of a customer's experience	• Low generalizability for defining a "typical experience" • Requires the mystery shoppers to be trained and articulate

The Parish Nurse Example

The remainder of this chapter details how a group of parish nurses took time to listen to those they serve and then developed collaborative solutions to respond to the VOC. Specifically, the following section will address how the parish nurses listened to the voice of parishioners by developing a survey, tabulating the results, and using the information gathered to create new collaborative relationships and programming options.

The W. K. Kellogg Foundation Project

In 1990, Lutheran General Health Care System received funding from the W. K. Kellogg Foundation for a 3-year evaluation project to describe and document the Parish Nurse Programs at Lutheran General Health Care System in the Chicagoland area and United Medical Center in the quad cities of Illinois/Iowa. The grant was completed in four phases. Phase I described how the parish nurse concept was operationally defined, interpreted, and implemented in 40 sites throughout Illinois. Phase II focused on the perceived needs of the parish nurse program as expressed by four key stakeholder groups: (a) representatives of the sponsoring institutions (Lutheran General Health Care System and United Medical Center), (b) the Kellogg Advisory Committee, (c) each congregation's leadership structure, and (d) each congregation. In particular, alignment of the stakeholders was examined. Phase III offered recommendations for the ongoing evaluation and documentation of parish nurse programs. Phase IV concentrated on the dissemination of the lessons learned as a result of the overall project. This chapter will use data collected from parishioners during the second phase of the grant to demonstrate the key principle of listening to the Voice of the Customer.

Listening to the Voice of the Parishioner

Every day, parish nurses listen to parishioners. This listening provides rich and detailed data, but it is often anecdotal information that has little generalizability. It was decided, therefore, to develop a survey that would obtain comprehensive and standardized feedback from parishioners along five dimensions. Table 9.2 presents the survey.

The first section of the survey used forced-choice responses (e.g., yes, no, and not sure) to obtain feedback on the parishioners' familiarity with the parish nurse program and its overall impact on the congregation. The second section consisted of 10 questions related to specific parish nursing services. Responses were either yes or no (i.e., respondents either used a service or they did not). Questions in the third section asked the respondents to indicate whether or not they would like selected parish nursing services to be offered more frequently in the future. Forced-choice responses of yes, no, and not sure were offered. In the fourth section, parishioners were asked to provide demographic information, including age, gender, marital status, and church membership. The final section allowed parishioners the opportunity to provide comments about the parish nurse program, share a story about their experiences with the program, and/or obtain further information about parish nursing by providing their name and address.

Parish nurses critiqued the initial draft of the survey. The final version was three pages long and was printed on yellow paper with large print so that elderly parishioners would have no difficulty reading the questions.

TABLE 9.2 Parish Nurse Program Parishioner Survey

We would like to know your thoughts about the health focus of our congregation. Please check the response that best describes your feelings about the following statements.

IN OUR CONGREGATION:

- *health awareness* is becoming a greater part of our church's everyday activities.
    Yes _____ No _____ Not sure _____

- we are becoming comfortable with the idea that a person's health results from the *interplay* of lifestyles, attitudes, faith and physical well-being.
    Yes _____ No _____ Not sure _____

- health and healing are becoming *explicit* parts of our church's mission.
    Yes _____ No _____ Not sure _____

How familiar are you with the Parish Nurse Program?
    Very familiar _____   Somewhat familiar _____
    Not very familiar _____   Not at all familiar _____

The Parish Nurse Program offers a variety of support services and activities to your congregation. We would like to know if you have ever used any of these services:

- I have read bulletin and newsletter articles on health topics provided by the parish nurse.
    Yes _____ No _____

- I have participated in a health screening activity; for example, blood pressure or cholesterol checks offered by the parish nurse.
    Yes _____ No _____

- I have attended a health education program or support group that was coordinated or presented by the parish nurse.
    Yes _____ No _____

- I have talked with the parish nurse about a personal matter such as medications, a new diagnosis, a relationship, or my overall health and well-being.
    Yes _____ No _____

- A member of my family has talked with the parish nurse about a personal matter such as medications, a new diagnosis, a relationship, or overall health and well-being.
    Yes _____ No _____

- The parish nurse has referred me to a physician, a group, or an organization in the congregation or community where I could go for further assistance.
    Yes _____ No _____

- I have suggested to a family member or friend that they might want to talk with the parish nurse about their health concerns.
    Yes _____ No _____

- I have participated as a volunteer from this congregation who provides service to poor, homeless, shut-ins, or bereaved.
    Yes _____ No _____

- A church volunteer has provided support to me during a time of personal need.
    Yes _____ No _____

- The parish nurse has helped me draw upon my spiritual strength in dealing with health issues.
    Yes _____ No _____

In the future, I would like the Parish Nurse Program to provide more articles on health topics in bulletins and newsletters.
    Yes _____ No _____ Not Sure _____

(continued)

TABLE 9.2 Continued

Health screening activities.
　　Yes ____No ____Not Sure ____
Health education programs or support groups.
　　Yes _•__No ____Not Sure ____
Opportunities for me to meet individually with the parish nurse.
　　Yes ____No ____Not Sure ____
Information on other community groups and organizations where I can go for further assistance.
　　Yes ____No ____Not Sure ____
Opportunities to participate as a volunteer.
　　Yes ____No ____Not Sure ____
Opportunities to discuss the relationship between my faith and health.
　　Yes ____No ____Not Sure ____

My age is: ____ 14-17____ 18-30____ 31-50____ 51-65____ 66-80____ over 80
I am a: ____ female____ male
I am currently: ____ single____ married____ separated/divorced____ widowed
I am a member of this church: ____ Yes____ No
This survey was completed at:
　____ a worship service
　____ a coffee or social hour
　____ a health education or support program
　____ a health education or support group
　____ a health screening
　____ home
　____ other (please specify: _____)

Please use the following space to provide comments on the Parish Nurse Program or to share a story about your experience with the parish nurse.

If you would like to know more about the Parish Nurse Program in your congregation, please print your name and address below.

　Name:

　Address:

　Phone:

Thank you for your time and cooperation!
Please return your completed survey to your parish nurse.

Data Collection

The initial idea was to distribute surveys to a random sample of parishioners from the 40 congregational mailing lists. However, it was decided that the cost and complexity of generating a random sample and distributing and collecting mailed surveys would not be justified. Therefore, a convenience sample was used, with parish nurses distributing and collecting the surveys. This technique does not allow generalizability to the congregations at large. However, such a method of data collection does yield valuable information about the perspective of parishioners.

Parish nurses distributed the questionnaires during fall 1992 at a variety of church functions, including blood drives, coffee or social hours, health education sessions, health screenings, support group meetings, and worship services. Some parish nurses also distributed questionnaires to parishioners during home visits. A total of 1,043 completed questionnaires were returned.

The forced-choice questions were coded and entered into a statistical software program for analysis. Descriptive statistics were prepared for the entire sample and for each individual congregation. Responses to the open-ended question documented rich and detailed stories. The data were analyzed qualitatively, using an editing-style methodology (Miller & Crabtree, 1992). Each comment was analyzed with respect to the actual words used by the writer. A key word or phrase that captured the "essence" of the writer's comment was used to establish categories. Individual comments were then aggregated into these categories. To minimize possible classification errors, the authors independently verified each other's work, resolving any discrepancies through consensus.

Survey Results and Parish Nurse Responses

This section will highlight only a few of the results of the parishioner study. Detail has been omitted in the interest of space, but the reader will get a feel for what types of data may be obtained by using these methods. Readers may consult Lloyd and Djupe (1994) for a more thorough description of the study results.

Respondent Profile

Of the 1,043 completed questionnaires, 92.5% were completed by congregational members. The nonmembers were affiliated with the churches in other ways. Of the respondents, 70% were female and 30% were male; 62% of the respondents were married. The age distribution was as follows: 8% were under 30 years old, 50% were between the ages of 31 and 65, 30% between the ages of 66 and 80, and 12% over the age of 80. The open-ended question was completed by 399 individuals (38% of the respondents). One hundred and fourteen individuals (10.9%) provided their name and address to obtain additional information about the parish nurse program.

Program Familiarity

Survey results suggested that 13% of respondents were not familiar with the parish nurse program. These results were verified by open-ended responses, in which some parishioners indicated they were not aware of the program or viewed it as underused or not needed. As a result, parish nurses have made a concerted effort to publicize their works verbally and in writing.

Use of Services

The most frequently used service, reported by 90% of respondents, was reading bulletin and newsletter articles on health topics. As a result, parish nurses continue to plan health articles for parish publications throughout the year.

Future Expectations

When asked to indicate the future importance of various services provided by the parish nurses, parishioners showed a strong preference for articles in bulletins and newsletters, education seminars and workshops, and health screenings. As a result of these findings, parish nurses continue to strengthen their written communications with their congregations and have increased their offerings of education seminars and workshops. In addition, many parish nurses have implemented the Congregational Health Screening Program, described in chapter 13, to meet the needs of their parishioners.

Interactive Situations With Parish Nurses

The open-ended question provided the opportunity to assess the impact the parish nurse program had on the lives of the parishioners. Within these comments were many rich stories that conveyed how the program affected individuals and their families. As shown in Table 9.3, the situation that most commonly resulted in interaction between an individual and a parish nurse was concern over the individual's health or the health of a family member. As a result of these findings, parish nurses make themselves available to discuss health concerns and other pertinent issues at a variety of church events.

Personal Traits of Parish Nurses

One of the major benefits of asking for written feedback is that it allows the reader to obtain very rich insights from respondents. In this study, parishioners commented on the personal traits and behaviors of the parish nurses. A total of 314 comments related to personal traits and behaviors were written. As seen in Table 9.4, the most frequently mentioned traits were "caring and compassionate." As a result of these findings, parish nurses have examined their personal traits. They use feedback from pastoral staff and other parish nurses to continue to grow in their roles.

Summary

Historically, the needs of congregations have been based on anecdotal information or input from individual parishioners. No general consensus or large-scale understanding has been traditionally sought. It is also relatively new to "listen to those served" rather than paternalistically determining the needs of a congregation.

As parish nurses listened to parishioners, they learned that parishioners tend to view health from a whole-person perspective. They don't just consider physical health, but their total well-being, which results from the interplay of physical, mental, and spiritual components. From the data collected, it is clear that parishioners are beginning to have an expanded definition of health and well-being, and they view the church as a natural partner in providing services aimed at improving health and well-being. The parish nurse is seen as a provider and facilitator of these services. Not only are individuals understanding health in a broader perspective, they also seem to be making lifestyle changes and taking a more active role in making health-related decisions.

TABLE 9.3 Reasons for Encounters Between Parish Nurses and Parishioners

Category	Number of Times Mentioned
Health concern for self or family member	27
Medical test or procedure	21
Relational or lifestyle issue	17
Attended a class, program, or group	15
Surgery or hospitalization of self or family member	15
Death or dying of loved one	10
Hypertension	10
Concern about an aging family member	8
Housing or living arrangement	5

TABLE 9.4 Parishioner Perspectives of Personal Traits of the Parish Nurse

Category	Number of Times Mentioned
Caring and compassionate	119
Available and accessible	45
Knowledgeable and professional	45
Helpful	36
Warm and friendly	20
Leader and valuable team member	19
Good listener	16
Spiritually filled	14

The parishioners described the services they value and use even in settings where many community services are already available. The parishioners clearly see a need for the services provided by the parish nurse. Parishioners found great value in having easy access to health care professionals who were able to answer questions or refer them to appropriate resources. Having educational activities take place in a familiar environment and having them supported by the pastor and leadership of the congregations were additional strengths.

Parishioners expressed a need for support on issues related to hospitalization, diagnosis of a health problem, management of a new medication, and particularly during times of grief and loss. In these situations, they need the ongoing support of a professional who can provide information and emotional support as well as direct them to appropriate resources. The parish nurse, as a trusted provider of services, may be the first point of contact for many hidden concerns such as substance abuse and domestic violence.

Lessons Learned

An excellent understanding of what parishioners value most about parish nursing came from listening to parishioners' stories and experiences. Parishioners were very willing to share their thoughts, feelings, perceptions, and experiences with parish nurses. Parishioners shared their stories in great detail even though they had to take time to write their responses. Therefore, focus groups and surveys may be effective means of listening to those served by the parish nurse. When surveys are used with parishioners, they may most effectively be distributed during functions held at the church rather than mailing the surveys to the individuals' homes. From the experience of this research, the personal contact achieved while distributing the surveys produced a much higher response rate than a mailing methodology.

Parish nurses can serve to link health and social services offered by community organizations and health care providers. This is currently happening, and in the future it will have even greater importance. This study has resulted in learning on the part of all involved, particularly the parish nurses. This learning will foster future collaboration. In particular, parish nurses learned two important lessons about data: the use of comparative data and the richness of stories.

First, the nurses learned how to use comparative data. A summary packet of the aggregate results of the parishioner questionnaire was distributed to each parish nurse. In addition, the individual congregation's summary statistics were given to that congregation's parish nurse. This allowed the parish nurse to view her practice in the context of the practice of other parish nurses. Parish nurses were encouraged to use these data as opportunities for improvement and synergy rather than as a formal or judgmental evaluation of their own program. As a result, parish nurses have collaborated with other parish nurses as well as with additional church and community groups.

Second, parish nurses saw the power of stories in generating rich data and also became aware of the need to analyze these stories for themes using qualitative methodologies. Each parish nurse was given the detailed written comments from the respondents in her congregation. Parish nurses have used these comments for planning and to identify opportunities for improvement.

Although many challenges remain for parish nurses, they have clearly demonstrated their commitment to listening and collaborating. Parish nurses are poised to continue to improve their practice and exceed the needs and expectations of the parishioners they serve.

References

Carey, R., & Lloyd, R. (1995). *Measuring quality improvement in health care: A guide to statistical process control applications*. New York: Quality Resources.

Chearney, L., & Cotter, M. (1991). *Real people real work: Parables on leadership in the 90s*. Knoxville, TN: SPC.

Deming, W. E. (1986). *Out of crisis*. Cambridge: MIT Press.

Dillman, D. (1978). *Mail and telephone surveys: The total design method*. New York: Wiley.

Hayes, B. (1992). *Measuring customer satisfaction*. Milwaukee, WI: ASQC Quality.

Kallestad, W., & Schey, S. (1994). *Total quality ministry*. Minneapolis, MN: Augsburg Fortress.

Kohn, A. (1986). *No contest: The case against competition*. Boston: Houghton Mifflin.

Kohn, A. (1993). *Punished by rewards: The trouble with gold stars, incentive plans, A's, praise, and other bribes*. Boston: Houghton Mifflin.

Lloyd, R. C., & Djupe, A. M. (1994). *Expanding our understanding of health and well-being: The parish nurse program*. Park Ridge, IL: National Parish Nurse Resource Center.

Ludwig-Beymer, P., Ryan, C. J., Johnson, N. J., Hennessy, K. A., Gattuso, M. C., Epsom, R., & Czurylo, K. T. (1993). Using patient perceptions to improve quality care. *Journal of Nursing Care Quality, 7*(2), 42-51.

Miller, W. L., & Crabtree, B. F. (1992). Primary care research: A multimethod typology and qualitative road map. In W. L. Crabtree & B. F. Miller (Eds.), *Doing qualitative research*. Newbury Park, CA: Sage.

Scherkenbach, W. W. (1991). *Deming's road to continual improvement*. Knoxville, TN: SPC.

Scholtes, P. (1993). *The team handbook: How to use teams to improve quality*. Madison, WI: Joiner.

Webb, E., Campbell, D., Schwartz, R., & Sechrest, L. (1969). *Unobtrusive measures: Nonreactive research in the social sciences*. Chicago: Rand McNally.

Westberg, G. (1987). *The parish nurse*. Park Ridge, IL: National Parish Nurse Resource Center.

10

The Congregation as a Workplace

Robert Cotton Fite

The Congregation:
Miserable and Glorious

When nurses become *parish* nurses, they join organizations they may have been familiar with since they were children. They understandably assume they know the lay of the land and just what to expect. For that very reason, they are frequently surprised, and sometimes disappointed, to find the congregation different than they expected. As they enter the practice of parish nursing ministry, therefore, it is a good idea for nurses to take a long look at their own expectations and some of the realities of congregational life.

Expectations

I recall with some amusement and a little embarrassment the expectations I took to the first parish I joined as a theological student in my early 20s. This, I believed, was going to be the community I had been looking for all my life, the place where I would be accepted and loved. It was the place where all the values that had drawn me to the church in the first place would be preached and practiced. We would stand up for what was right, we would bring God's love more fully into the world, and those who had doubts about all this would be carried along and eventually converted to believe as I did.

I am sure those expectations were not conscious, but I suspect if anyone had scratched very deeply, they would have found a very idealistic and quite judgmental young man beneath the smooth facade. Life and many gracious people tempered and hopefully humanized my expectations of self and my fellow congregants, but some of those deeply ingrained wishes still roam around in my psyche. When I become overly disappointed or discouraged with my pastor's performance, the old wish for a perfect mother or father reasserts itself. Do I expect that he or she will be any less human than

I? Certainly not in my rational mind, but at those other levels . . . oh, I do wish I could find just the right pastor and just the right congregation!

The point of the story is that we bring both positive and negative, realistic and unrealistic expectations to our involvement in church and synagogue. It seems a natural process. Early experiences with a wonderfully warm church school teacher or rabbi or endlessly long, boring sermons color our memories, but church and synagogue also stand as the repository of our greatest hopes and greatest fears. The very human psychological phenomenon of projection usually works overtime when it comes to church. We can easily load it up with all the things we hate about the world (and ourselves) as well as all the things we want to be true.

As a parish nurse, it is important that you examine your expectations so that you avoid behaving in ways that will finally disappoint you and undermine or diminish your effectiveness. A good way to bring some of the less obvious expectations to the surface is by recalling as many stories as possible about your early religious involvement and asking a series of questions: What are the stories you cherish? What memories continue to cause you pain, sadness, or anger? What do you really expect of other members of the staff? What does this role of parish nurse really mean to you? Try writing down everything that comes to mind without deciding for the time being if it is realistic or unrealistic, good or bad. And then, with a healthy dose of humor, put stars next to those you need to keep an eye on. The unrealistic wishes and fears probably cannot be eliminated, but they can be managed. And that is plenty good enough.

Understanding the Congregation

Resources exist to help us understand and appreciate the particular nature of congregational life, and they are well worth exploring. In many respects, congregations resemble multigenerational family systems. Edwin Friedman's (1985) very helpful book *Generation to Generation* describes the dynamics of family systems as well as the dynamics of congregations and provides guidance in moving them toward healing and wholeness. The Alban Institute (4550 Montgomery Avenue, Suite 423 North, Bethesda, MD 20814) is another resource devoted to understanding the dynamics of congregational life and enhancing its effectiveness. Its publications are well worth exploring.

The first thing to remember is that just like your family, the congregation has a history, and that history continues to shape the life of the congregation. There may be grandparents who sacrificed a great deal to establish the church and who set the tone for all who followed. They may have been liberal or conservative, strict or permissive, and although successive generations of parishioners have modified the patterns set by the founding parents, that history is still remembered and is still relevant. Some congregations have dark periods of their history that are referred to in hushed tones because of the shame attached to someone's behavior. Very much like the family secret of an uncle who was alcoholic and committed suicide, which continues to shame the family, episodes in parish life that are kept secret continue to influence the quality of congregational life.

When it comes to congregational life, what you see is usually not what you get; there is usually more to it. It is just like meeting a person for the first time: not that first impressions are entirely wrong, there is just usually more to that person. Just as understanding another person's personal history, the good parts as well as the bad, enhances your understanding and appreciation for that person, understanding a congregation's history can deepen your understanding of present dynamics and enhance your ability to work effectively with that congregation.

Anyone who chooses to work with and in a congregation should take the time to learn about that congregation's history. I remember spending several days with my father as he entered his 80s, asking him to tell me the stories of how he grew up. In addition to the sheer enjoyment of his storytelling, I gained an appreciation for him I would surely have missed had I not learned more about him. Some of the kinks in our relationship remained until his death, but they loosened some and the warmth flowed more freely between us. Whether it is our parents or our congregation, we need to listen to the stories.

In the history of most congregations, there are glorious eras as well as miserable ones. But they are all important, and in God's economy, the whole story must be told for the whole community to be redeemed.

The second thing to remember is that every congregation has a culture shaped by both its history and its present environment. The culture in our home has to do with the way we spend our time, the way we clean the house, the way we invite others into our environment. It has to do with the expectations we hold for each other, the way we deal with conflict, and the way we express affection. It is the same with the congregation. Some congregations are very formal; others are more relaxed. Some welcome newcomers enthusiastically; others seem almost suspicious of new people. How conflict is handled, how money is talked about, how children are treated—these factors and a hundred more make up the culture of a congregation.

Whether we like them or not, cultures need to be understood and respected if we are going to enter them. Cultures can be influenced and destructive patterns can be replaced by more constructive ones, but change occurs most readily when present patterns are understood for what they mean to those who embrace them. I recall the struggle in my own congregation as we tried to move from a tradition of the pastor spending endless hours counseling troubled individuals to one in which the pastor facilitated people getting the professional help they needed and trained lay people to minister more effectively to each other. We had to appreciate the meaning of that very personalized care from the pastor before we could help our congregation accept a different and often more effective type of pastoral care. In the process of change, some people were confused, others were angered, and a few even left. Organizational cultures are powerful realities, and we ignore them at our peril.

Finally, every congregation has a polity, a set of rules that governs its life. We had best learn what they are! The formal rules may be apparent. How people are elected to the council or vestry, who presides at council meetings, how long they serve—these and many other rules are spelled out in formal documents by the congregation and the religious body of which it is a part. But there is an informal polity too. Who speaks to whom, who *really* makes decisions, what is expected of men, what is expected of women are all part of the informal and unwritten polity of a congregation. Some of the "rules" may be quite healthy (i.e., open and empowering); others may contribute to the less healthy aspects of the congregation. The point again is to become a good student of the congregation's polity so you can get things done with minimal frustration and, in time, so you can help modify some of the less constructive aspects of the congregation's way of doing business.

Historical Sources

A thorough examination of your expectations and an analysis of the congregation may result in some disappointments. Honest scrutiny of reality has a way of doing that. But if we look caringly enough, we will recognize the light as well as the darkness in the human condition and perhaps even the traces of God's redemptive love. The congregation is surely a fragile instrument of God's love, but then, it has never been any different. Old and New Testament scripture record in painful detail the petty squabbles and more serious divisions among God's people. They were faithless more frequently than they were faithful. As Exodus and I Corinthians make painfully clear, neither Moses nor Paul had an easy time of it.

Take I Corinthians, for example. Without worrying here about some of the literary and textual questions regarding this epistle, it is clear that Paul was deeply distressed about this Christian community. There were serious charges of moral laxity as well as less serious but persistent concerns about destructive behaviors we would quickly recognize in our own congregations.

In I Corinthians 12, Paul alludes to the competition for spiritual supremacy that characterized some in the community. These Christians clearly believed they had a straight line to the Almighty and that their ecstatic but unintelligible utterances were proof of their spiritual superiority. Self-righteousness and the arrogant claim of divine inspiration are as old as human consciousness, and they caused as much dissension in the 1st century as they do in the 20th. The wonderful thing about this chapter is the way Paul responds. He spells out a theology of organizational life that continues to guide us: "Now there are varieties of gifts, but the same Spirit; and there are varieties of activities, but it is the same God who activates all of them in everyone. To each is given the manifestation of the Spirit for the common good" (I Cor. 12:4-7).

Do not stop with the above or this chapter, but read the whole epistle. It will quickly normalize your concerns about the deplorable behavior of some in your congregation. It will also give you some principles for building a healthy congregation. Look at just the few lines quoted above. Paul first affirms the principle of diversity. We are not all alike, and we bring different gifts to the community. But we are all needed: in the congregation, in the community, in the nation, and on the planet. Later in the chapter, he uses the metaphor of the human body to illustrate the absurdity of claiming that we do not need each other. I think with gratitude of the mentally ill and sometimes disruptive man who comes to the Eucharist I celebrate Wednesday mornings in my parish. He is sometimes inappropriate and often awkward in his movements, but the simple warmth and enthusiastic greeting he brings to those who gather around the altar each week makes a difference in the way we approach the world that day.

Another principle affirmed the source of the gifts. There are not many gods; there are many expressions of one God. And the marks of the one God are clear: justice, reconciliation, redemption, peace, and empowering love. There is little need to promote our god over someone else's god. Finally in this passage is the principle of community.

The gifts of each are for the "common good." They are not for selfish hoarding or for the accrual of personal power. They are for the common good. Pretty simple. If congregations, communities, and nations could live by these principles, our planet would be in far less danger of destroying itself.

The lesson in looking to historical sources is that not much has changed. The process is much the same. Congregations can be both miserable and glorious. And there is little mystery to what makes them the healing communities we would like them to be. It is a slightly more difficult task to be truly open to and an instrument of that healing.

Getting a Good Start

Voluntary organizations are notoriously poor at writing good job descriptions, and the church is no exception. Because parish nursing is a relatively new expression of ministry, most congregations have little experience in spelling out their expectations for the parish nurse. Nothing, however, could be more important than the time and energy spent at the beginning of this ministry to write a contract that answers three important questions:

- What is your job? (a clear job description)
- To whom are you responsible? (clear accountability)
- Where do you fit in the overall ministry? (role clarity)

Congregations need to remember that contracts that answer these three questions are always works in progress. There is no need for the perfect document; there is only a need for a clear document that is regularly reviewed and revised in light of experience. Some congregations launch the parish nurse with something as skimpy as "We know you'll know what to do and will fit in just fine. We're so glad to have you here!" Parish nurses who think that kind of "contract" gives them freedom should think again. It is a pretty good recipe for significant conflict and real disappointments. These can, however, be avoided.

A clear job description involves spelling out the kinds of activities and outcomes the congregation is expecting from the parish nurse. It is true that congregations have little experience with this ministry, so the parish nurse can and should help formulate these expectations. The process may become quite innovative as nurse and congregational committee begin to reveal their dreams about this ministry. But it is probably a good idea to err on the conservative side at first, indicating those expectations that are fundamental and those that are on the wish list. Voluntary organizations like the church are good at creating 60 hours a week of expectations for a 30-hour-a-week job. Dream a little, but do not create an undoable job for yourself.

The next question to be answered is "to whom are you responsible?" In some ways this needs to be the first question, rather than the second, so that the right person or persons can help shape the job description. The importance of answering this question involves a lot of self-interest. It is important, when a few people in the congregation begin complaining, "Why are we paying this nurse all this money? Do we really need her?" for the chair of the parish nurse committee to step up and explain exactly what the parish nurse has been asked to do and what she is in fact doing. Everyone works better when there is clear accountability within the organization. When the parish nurse is confused and struggling, a frank conversation with the person or persons to whom she is accountable can be a wonderful support. Evaluations should be carried out on a regular basis and a written program report should go to the whole congregation. Clear accountability builds joint ownership of the ministry and guards against sneak attacks from the chronically disgruntled.

The final question has to do with role clarity. Where does the parish nurse really fit in? Even though there may be a very small congregational staff (paid and volunteer), they will be far more effective and more fulfilled if they operate as a team rather than as lone rangers. Many functions overlap in ministering to a congregation, and noses can quickly get out of joint if someone seems to be edging in on someone else's domain. For instance, how does the parish nurse's pastoral role (listening, comforting, confronting, supporting, guiding) relate to the pastor's? How will the decision be made as to who carries the primary role with regard to shut-ins, the seriously ill, malcontents, the prestigious and less prestigious members, those who are dying?

There are probably no easy answers to questions of role clarity. They have to emerge out of experience. The answers can only be found if there is regular, open communication between all the team members. Being sure this kind of communication is built in from the start may help avoid painful conflicts down the road. It takes time and intentionality for this to happen.

Like most things, getting a good start is important. It takes some time and usually some discomfort to build a good foundation, but like the house built on rock, it can withstand the storms that will inevitably come.

Pity the Poor Pastor/Rabbi/Priest

There are few jobs more difficult to do well (and stay personally healthy in!) than that of the professional leader of a congregation. But the reasons are not what most think. There are, of course, long hours and many demands, and the pay usually is not great, but that is true of many responsible jobs today. The difficulty is in the symbolic role the pastor, rabbi, or priest inevitably plays in the congregation. He or she becomes the one who psychologically carries all the hopes and fears of a people. People tend to project fragments of themselves on their pastor. If there is a part of ourselves we cannot stand, we often look for some hint of it in our pastor and attack it with the same level of intensity and frustration with which we have tried to root it out of ourselves. If there are positive qualities we desperately seek for ourselves, we frequently project those and idealize the pastor in flattering, yet unrealistic, ways.

The point is that it is often difficult for a pastor to be sure of just who he or she is and to retain a "true self." A false self, either unrealistically critical and depreciated or idealistically inflated, is a constant temptation. Given the fact that all pastors come to their position with mixed motivations (only a fool would claim an absolute purity of "call"), it is a career-long struggle to retain a degree of personal authenticity and professional integrity.

The reason the parish nurse needs to understand the dynamics of the pastorate is that this is the person or persons who will become the nurse's most important professional colleague(s). The parish nurse needs to form (and continually reform) the most honest and compassionate appraisal possible of the pastor. The parish nurse can become an invaluable ally to the pastor if she is capable of being honest, loyal, and supportive.

There are always possibilities for partnership in this professional relationship. There are also opportunities for unhealthy competition and personal animosity, and no one wins when that happens. By understanding the difficult dynamics that attach to the pastoral role, the parish nurse may be able to recognize when she needs to walk gently as well as when she needs to speak and act boldly.

Contagious Diseases

There are any number of destructive congregational dynamics of which parish nurses need to be aware. Most of them derive from a family systems understanding of congregational life and should be recognizable from the nurse's experience with her own family. A good inoculation against these congregational diseases consists of an understanding of the process and a firm resolve not to contribute to the illness.

The first is triangulation. It is a normal human tendency, but it is particularly destructive in congregational life. People who have a beef with the pastor (or for that matter, anyone else important to them) frequently form an alliance with a third person based on their feud with the former. And the parish nurse is the ideal person with whom to form that unholy alliance. "The pastor doesn't seem able to get around to see the old people anymore, does he? Thank heavens for you!" "I'd really rather talk to you than the pastor. She's so busy all the time." The parish nurse may be the first one parishioners come to with complaints. How she deals with them becomes critical to avoiding a destructive professional undertow in the leadership of the congregation. Possible responses to the triangulating comments noted above might be: "I'm always glad to see you, but it sounds like you have some unhappiness with the pastor. I hope you'll discuss that with him." "You're right, the pastor is very busy. But I know she also wants to be available to anyone who needs to talk to her."

The second is scapegoating. When an organization is having trouble (raising money, getting enough member participation), it frequently looks around for someone to blame—and that might as well be the parish nurse as anyone else. The best way to avoid being scapegoated is to be sure you have a clear contract and a solid relationship with your sponsoring body (ideally, a congregational committee). The pastor may also become the scapegoat, and then it becomes the parish nurse's responsibility to become a force calling for a more balanced appraisal of the problem.

There are any number of destructive dynamics that may have a contagious quality to them. Probably the most insidious and most characteristic of the congregation is the messianic imitation syndrome. Its symptoms are irritability, a general sense of exhaustion, and a certain indignation that others do not share the same depth of commitment as those with the illness. Given the theological underpinnings of the congregational culture and the very human wish to save ourselves through saving the world, it is not surprising that those in leadership positions are particularly vulnerable to this condition.

Relatively mild cases are successfully treated with a sense of humor, a good dose of recreation, and the recognition that no matter how hard we try to save them, some of our brethren are going to drown. More serious cases involve a characterological commitment (life-long, pervasive pattern) to saving the world. Usually, the most that can be hoped for in these cases is a moderating of symptoms. It is wise to maintain firm boundaries between yourself and these people, sometimes a difficult task when they are in top leadership positions.

Working the System:
Communications, Power, and Conflict

In addition to being a competent nurse and a compassionate person, the parish nurse must also know how to work the system. Although that may initially sound manipulative and unworthy of one with such a high calling, the parish nurse needs to remember that the health of the congregation can be as important a concern as the health of individual congregants. There are three aspects of the system the parish nurse needs to monitor and help manage.

Communication is at the heart of congregational life and the parish nurse needs to take its pulse regularly. Is there clear and consistent communication from the leadership (lay and ordained) to the rest of the flock? Is there free and open communication from the flock to the leadership? Many who have entered leadership positions have observed that that was the last day their troops spoke honestly to them. The freedom to communicate questions, concerns, and criticisms to leadership is what makes good leadership great. But it is only the healthiest of congregations that achieves this kind of flow. Leadership must be proactive in seeking feedback, and it must be willing to hear it in its most distorted and irritating forms. The parish nurse can be instrumental in helping develop channels of good communication and in removing some of the obstacles to its steady flow. Taking a thorough assessment of congregational communications may be one of the parish nurse's first interventions, and if she reports her findings to a representative committee, she may amplify the benefit of her assessment.

Communication is, however, more than a hierarchical reality. It is multilayered and multidirectional. When it is good, people feel nurtured by informal conversations. They feel less inclined to hide the embarrassing dimensions of their lives (loss of a job, a marital separation, a teenager in a drug rehab program) and more inclined to share the real joys, knowing that, whatever the reality, they will be understood and appreciated.

Good communication does not happen all at once. It develops gradually as people learn they can trust one another to listen to and respect what is said. That is why gossip and triangulations are such destructive mechanisms. They destroy trust and create the isolation that is the antithesis of community.

People called to ministry are rarely comfortable with *power,* and as a result they frequently misuse it. But power, personal and organizational, is as natural a part of the human experience as eating and breathing. It is how we build community, provide healing, and create the structures and relationships that give meaning to our lives. Because there are so many examples in this society of the misuse of power, we sometimes think of it as having no place in congregational life. But it is critical for the creation of a healthy congregation.

If they are effective and clinically competent, parish nurses will gradually realize they have accumulated a great deal of power. They accumulate power because they have cared enough to do their homework, listened carefully enough to hear the deeper pain hidden behind defensive reassurances ("everything's just fine, thanks"), and spoken out of an authentic concern for another. They accumulate power as they plan their initiatives carefully, take time to get to know those with whom they do business, and recognize the limits of their ability to change the world. They accumulate power as they work through appropriate committees, involve others in planning important tasks, and applaud their accomplishments. They accumulate power as they relinquish the need to control others and recall over and over again that the power of love rarely comes without some pain.

Finally, *conflict.* Most of us live our lives tiptoeing around conflict, doing our best to avoid or at least to minimize it. So many human fears are attached to conflict! And no wonder. We have all seen and perhaps experienced the destructive power of violence (verbal or physical) or have been shamed by our own expressions of anger. But the reality is that conflict is a natural and potentially creative part of any relationship and every organization. Rage and destructive conflict are generated not by the normal expression of differences but by their suppression.

Congregations are notable in their reluctance to engage conflict creatively. We have all absorbed theological and spiritual distortions that suggest that conflict is inherently ungodly, but these are merely the flimsy defenses we construct to protect ourselves from the rigors of reality.

The parish nurse must learn not only to transcend her own difficulties with conflict but to assist individuals and committees within the congregation to do so as well. There is a large body of literature dealing with conflict management, and it is well worth making it the focus of a few adult study groups. There are also some simple guidelines that can be practiced on a daily basis. When the conflict is interpersonal (one on one), it always goes better when people speak in the first person. "I felt hurt when you made the decision without consulting me" is preferable to "You were selfish not to include me in the decision." Empathic listening (not an easy thing to do when you are hurt and angry) can go a long way to helping someone own up to their part of the problem.

Organizational conflict that is unresolved and/or unattended to can demoralize a congregation. One of the most important functions of leadership is to name the conflict and create environments safe enough for issues to be addressed. Safety is created when people know they will have a chance to express themselves and when clarity, rather than agreement, is the goal. Differences will remain, but mutual respect built on understanding can make the differences not only tolerable, but creative.

Scripture provides the simplest (and most challenging) guideline for the management of conflict. The sixth chapter of Micah is an excellent source: "And what does the Lord require of you but to do justice, and to love kindness, and to walk humbly with your God?" (6:8). *Doing justice* means to look to principle rather than position when negotiating differences. *Loving kindness* means to remember that people matter and that relationships are essential. *Walking humbly* means remembering that we may learn from the opposition, and that because we are safe in God, we can afford to be wrong.

Surviving and Thriving

Up to this point, we have focused on the organizational and systemic issues a parish nurse must learn to keep her eye on. The difference between surviving and thriving in such a position is often determined by the parish nurse's ability to sidestep or neutralize a congregation's pathology (and every congregation has some!) and to nudge the community in the direction of greater health.

But there is another dimension, equally as important, which the parish nurse must keep her eye on as well—the very personal dimension of her self. The parish nurse can be professionally competent and organizationally adept, but if she ignores her self, there will be little standing between her and burnout.

Ministries such as parish nursing call for a high degree of self-knowledge. Parish nurses must know their strengths and weaknesses and have developed strategies for managing them effectively. If there is a redemptive dimension to the ministry, the parish nurse will grow along with her people, and some of those weaknesses may be rediscovered as strengths.

Every parish nurse should make her own list of personal issues to monitor. Here is a starter list that can be edited to fit personal awareness.

- Keep track of your humor meter. When it begins to dip into the minus category, it is a sure sign that you are taking yourself too seriously and are probably trying too hard. You have lost the invaluable perspective that, contrary to popular opinion, we are safe in God's love and the future of the world is not up to us. Grace flows more freely when we are laughing.

- Watch for the build up of anger and resentment (another humor depressant). Anger is a wonderful warning sign that we are hurting, and it may generate the energy necessary to help us right some wrongs to ourselves or others. When it goes underground, however, it depletes our energy and sours our spirituality.

- Be open and honest in your prayer life. Christianity, Judaism, and Islam all include the self-examination that in 12-step programs is called "taking a moral inventory." Guilt, like anger, is a normal and healthy part of living. It is the internal compass that lets us know when we have violated ourselves or another or have veered off in the wrong direction. Nothing impairs a person's creativity and initiative likthe corrosive power of guilt. Let guilt guide you to where healing takes place. Do what you need to do and get on with it.

- Attend to your own narcissistic needs. Narcissism has gotten a bad name in recent years, but there are healthy and unhealthy types of narcissism. If you are not discovering enough love for your self (healthy narcissism), you will manipulate others to give what you cannot find (the unhealthy type). God admonished us to love ourselves, and without self-love, we have little to give others.

- Build self-care into your schedule—not as the time left over when everything else is done but as an essential part of your life. Most Americans are running around frantically seeking a good time, but few know how to balance the demands of their lives with opportunities to renew themselves. Modeling *balance* may be the greatest gift the parish nurse can offer. Balance can mean any number of things. It means recognizing limits, learning to say no. It means taking time for silence and exercise and good nutrition. It means finding time to play. It means attending to important relationships.

- Nurture your own faith and spirituality. Without a working faith and a healing spirituality, your uniqueness as a parish nurse will not be fully realized. Everyone must find his or her own way to grow this dimension of life, but all can benefit from a spiritual companion or director, someone with maturity and wisdom who loves us just for being ourselves.

- Finally, practice humility, the art of becoming totally human. So many things may contribute: a sense of humor, pain, failure, success, people who forgive us when we have really messed up, an awareness that we are cherished for no other reason than that we are ourselves.

Reference

Friedman, E. H. (1985). *Generation to generation: Family process in church and synagogue.* New York: Guilford.

11

Team Ministry in the Congregation

Leroy Joesten

Nurses who have had clinical experience in a hospital setting are usually familiar with the multidisciplinary team concept. The parish nurse needs to reflect on this hospital experience of *team* and translate it into the parish setting. Congregations are expanding their thinking about the nature of ministry and the nature of health. Even congregations that agree with the idea that communities of faith can be places of whole person health and healing and that the profession of nursing has a legitimate role in the church structure to promote that idea may not immediately or unquestioningly accept a nurse as a member of the church staff. Although the concept is gaining popularity among nurses, congregations, and health care institutions, parish nursing is still in its infancy. This chapter explores some of the issues that surround a nurse as she becomes part of a congregational staff.

Team Concept in Health Care

Although there is evidence that a team concept was already emerging in health care at the turn of the century, it was not until after World War II that it experienced its most dramatic expansion. The idea of team had flourished for decades in the mental health field, but it was not until after World War II that what was commonly accepted in the mental health field made its way into other health care settings.

Three factors are often cited as the key contributors to the general acceptance of interdisciplinary teams in health care. First, after World War II, there was a rapid expansion of hospitals and hospital-centered medicine (Lecca & McNeil, 1985). Funds were readily available for capital investments and also for a wide array of services that this fertile environment fostered. A second factor was the dramatic advance in medical technology. Not only did this phenomenon contribute to specialization among physicians, it helped create a vast assortment of other health care professionals as well. A third factor was a broader understanding of health. Individuals became more active in their health care decisions. Meredith McGuire (1988) has documented the multiple ways in which many average Americans are using a variety of conventional and unconventional methods in an effort to cure their ills or promote health.

Changes in Health Care Delivery

Even the casual observer is aware of the dramatic shift in health care delivery away from inpatient settings to community-based, outpatient services. Managed care continues to set tight limits on reimbursement for health services. As more and more services go unreimbursed by government entitlement programs, private insurers, or managed care plans, we have witnessed hospital closings, shorter patient stays, cost-containment measures, and staff shortages.

The reasons for this shift are numerous. First, high-tech medicine, even though it has considerable glamour, benefits relatively few people in our society. Granger Westberg's zeal for promoting whole-person health centers and parish nurse programs has been fueled by the fact that a small percentage of the population absorbs most of our health care dollars today. Second, high-tech medicine is very expensive. Hospitals often stake their reputations on having the finest state-of-the-art facilities to attract the most excellent staff and an ample number of clients who will benefit from such services.

Third, we know that the most dramatic improvements worldwide within this century in life expectancy and infant mortality are the result of improved sanitation, hygiene, nutrition, and the discovery of antibiotics. James Mason (1990), former assistant secretary for health in the U.S. Department of Health and Human Services, said at a Carter Center for Disease Control consultation that "we can become much healthier people by making more effective use of what we already know about prevention and intervention of disease" (p. 24).

Changes in Congregational Life

Just as there have been major shifts in health care delivery, major changes have also occurred in the church in recent years. One major shift has been the greater mobility of congregants. Just as shorter patient stays influence the ways in which hospitals deploy their resources, so the movement of parishioners from one community to another has required churches to develop new techniques in mobilizing resources and getting to know their members.

Shortages of ordained clergy in some denominations have resulted in training programs for laity. The "priesthood of all believers" is more than a theological concept, it is the very means of survival for many congregations and the only assurance that ministry will continue.

At the start of this decade, the authors of *Megatrends 2000* (Naisbitt & Aburdene, 1990) noted that American baby boomers who rejected organized religion in the 1970s were returning to church. However, they were not necessarily returning to the church or denomination of their childhood. Interdenominational marriages may also contribute to the ease with which couples or individuals "shop" for a church home.

These issues, along with the varying degrees of financial concerns that many churches face, have forced congregations to rethink their mission and to find more effective ways to minister to their congregants.

The Church's Response

Religious institutions have long invested in health care. As we experience a shift in the delivery of health care services, churches are reevaluating their role in caring for the sick, injured, and dying. Indeed, many religiously oriented hospitals have been sold to nonsectarian groups. Others have merged with neighboring institutions; others, as stated earlier, have simply closed.

What is the church's role in health today? One response has been that congregations, which are community based, have picked up the banner of health promotion from the religiously affiliated hospitals that are more immediately identified with the critically ill. There is the understanding that congregations are a potential source of health through being a healing and sustaining community (Solari-Twadell, 1997, p. 5). Within these sustaining communities, there is an emphasis on team ministry within congregations, with health care shifting from acute care settings to community settings. As these forces merge, the nurse is becoming a leading figure. The parish nurse concept is one model where churches can cooperatively work with health care institutions to address the needs of their parishioners.

Team Concept in Congregations

If it has been only recently that the general health care needs of individuals have been shared among many different health professionals, it has been even more recently that a team concept of ministry has arisen within congregations. Different disciplines within church structures have been long-standing, including specialized orders of nuns in the Roman Catholic tradition and deaconesses in the Protestant tradition. However, in the past 20 years, more disciplines have become involved in the ministry of the congregation, specifically youth ministers, ministers of music and Christian education, and so on.

Now, more than ever, congregations of all stripes boast a shared ministry, or as the health setting calls it, "team ministry." However, what is true in the health setting regarding team is also true in congregational structures: namely, that the involvement of a number of professionals (on a staff) does not automatically ensure a team approach.

The definition of *team* as it is used here is "a functioning unit, composed of individuals with varied and specialized training, who coordinate their activities to provide services to a client or group of clients" (Durmis & Golin, 1979, p. 3). This definition suggests three features of a team that have relevance for the parish nurse, as well as other members of the congregational team: role, goal, and organization.

Role

I liken the experience of nurses trying to define or justify their role in the parish setting to that of community ministers who have had to define or justify their role in the medical setting as chaplains. That process has not been an easy one, and there are many who remain unconvinced that clergy have a valid role to play in the health care setting.

It used to be common that chaplains in hospitals were either retired ministers or those who were said to be ineffective in pastoring congregations. Their role was usually defined in very narrow terms that emphasized overtly religious acts, such as administration of sacraments, prayer, and use of scripture. Frequently, clergy were thought of as "in the way" or as obstacles to primary medical care for patients.

There are two things that I believe help to define one's role. The first is training, and the second is expectation. In an effort to gain more respect from other professionals, movements developed within mental health institutions, hospital settings, and in other areas that gave ministers more in-depth, specialized training in the behavioral sciences. Pastoral care as a clinical specialty has its roots as early as the 1920s, through the pioneering leadership of Anton Boison and Richard Cabot (Holifield, 1983).

The clinical pastoral education movement did expand the repertoire of helping skills that clergy possessed to complement their appreciation for the rituals and symbols of their faith tradition. As clergy's clinical skills in listening and counseling increased, their role became more blurred with the role of other professionals who not infrequently felt themselves in competition with the chaplain. Chaplains were challenged to define their roles and claim their uniqueness as clergy, pushing them evermore toward those behaviors that were more overtly religious. There remains a tension for chaplains between a narrow, limited focus and a more comprehensive, whole-person understanding of ministry, between the values and practices of their faith tradition and the technologically sophisticated world of hospitals (Holst, 1985, pp. 12-27).

Over the past 20 years, the role of the chaplain in the acute care setting has become much more accepted. The chaplain has become an important member of the multidisciplinary team and the spiritual needs of patients are becoming better recognized and addressed. The recent work of physicians such as Larry Dossey (1993), Herbert Benson (1996), and David and Susan Larson (1991) has served to reinforce the importance of pastoral services in a medical setting.

Many nurses who find themselves on congregational staffs feel a similar tension in the definition of their role. The traditional role for nurses has been more task oriented. The nurses with whom I work seem attracted to parish nursing because it is not so task oriented. They feel they can be more themselves. Their work is more relational and viewed to be ministry in a way that conventional nursing often is not. As parish nurses, they can more unapologetically give expression to their faith within the context of their work by addressing the whole person. It is true that the parish setting may grant greater liberty to nurses to give expression to their faith and to do those things that in the past were limited to ordained clergy, such as prayer and the sacraments. But is this what the congregations in general or specific congregants actually expect from their nurse? Often, parish nurses are challenged to claim those skills and abilities for which they are trained and that make them uniquely nurses. This tension continues to exist.

Various approaches to the training of parish nurses are developing across the country. There are formalized advanced degrees and continuing education programs along with institutionally based in-services. In the Advocate Health Care program, an in-service component has been built into the role. After orientation, the parish nurses regularly come together for ongoing educational and support activities. A "faculty" of chaplains, nurse educators, and physicians coordinates these activities. This faculty also has the opportunity to model the team approach to the parish nurses, pastors, and congregational members.

Along with training, expectations also help define one's role. These expectations are both external and internal. External expectations are those placed on the nurse by other people. Just as patients in a hospital expect certain behaviors from a chaplain because of their experience with clergy in a congregational setting, so persons in a congregation will expect certain things of nurses because of their experience with nurses in a medical setting. Hospital patients may be chagrined if a chaplain doesn't pray with them; a parishioner may be surprised if the parish nurse offers to pray with them. Just as patients in a hospital may be frustrated if a chaplain focuses more on their feelings than on their religious presuppositions, a parishioner may be disenchanted with a nurse if she doesn't seem knowledgeable about a particular physical condition.

On the one hand, nurses must be able to respond to the specific expectations parishioners might have of them; yet on the other hand, nurses must exceed those expectations in the quest for a more whole person understanding of the individual. It is not unusual for individuals to come to a parish nurse with a presenting physical concern only to find that the majority of their time with the nurse is spent talking about loneliness, older parents, or a troubled marriage.

There are also internal expectations with which parish nurses live. As much as they try to be free of the limits of a traditional understanding of nursing, they frequently seem to be victims of it. They struggle against the need to be expert or knowledgeable in all phases of health. Their role as a representative of the church carries with it additional burdens. A nurse may believe that a parishioner's attitude toward the church will be determined by how well she meets their needs. Not wanting to be an offense to parishioners, the nurse may find it difficult to set limits on the many demands that people make on her. People can be as demanding, unreasonable, or manipulative in a congregational environment as they can be in a hospital context. Nurses need support in saying no and in setting limits with congregants on the basis of time, limited capability, or availability.

The Advocate Parish Nurse Program reserves time for the nurses to openly discuss their feelings about and frustrations and struggles with internal and external expectations and how they are affected by them. Specific case presentations by the nurses form part of the foundation for this discussion.

Goal

Inherent in any group of professionals coordinating their activities is the issue of congruence between each person's role and the institution's mission or sense of purpose. Just as all hospitals have an assumed common purpose yet adopt individualized ways of articulating that purpose, so do congregations have a common calling yet distinctive ways of expressing their mission. Such definitions of objectives can be a reflection of the congregation's surrounding community, the makeup of its constituents, and its ethnic and theological heritage. Just as congregational members must be aware and feel comfortable with the goals and directions of their church, the parish nurse also needs to have a clear sense of the goals and mission of the congregation in which she works and her subsequent role in the team ministry.

In his book *Congregation: Stories and Structures,* the late James Hopewell (1987) identifies four ways in which congregational cultures can be defined, each way implying a different goal or mission. Hopewell refers to these as contextual, mechanistic, organic, and symbolic.

Contextualism sees God's saving activity in the world at large. In the 1960s, under the watchful eye of sociologists like Peter Berger (1967) and Gibson Winter (1961), spurred by the spirit of ecumenism, congregations reached out to the broader community not to bring in more members, but to participate in God's work toward full creation. The analogy that Hopewell uses is that of house hunting. Many people select the home in which they want to live as much on the basis of the community as on the house itself. People may be more concerned about the school system, transportation, or shopping than the style or architecture of the house. The church's role in the world is still a central concern for many congregations as they define their life and work today.

In Hopewell's opinion, the appeal of contextual studies waned in the 1970s and was replaced by mechanistic and organic studies of congregations. To follow the house-hunting analogy, the desirability of a house is conditioned by its serviceability. How well do things in the house work? What is the cost to maintain it? This emphasis is best exemplified by the "church growth" movement. Here the goal is growth in size of membership. God's saving activity is seen in individual souls, and the church prospers as souls are added to the kingdom—as evidenced by the numerical enlargement of the congregation. The congregation as a "machine" is promoted by techniques such as annual reports that collect data about money, membership, and meetings. Whereas the mechanistic approach values homogeneity, the organic approach stresses heterogeneity. Differences are welcomed as people see potential growth in a mixture of values, backgrounds, and interests. As an organism, the local church grows not externally but internally. What is it that makes a house a home? It is that same difference that helps distinguish the organic approach from the mechanistic one. Whether or not a church is doing what it is meant to do is measured by the closeness between its members.

The fourth way in which a congregational culture can be defined is the symbolic understanding of church culture. The symbolic outlook focuses upon a congregation's identity, as revealed through the collective and individual stories of its members. Here the goal is not so much outreach, growth, or closeness as the discovery of a particular congregation's views, values, and motivations. Hopewell's book elaborates a method for making this discovery. Yet another approach for understanding the culture of a congregation comes from systems theory. Edwin Friedman (1985), in *Generation to Generation,* described congregational life as three interlocking family systems: each family unit within the congregation, the clergyperson's own family, and the entire congregation as a family.

These various approaches can be helpful to parish nurses and clergy as they attempt to better understand the culture within the congregation, their goals and mission, and their ways of interacting together.

Organization

The best-trained individuals with the noblest of goals will not function as a team unless there is a coordinated effort by the staff and congregational leadership. Teamwork requires an administration that recognizes the unique contribution of each team member and keeps the congregation's goals in proper focus. At least three ingredients are fundamental for a healthy administration of team: communication, respect, and accountability.

We observe great diversity in communication methodologies among the congregations in the Advocate Parish Nurse Program. These differing methods are usually the product of both denominational idiosyncrasies and the leadership style of the congregation's senior minister. The most satisfying communication method for our parish nurses is one where there is ample opportunity for face-to-face conversation with all members of the pastoral staff. Those who conduct staff meetings on a regular basis promote a feeling of shared ministry that reduces each individual's sense of isolation and subsequent uncertainty about his or her role.

Meetings can be a bane or a blessing, depending on how the time is orchestrated. The kinds of meetings that seem most appreciated are those that are the congregational team's version of a traditional multidisciplinary team meeting in the hospital setting. Usually conducted on a weekly basis, these meetings allow each staff member the opportunity to discuss congregants who are ill or going through a personal crisis; a particular concern or problem may also be posed. Meeting discussions may range from who is hospitalized or shut in to suspected elder abuse or neglect, evidence of a strained marital relationship, someone's abuse of alcohol or drugs, or a member's inability to care for him- or herself alone anymore.

Experiences, individual perceptions of the concern, and suggestions for follow-up are contributed by all members of the pastoral team. The highest of professional standards regarding confidentiality is demanded. Unlike a hospital staff meeting, where the team members generally have no other association with the subjects of concern outside of the institution, a congregational staff meeting concerns itself with the problems of people who may be well known in a variety of settings by, possibly, every staff person. Improper discussion of highly personal information outside of the staff meeting can be detrimental to the person being discussed and to the total ministry of the congregation. Where the size of the staff is smaller, this concern is reduced but by no means eliminated.

Respect for the valid contribution of each staff person is essential. The effectiveness with which a staff member is able to relate to a congregant may have less to do with role or responsibility than with personality. Even pastors who theoretically support a nurse being part of the church staff may resent that same nurse's ability to relate to a favored parishioner. At other times, the nurse may be the staff person who is saddled with the hostile parishioner, the troublemaker who constantly criticizes the way the church is run. Both responses are indicators of disrespect.

Respect for other team members recognizes both the professional status and the human qualities that people can possess. Close working relationships bring to the surface the certainties or insecurities people have about either their training or ability to relate meaningfully with others. Nurses, as well as clergy, may well receive negative feedback from peers or congregants regarding the way they responded in a particular situation. An atmosphere that encourages expression of both negative and positive feedback from peers is one that respects our incompleteness as God's creatures and provides an opportunity for personal and professional growth to occur.

Accountability is also important for effective team work. This includes some formal mechanisms for evaluation of one's efforts. Nurses who have come out of hospital settings are accustomed to routine annual evaluations by their manager. Church structures may be less formal about evaluations. Most of the congregations in our program have health committees that include several parishioners as congregational representatives. These committees help assess health needs of the congregation and give general guidance and support to program activities. Some churches also use the health committee in the evaluation process of the parish nurse.

A formal evaluation of the nurse, similar to that of every staff nurse, is an important process for the parish nurse and pastor. There are varying degrees of comfort with such a formal process. Some pastors and health committees have been very imaginative in developing evaluative instruments. Effective use of the evaluation also helps set appropriate and realizable goals for the forthcoming year. Nurses in congregations whose pastors take this exercise seriously feel affirmed in their efforts and very much a part of the church's total ministry.

Conclusion

I have enjoyed working with nurses in a hospital setting for many years. I have also had the pleasure of working with nurses who are in a congregational setting. I have been inspired by the idealism with which nurses have approached their efforts to help congregations achieve greater health, and I have been moved by the seriousness with which they take their own spiritual growth. I feel privileged to have been included in their struggles to more fully integrate their faith into their identity as nurses. Parish nursing provides a unique opportunity for such integration. As I have seen some of their idealism of congregations and professional church work fade, I have witnessed a deeper sensitivity in them to their own and other people's humanness. They have come to realize in new and deeper ways that life is a journey that is often marked by unexpected detours. The path to health is not measured by perfection but by faithfulness and persistence. Health is also measured not only by what one gains but by what one surrenders. Health is aided by others who are willing to walk with us without condemnation or prejudice. There is no question that the parish nurse's skills and sensitivity are a rich resource for any congregational staff. The parish nurse concept is still young. I am grateful for the opportunity to have worked in an innovative way with nurses who are, before anything else, people of conviction and compassion.

References

Benson, H. (1996). *Timeless healing: The power and biology of belief.* New York: Scribner.

Berger, P. L. (1967). *The sacred canopy.* Garden City, NJ: Doubleday.

Dossey, L. (1993). *Healing words: The power of prayer and the practice of medicine.* San Francisco: Harper.

Durmis, A. J., & Golin, A. K. (1979). *The interdisciplinary health care team.* Germantown, MD: Aspen Systems.

Friedman, E. (1985). *Generation to generation.* New York: Guilford.

Holifield, B. (1983). *A history of pastoral care in America.* Nashville, TN: Abingdon.

Holst, L. (Ed.). (1985). *Hospital ministry: The role of the chaplain today.* New York: Crossroad.

Hopewell, J. F. (1987). *Congregation: Stories and structures.* Philadelphia: Fortress.

Larson, D. B., & Larson, S. S. (1991). Religious commitment and health: Valuing the relationship. *Second Opinion, 17*(1), 27-40.

Lecca, P. J., & McNeil, J. S. (Eds.). (1985). *Interdisciplinary team practice, issues and trends.* New York: Praeger.

Mason, J. O. (1990). Health care in the U.S.: Facts and choices. *Second Opinion, 13,* 22-29.

McGuire, M. (1988). *Ritual healing in suburban America.* New Brunswick, NJ: Rutgers University Press.

Naisbitt, J., & Aburdene, P. (1990). *Megatrends 2000.* New York: William Morrow.

Solari-Twadell, P. A. (1997). The caring congregations: A health place. *Journal of Christian Nursing, 14*(1), 4-9.

Winter, G. (1961). *The suburban captivity of the churches.* Garden City, NJ: Doubleday.

12

Parish Nurse and Physician Relationship in Serving the Congregation

Greg Kirschner

It is possible that the title of this chapter will elicit two polarized responses during a survey of the table of contents. Perhaps the reader will react with an "Of course there needs to be physician input into this program!" Alternatively, a reader might note that "physicians are always muscling in on programs where they are not necessary, especially when it involves nurses!" This healthy tension has contributed to the enjoyment I have experienced in working with the parish nurse program at Lutheran General Hospital. This chapter is written out of my personal experience and intended to serve as a guide to the potential relationship that a physician may have with a parish nurse program. The primary focus is the administrative capacity in which a physician may serve such a program, with comment as well on the role of the physician in a community or congregation with a parish nurse. The benefits for the program gained by physician involvement, as well as benefits for those physicians who choose to become involved, are highlighted. Potential pitfalls for the physician and the parish nurse are also revealed.

Roles Not Chosen

Before describing the various responsibilities that physicians such as myself may choose to accept in a parish nurse program, I am compelled to outline two roles I have personally chosen not to pursue—and in fact have not been offered. The first is that of *Leader/Organizer/Captain of the Ship*. The administrative structure of the parish nurse program has clearly called for an interdisciplinary team approach in which the physician is an integral part but *not* the central focus, or the key player. This congregationally based, wellness-oriented hybrid of theology and community medicine contrasts sharply with the hospital settings in which most physicians serve in leadership capacities. In fact, placing a physician in the key leadership role in a parish nurse program could subtly point away from a wellness orientation. Thus, I have found myself comfortably serving in an advisory, facilitative capacity—and enjoying it thoroughly. As a family physician, I am accustomed to working in partnership with patients, families, and a variety of health care providers in such a team approach.

The second role I have attempted to avoid is that of *Sole Physician to Needy Parishioners*. Although the provision of direct hands-on patient care services by a physician is possible and on occasion appropriate, the parish nurse program functions in a broad community, covering a wide geographic area. Those patients requiring physician services may be best treated by physicians in other specialty backgrounds, geographic locales, or practice arrangements. I have enjoyed seeing patients referred through the parish nurse program, but I do not view this as a function of my administrative role—rather as one arising from my role as a community doctor.

Administrative Roles

In the Lutheran General Hospital Advocate Health Care Parish Nurse Program, family physicians have served administratively in five basic capacities. These include:

1. *Steering committee member* (Holst, 1987, p. 15). Having offered a disclaimer about my personal desire to not be a central leadership figure, I will say that physicians have played an important part in providing direction to the development of the parish nurse program. Historically, this role was probably most important in the early years of the program, as the scope of the program was being determined and resource assessment was critical. A physician may be particularly able to provide guidance in the manner in which a community-based program can interrelate with traditional medical services. Physicians may be particularly aware of sensitive "political" areas in the medical community at large and are often familiar with liability concerns.

Additionally, the presence of a physician on the steering committee helps provide credibility for those who believe that physician input is essential to any medical program. We hope this type of figurehead representation is diminishing in importance, but it can, on occasion, be critical, not only when negotiating with hospital-based personnel but with parish pastors and wellness committees.

As in all roles, the exact function will be determined by many factors, including personal desires. Representation on the steering committee does offer the interested physician the opportunity to influence the direction of the program, as well as dealing with day-to-day operations in a limited fashion.

2. *Parish nurse faculty member* (Holst, 1987, p. 14). In this capacity, the physician works with the interdisciplinary staff to develop appropriate educational opportunities for the nurses. This function includes the joint supervision of the continuing education program to ensure that program goals are being advanced with regard to nurse development.

Historically, the practical form of this role at Lutheran General Hospital has included monthly planning meetings with the other faculty members as well as quarterly meetings with the parish nurses. During the latter, topics of current medical interest to the nurses are addressed, with ample opportunity for questions and answers. These sessions have served not only to update the nurses' medical knowledge but as opportunities of mutual encouragement in the philosophy of the parish nurse program as it relates to traditional physician services.

3. *Emergency resource.* Physician availability as an emergency phone resource provides urgent consultative backup for nurses faced with challenging clinical situations. Having made myself available by phone to nurses for several years, I am struck by the scope and appropriateness of their concerns. I am also impressed by their considerable problem-solving skills, with which they have often handled the issue properly prior to the call. The nurses have indicated informally that this backup function, although rarely used, is an important provision of the faculty.

4. *Referral resource.* Perhaps the most frequent contact I have had with parish nurses has related to the appropriate choice of "the next step" in a given clinical situation. Nurses may need guidance in recommending the most suitable category of specialty referral. They have requested my opinion regarding diagnostic workups or therapeutic plans for their parishioners.

Quite commonly, the nurses have requested assistance in the identification of physicians who are sensitive to the theology of the parishioner in question. For example, they may be aware of a patient with hypertension in need of a new primary care internist or family physician but who now wants a physician with a truly whole-person approach. Unfortunately, this type of request is often more difficult to define and has a limited array of possible solutions. The identification of a physician as wholistic is highly subjective. The term wholistic may even be shunned by physicians who in reality are practicing a highly integrated form of whole-person health care.

Throughout this referral process, a physician in an administrative capacity must be aware of the political sensitivities of the medical community. For example, I have attempted to avoid favoritism to my own multispecialty group members and to offer nurses at least two alternatives for referral, if possible, when "a name" is requested.

Rarely, this role, as well as that of emergency resource, has included the urgent provision of hands-on clinical services. As a family physician accustomed to the role of primary care physician or physician of first contact, this function comes naturally. However, in part to avoid accusations of self-serving behavior and, more important, to keep the program focused on a community-based, wellness-oriented agenda, I have avoided automatically taking each potential referral. I believe this has helped my credibility with the parish nurses, as well as with the members of our hospital's medical staff familiar with the program. I do enjoy patient care, however, and the excitement of caring for this patient population is considerable, as I will discuss later in this chapter.

5. *Resource for educational programming.* The parish nurses are truly experts in seeking out community resources for educational programs in their respective congre-

gations. Physicians have made themselves available as a physician speaker resource if there is a request for such presentations.

In the past I have held a full-time position on the faculty of the Family Practice Residency Program at Lutheran General Hospital and coordinated the family practice residents' experiences in community medicine. An exciting opportunity has developed to give the residents exposure to community education by linking them up with parishes looking for physician speakers. I have personally supervised residents in the development of such programs and provided formal feedback on the quality of their presentation. Not all physicians in training would feel comfortable or be appropriate for the congregational setting, but for others it has proven a valuable educational activity.

At the same time, residents have given high-quality presentations in the congregations on topics such as men's health and adult health maintenance. This collaborative relationship thus meets goals for both the parish and the sponsoring hospital.

Potential Pitfalls

The administrative relationship I have described is unique among my responsibilities. Although the fluid, team-oriented approach is used in other settings, it takes on a different meaning in a program focused outside the hospital on the activities of congregations and nurses. For physicians involved in such activity, the ability to work closely with nurses and pastors through novel and sometimes challenging ideas requires relinquishing some control, as mentioned in the opening of this chapter.

In addition, the parish nurse program can have a tendency to "fall out" as an add-on activity or responsibility for the physician. That is, as physicians volunteer their time to work on such a program, there can be a tendency to "leave this commitment to last," as important as it might be personally to the physician. This can be a liability for the parish nurse, who may be depending on the physician for the completion of certain tasks in a timely fashion.

A brief word to those physicians working for other employers. It is certainly probable that your employer will hold you accountable for the time you spend working in conjunction with a parish nurse program in an administrative capacity, unless it is entirely on your personal time. This calls for careful attention to the manner in which your involvement in the parish nurse program meets your employer's expectations—that is, how a parish nurse program advances your employer's goals. Our faculty group has come to understand my involvement in the parish nurse program as important to institutional objectives, as a unique referral source, and as an avenue of achieving educational goals for the residency. Such a sponsorship is critical for sustaining activity. I periodically update the other faculty on developments in the parish nurse program and highlight all resident educational opportunities that have resulted from the program.

Role of the Community Physician

I wish to comment on my involvement as a health care provider to patients from congregations with parish nurses. By way of example, consider the case of Mr. and

Mrs. D. Referred by a parish nurse, this couple was looking for a new primary care physician and lived near our office. Mrs. D. first presented for follow-up and ultimately required relatively minor surgery. Mr. D. initially presented with an acute attack of gouty arthritis. During the ensuing months, I came to know this couple quite well, although there were no explicit conversations regarding their expectations of me, and I had little insight into the extent of their involvement in the local congregation. However, on one occasion I inquired of Mr. D. "how he maintained the obviously positive outlook he had on life." He quickly responded with a clear explanation of the importance of his Christian religious beliefs for "the hope that was within him." It was a remarkable doctor-patient office interaction. It achieved greater significance only a few weeks later when, on Christmas Eve, I had to inform him and his wife that he had probable metastatic cancer. During the few remaining days of his life, in a time of rapid deterioration in his health, we were faced with addressing questions of life support, pain management, and the uncertainty of the underlying primary cancer site. The previous conversation related to his belief system, coupled with the ongoing support of his parish pastor and parish nurse, opened up our conversations to a level of honesty and openness that was desirable for such serious decision making. His family fully participated, particularly as he became unable. Mr. D. chose to forego life support measures and died within 2 weeks. Personnel from my office who chose to attend the funeral services were visibly moved by the deep faith of this family and the supportive structure of the church community. Nearly 3 years later, I continue to care for his wife, who has recently again referred another family for care.

The case of Mr. and Mrs. D. represents for me much of the positive work the parish nurse program can do when working with the traditional medical community. Beginning with the referral of a family whose care had "fallen into the cracks" of medicine, the parish nurse facilitated the most appropriate management I could have imagined for a patient with the type of malignancy exhibited by Mr. D. Although the outcome of death was not prevented, the manner in which his last days were spent was significantly altered by the presence of a committed parish nurse and parish pastor, working together with the patient's primary physician.

The character of my practice has changed through my involvement with the parish nurse program. Through referrals of patients such as Mr. and Mrs. D., and through subsequent patient-to-patient referrals, a significant percentage of those patients forming my practice now could be characterized as truly interested in a whole-person approach to their health. That is, these patients are seeking to understand their health as related to the physical, mental, and spiritual dimensions of their lives, and they appreciate a need to integrate these areas into the medical care they receive through their family doctor. I have also come to care for a number of parish nurses and parish pastors. I am challenged regularly by patients to explain my own religious beliefs or my thoughts on such difficult issues as life support measures or abortion. In turn, my ability to inquire sensitively about a patient's spiritual outlook and its relation to his or her health is improving, albeit slowly. I may urge patients to have their parish nurse check their blood pressure and refer others to explore the counseling resources through their congregation.

My involvement in the parish nurse program has, to date, been personally and professionally rewarding. Most of all, I have witnessed the tangible benefits the program has had in my own community, with my own patients! Opportunities for physician involvement in parish nurse programs are increasing, and I am sure that new models of physician involvement will be attempted. How could a physician not choose to be involved if asked?

Reference

Holst, L. (1987). The parish nurse. *Chronicle of Pastoral Care, 7*(1).

13

Parish Nurse–Physician Partnerships

A Continuum of Care

Patti Ludwig-Beymer
H. Scott Sarran

Mrs. Z is an 85-year-old woman who lives alone. She regularly attends church and one day stops after services to have her blood pressure checked by Ms. Smith, a parish nurse. This is her first interaction with the parish nurse. Ms. Smith finds that Mrs. Z's blood pressure is 172/96. "Oh, that's not bad for me," says Mrs. Z. Ms. Smith talks to Mrs. Z about her health. Mrs. Z says, "I have a touch of sugar, but who doesn't at this age? The worst thing is the horrible leg ulcer. And who can keep up with all the things they're doing with me? I have a dozen pills to take for this or that."

Ms. Smith arranges to meet with Mrs. Z in her parish nurse office on Monday. There, Ms. Smith attempts to sort through the myriad of medications and instructions that Ms. Z has been given by three separate physicians and a home health nurse. With Mrs. Z's permission, Ms. Smith calls each of the physicians to discuss Mrs. Z's hypertension, her out-of-control blood sugar, and her lack of understanding of what she must do to stay healthy. The physician office staff personnel, who are not familiar with Ms. Smith or with the concept of the parish nurse, give low priority to the messages. None of Ms. Smith's calls are returned. Ms. Smith also calls the home health agency responsible for sending the nurse who has been visiting Mrs. Z for her leg ulcer. She is unable to speak to the nurse who has made the visits and is told that no one can discuss the case with her.

The following week, Ms. Smith again checks Mrs. Z's blood pressure. It has risen to 186/100. With Mrs. Z, she again calls the physician's office. This time, she successfully arranges for an appointment for Mrs. Z to be seen on Wednesday. She arranges for a volunteer to provide transportation for Mrs. Z. But when the volunteer arrives at Mrs. Z's house to transport her to the doctor's office, no one is home. Ms. Smith is puzzled. On a hunch, she calls the local hospital and learns that Mrs. Z is indeed a patient there.

Although she calls the nurse's station, no information is given to her. Ms. Smith visits Mrs. Z at the hospital. "I'm so glad to see you," says Mrs. Z, "Maybe you can explain what's happening to me!"

As described in the vignette above, parish nurses are accustomed to functioning in the patchwork quilt of sickness and wellness services we know as "health care" in the United States. Parish nurses are very familiar with the defects inherent in the current system: the emphasis on individual illness and episodes of care; the lack of communication between providers; the fragmented, bureaucratic, and complicated care.

However, just as the practice of parish nursing is evolving, so too is the health care delivery system. One of the trends in health care is the movement toward developing population-based care. Integrated delivery networks (IDNs) pull together various levels of patient care services in multiple settings. They develop continuums of care designed to improve the health status of defined populations (Ludwig-Beymer, 1994; Ummel, Schaffner, Smith, & Ludwig-Beymer, 1995). As defined by Evashwick (1987), a continuum of care is

> an integrated, client-oriented system of care composed of both services and integrating mechanisms that guides and tracks clients over time through a comprehensive array of health, mental health, and social services. (p. 23)

Such a seamless system of care is viewed as an effective model for linking the delivery and financing of health care, with all providers aligned under a common set of incentives, to manage care in a high-quality and cost-effective manner.

Reimbursement mechanisms for health care are also changing. In a capitated payment system, health care providers are reimbursed a set amount per member per month, regardless of utilization. Like integrated delivery networks, capitation can result in the improvement of the health status of individuals. Under capitation, providers (typically physicians) gain incentive to keep people healthy and improve the health status of their panel of patients.

The parish nurse is in a prime position to assist in improving the health status of individuals, families, and groups. To improve the health of specific populations, true collaboration and partnership must be present. The parish nurse may form effective partnerships with physicians within a continuum of care by serving target populations, providing health promotion and disease prevention services, extending care management tools, increasing the client's ability to form partnerships, facilitating referrals, and forming spiritual partnerships. Each aspect of partnership is described below. In addition, challenges and opportunities, including mechanisms to allow for exchanging information, measuring effectiveness, and reexamining practices are discussed.

Partnerships

Serving Target Populations

In today's evolving health care arena, partnerships are more important than ever. Physicians who take on full financial risk through a capitated payment system are particularly interested in partnerships. Rather than creating duplicative services, partnerships must be forged. Physicians are seeking to become partners in new ways with community agencies for community-based services.

A partnership typically involves two or more people associated in some common activity. Partners cooperate with one another in a venture, occupation, or challenge. Partners typically have equal status and a certain independence but also have unspoken or formal obligations to each other. Often, partners share resources and risks. Partners do not typically duplicate each other's services. Instead, they augment each other.

The parish nurse is in an ideal position to form partnerships with physicians and IDNs to improve the health status of defined populations. Parish nursing has always been a population-based practice. The religious institution (church, synagogue, or mosque) has been viewed as a faith community, situated within the context of a larger community. Practicing as part of the continuum of care, in partnership with community-based physicians and IDNs, will further enhance the concept of population-based care.

The seven functions of the parish nurse fit well within this partnership. In their function as health educator, parish nurses educate their congregations in many ways. They post notices on bulletin boards, write articles for newsletters and church bulletins, schedule and/or present wellness and disease management classes, and plan and implement health screenings. Physicians may refer their patients to these services and feel secure that the patients are receiving the wellness education and general health education that they need and deserve. In addition, group visits for individuals with chronic disease may be facilitated by parish nurses. Such group visits may involve ongoing education provided by a variety of professionals (including physicians, nurses, respiratory care practitioners, dietitians, and social workers), "sharing sessions" provided by clients, prayer, and emotional support for clients and families. Parish nurses, in their function as developer of support groups, have experience in referring people to and establishing support groups that is transferable to other types of group sessions. These group visits may be very beneficial for clients who wish to learn more about their condition, make life changes appropriate to their situation, and live whole within the confines of their conditions.

Parish nurses function as personal health counselors. Parish nurses see individual clients when they are well. They see clients with chronic disease and acute conditions. They see clients before planned surgeries and during their recovery phase. They see clients when they are dying. In short, they see clients in all degrees of wellness and illness. Parish nurses often help clients deal with the everyday living alterations made necessary by chronic health conditions. They help clients modify their homes and their daily activities so that clients are better able to manage their care in their homes. Physicians may request assistance from parish nurses in gathering data from patients. They may also collaborate with parish nurses so that the treatment plan is better followed by the client.

The parish nurse functions as a *coordinator of volunteers,* mobilizing the faith community to meet the needs of parishioners and other community members. Again, this may prove to be very helpful to physicians. Volunteers routinely transport clients to physician offices, pick up prescription drugs, purchase groceries, and provide other important services. The other functions of the parish nurse will be discussed later in this chapter.

Providing Health Promotion and
Disease Prevention Services

Health promotion activities have as their goal enhancing positive health and preventing illness through health education, prevention, and health protection. Several of
the parish nurse's functions, such as health educator, personal health counselor, integrator of faith and health, and advocate are aimed at health promotion. Disease prevention,
on the other hand, encompasses strategies that inhibit the development of disease or
interrupt or slow the disease's progression. Again, parish nurses have been proactive in
this area. For example, parish nurses conduct blood pressure screenings and often
organize extensive health screening services.

As financial incentives in health care change, it is becoming increasingly important
to keep people well rather than treating them after an illness has occurred. Parish nurses
have always identified keeping people well as a high priority and have incorporated
health promotion and disease prevention activities into their work. They bring that
expertise to their partnerships with physicians and their practice within the continuum
of care.

Parish nurses may also strengthen and enhance their health promotion and disease
prevention activities. The parish nurse often visits a client at home. During the visit, the
parish nurse might appropriately assess the house for safety. This is especially important
for the elderly and chronically ill, who are considered high-risk populations. Based on
the nurse's findings, appropriate educational interventions may be started. For example,
the nurse may visit a parishioner and notice dim lighting and unsecured area rugs, both
of which increase the risk of falls. The nurse is in an ideal position to discuss these
situations with the parishioner, provide education and support to the client and family,
and even mobilize parish resources to intervene if needed. Or the nurse may notice that
assistive devices such as handrails and a shower seat are needed for safety reasons. The
parish nurse may communicate this to the physician, who may then write a prescription
to procure the necessary devices.

Extending Care Management Tools

To optimize health, tools that assist clinicians in managing patient care need to exist
across the continuum. Such tools may include clinical care pathways, standing orders,
assessment and documentation forms, and patient education materials. In a true continuum, it is not enough to manage the acute phase of a person's illness. Instead, the whole
life of a person must be considered. Nurses have long been concerned with the whole
person. The American Nurses Association (1985) definition of nursing emphasizes this
point: "Nursing is defined as the diagnosis and treatment of human responses to actual
or potential health problems" (p. iv).

The work of parish nurses has always been oriented toward the whole person and
has emphasized wellness promotion and disease prevention as well as illness management. As indicated above, parish nurses prepare parishioners for surgery and hospitalization, visit the sick, and provide ongoing family support. In addition, parish nurses have
been instrumental in easing the return of hospitalized parishioners back into the com-

munity. As such, parish nurses are in an ideal position to extend care management tools and advocate for appropriate care to be available before, during, and after an illness.

Parish nurses are also in a position to collaborate on clinical improvement efforts (Ludwig-Beymer, Welsh, & Micek, 1998). First, because of their work in the community, parish nurses may identify clinical processes in need of improvement. For example, does the parish nurse notice that clients consistently feel unprepared for and frightened of a particular test or procedure? If so, then the parish nurse as a health advocate identifies this as a concern for this population. A fully functioning integrated delivery system needs this type of feedback. Second, the parish nurse may participate on multidisciplinary teams to design clinical improvement products. Parish nurses possess valuable information about clients and processes. These must be shared with other care providers. Third, parish nurses may plan and implement clinical improvement programs. Fourth, the parish nurse may develop and use patient education materials with her distinct population. Fifth, the parish nurse may assist in evaluating the effectiveness of clinical improvement efforts. Measurement of outcomes of care will be discussed in greater detail later in this chapter. Sixth, the parish nurse may play an important role in revising the products as necessary.

Increasing the Client's Ability to
Form Partnerships

Health care is moving from a historically paternalistic attitude to one that endorses and expects partnerships between patients and clinicians. Particularly for chronic diseases such as asthma, diabetes mellitus, hypertension, and cardiac conditions, patients and family members are becoming full members of the health care team, involved in decisions about care. Physicians are anxious to form more effective partnerships with their patients but lack the time and resources to make it happen in a consistent fashion. Enter parish nursing.

Parish nurses have long fostered empowerment and accountability in their clients. Clients are taught how to become partners with physicians and other clinicians in their care, and this behavior is modeled by the parish nurse. An excellent example of this empowerment is Congregational Health Services (Solari-Twadell, Truty, & Ryan, 1994). Although Congregational Health Services can be coordinated by the parish nurse, the services involve a multidisciplinary team, including physicians. In this program, parishioners learn about medical terms and laboratory tests, how to work with physicians, how to take responsibility for their behaviors, and how to modify their behaviors for a healthier life. In addition, they receive a portable personal health record. Physicians report that many patients bring the health record to office visits with them. Both physicians and patients find this continuity of care to be helpful.

Management of chronic diseases requires a partnership between care providers, clients, and families. Parish nurses are in an ideal position to help clients enhance their chronic disease self-management skills. For example, the parish nurse may emphasize the importance of glucose monitoring for an individual with newly diagnosed diabetes mellitus. She may also assist the client with documenting and interpreting the results. Physicians may collaborate with parish nurses so that the treatment regime they design is individualized and thus better followed by the client. With proper communication, parish nurses are in a position to support and augment physician-directed aspects of the treatment plan.

Changing financial incentives are also affecting the move toward health care consumer empowerment. We are moving from an era of fee-for-service, when more care was viewed as better, to a time of capitation, when less care may be preferred. In a continuum of care, timely and appropriate care must be ensured. When the client becomes a partner with his or her provider, appropriate and timely care is more likely to happen. Parish nurses are in an ideal position to educate the public about these changes. They are trusted members of the community and can address the complex issue of "does more care always mean better care?" with their constituencies. In addition, they may educate clients about the roles they have to play in their own health.

Facilitator of Referrals and
Health Advocate

The parish nurse functions as a referral source and advocate. Because of the complexity of care, referrals are ever present in health care. Referrals are a special issue within a continuum of care, as each referral potentially fragments the care received by the client. Hand-offs must occur smoothly, so that the recipient of care experiences continuity of care rather than fragmentation. Parish nurses help to provide this continuity. Parish nurses have a long history of making referrals to health care providers, health agencies, and social service agencies. Community members frequently come to the parish nurse requesting referrals to physicians and other providers of care. When the nurse works in true partnership with specific physicians and knows the ways in which they practice, she will feel very comfortable providing these referrals. In addition, physician offices cannot possibly know all of the community resources available. Parish nurses, however, are very knowledgeable about existing resources. Because the parish nurse functions in the community and knows it so well, she can be a resource for the physician. She serves as a two-way conduit of information, taking information from the IDN to the community and information from the community to the IDN. Parish nurses as health advocates are in an ideal position to link clients to appropriate referrals, coordinate referrals, and assist clients and families through the referral process.

Forming Spiritual Partnerships

The parish nurse serves as an integrator of faith and health. Churches are becoming aware of their role in keeping people healthy and are viewing themselves as essential links in health care. Parishioners are viewing health in terms of the whole person and are describing health in terms of physical, mental, and spiritual components. Churches want to contribute to healthier communities (Wylie, 1990).

Physicians, too, are viewing health as more than the absence of disease and are acknowledging the complexity of wellness. They are accepting the role that spirituality and faith play in the well-being of their patients. They are aware of the research that links church attendance and spirituality to better control of hypertension, healthier behaviors in college students, lower suicide rates, diminished pain in patients with cancer, and fewer psychological disorders when encountering significant levels of stress (Larson, 1996).

Physicians may view parish nurses as resources as they grow in their recognition of spirituality. In addition, parish nurses may feel comfortable referring clients to physicians who are able and willing to discuss spiritual issues with their patients.

Challenges and Opportunities

Building the partnership described above is possible but takes time and effort from all parties involved. Ensuring the allotment of that time is a challenge. Exchanging information, measuring effectiveness, and reexamining practices are three challenges and opportunities that exist in this area.

Exchanging Information

An important communication link that fosters partnership is that between defined users who share common information sets. The information sets may include client, clinical, financial, and outcomes data. An essential part of any continuum is this exchange of information. Clients are often frustrated by the need to repeat information. Clinicians are frustrated by the lack of pertinent, readily available clinical and demographic data. For example, the parish nurse may possess and document important information about a parishioner, yet that information is not available to other health care providers.

Ideally, the parish nurse should be linked with other providers in an integrated information system. A variety of providers should share a common database that contains demographic and clinical information. The parish nurse should have access to referral information and should be able to make referrals electronically. The parish nurse should share her information electronically and should also receive information electronically. For example, she should be notified immediately when a parishioner is admitted to the hospital so that she can visit or arrange a visit for that parishioner.

Unfortunately, there are no quick fixes when it comes to this information exchange. A health information network remains a dream of the future. However, even now, the parish nurse and physician are putting communication strategies into place. Telephone calls are generated. In addition, faxes and electronic mail are used. All of these require a mutual understanding of roles and a healthy respect for what each partner has to offer to improve the health of clients.

Measuring Effectiveness

Programs can no longer exist if they are unable to measure and document their effectiveness. Within a continuum of care, both micromeasures (measurement of the individual parts of the IDN) and macromeasures (measurement of the IDN as a whole) are needed. Thus, parish nurses must examine outcomes that result from a person's interaction with parish nursing services. Parish nurses are beginning to examine and describe their practice. However, longitudinal studies that examine the impact of parish nursing services over time are lacking. One such set of studies is being conducted using the population served by the congregational health program (Solari-Twadell, Truty, Ludwig-Beymer, See, & Yang, 1995; Solari-Twadell, Truty, & See, 1994; Truty, Solari-Twadell, Ludwig-Beymer, Yang, & Dunn, 1996). These studies examine changes in health status and physical parameters such as weight, blood pressure, and cholesterol level. Additional large-scale studies are needed to examine the outcomes of all aspects of parish nursing practice. In addition, the overall outcome of patient care within an IDN must be examined.

Reexamining Practice

Modifications in practice are needed to make the parish nurse–physician partnership a reality within a continuum of care. Both the IDN and the parish nurse may need to change.

The IDN needs to consider or reexamine parish nursing. It needs to answer several questions: "What is parish nursing?" "What could parish nursing be?" "What does parish nursing have to offer the IDN?" and "How can parish nursing function within the IDN?" The IDN must develop a partnership with the church in continuing to provide parish nurses' salaries and assist parish nurses to develop the skills needed to practice in a complex health system, tell their stories effectively, and document their effectiveness.

The parish nurse must carefully consider partnership with a for-profit IDN. Historically, for-profit health care systems have been unwilling to provide ongoing support programs that do not contribute to the financial viability of the organization. This places parish nurses in a precarious position. It may take years, if ever, for parish nursing to reach financial viability. Caution is called for in these relationships.

For parish nurses, revisions are needed in the way they practice within an IDN. They are risk takers who are willing to forge new paths and new relationships. Often, they are accustomed to "going it alone." Parish nurses network well with others, particularly in social services, but they have not for the most part been well integrated within the health system. In addition, parish nurses may have left nursing in more traditional settings to avoid the formal structure of health care, including documentation and measurement. However, for the good of the communities they serve, as well as professional accountability, parish nurses need to address the documentation and measurement issues.

Partnerships between physicians and parish nurses are relatively unexplored. Yet, such partnerships can be very effective, especially in the management of clients with complex and chronic conditions. Parish nurses need to work as team members, contributing their understanding of individuals, family, and community to the health care team. Parish nurses will need to standardize their roles in education and screening and expand their role in identifying high-risk groups and individuals. Most of all, they need to continue to do what they do so well: consider the needs of their parishioners and serve as advocate, educator, and counselor for them.

Clearly, health care in the future will be different from the sickness services offered today. A continuum of care, providing an array of appropriate services at the right place, the right time, and the right cost, is in our future. The parish nurse is in a position to play an important role in partnership with physicians within the continuum of care. We must tap the skill and expertise of the parish nurse for the good of individuals, families, and communities. How we harness the creativity, flexibility, and dedication inherent in the parish nurse role is up to us.

Now consider a vignette that can be a true partnership between the parish nurse and the physician within a continuum of care.

Ms. Smith is a parish nurse and Dr. Jones is a primary care physician practicing within an integrated delivery system. Mrs. Z is an 85-year-old woman who lives alone. She has enrolled in a Medicare HMO and has selected a new primary care physician. On her first visit to her physician, Dr. Jones, she mentions that she regularly attends church. Dr. Jones asks her if she has ever sought out the services of Ms. Smith, the parish nurse at that congregation. Mrs. Z responds, "I know about her. She checks blood pressures after services. But I thought she was just for sick people." Dr. Jones encourages Mrs. Z to get to know the parish nurse. He also sends a brief e-mail message to Ms. Smith indicating that Mrs. Z is a complex patient who could benefit from interacting with the parish nurse. He attaches a health history and his physical findings.

When she receives the message, Ms. Smith telephones Mrs. Z, inviting her to stop by her office. The following week, Mrs. Z stops in after services to have her blood pressure checked by Ms. Smith. Ms. Smith tells Mrs. Z she is glad to meet her and lets her know that Dr. Jones has suggested they work together on her health issues. Ms. Smith finds that Mrs. Z's blood pressure is 172/96. "Oh, that's not bad for me," says Mrs. Z. Ms. Smith asks Mrs. Z about her health. Mrs. Z says, "I have a touch of sugar, but who doesn't at this age? The worst thing is the horrible leg ulcer. And who can keep up with all the things they're doing with me? I have a dozen pills to take for this or that." Ms. Smith compares Mrs. Z's perception of her health to the history and physical sent by Dr. Jones. She notes that Mrs. Z's blood pressure is elevated and that both her hemoglobin and cholesterol levels are elevated.

Ms. Smith arranges to meet with Mrs. Z in her office on Monday. There, Ms. Smith sorts through the myriad of medications and instructions that Ms. Z has been given by three previous physicians and a home health nurse. Because Ms. Smith has a copy of Mrs. Z's medical record, she knows which medications are current and which should be discarded. She also knows that home health care is not warranted at this time. Ms. Smith reviews the medications with Mrs. Z and provides some basic information about them. She then assesses Mrs. Z's diet and finds that Mrs. Z is confused about meal planning for her diabetes. With Mrs. Z's permission, Ms. Smith calls Dr. Jones to request a consult with the diabetic educator for nutritional counseling. The physician makes the referral, and Ms. Smith arranges for transportation for Mrs. Z to attend the session.

The following week, Ms. Smith again checks Mrs. Z's blood pressure. It has dropped to 148/90. Ms. Smith congratulates Mrs. Z and again reviews her medications and diet with her. Later, Ms. Smith e-mails her findings to Dr. Jones. They agree that Ms. Smith will follow Mrs. Z weekly and that Mrs. Z will return to Dr. Jones in three months. Mrs. Z calls Ms. Smith during the week. "I want to thank you for all your help," she says. "I've never felt better!"

References

American Nurses Association. (1985). *Code for nurses.* Washington, DC: Author.

Evashwick, C. J. (1987). Definition of the continuum of care. In C. J. Evashwick & L. J. Weiss (Eds.), *Managing the continuum of care.* Gaithersburg, MD: Aspen.

Larson, D. (1996, November 8). *Making the care for religion in clinical care: A look back.* Paper presented at the "Spiritual Care Research: What We Are Learning" Mayo Medical Center Conference, Rochester, MN.

Ludwig-Beymer, P. (1994). Developing a continuum of care: A nurse's perspective. *Nursing Spectrum, 7*(10), 11.

Ludwig-Beymer, P., Welsh, C., & Micek, W. T. (1998). Parish nursing's role in clinical quality improvement. *Journal of Christian Nursing, 15*(1), 28-31.

Solari-Twadell, A., Truty, L., Ludwig-Beymer, P., See, C., & Yang, J. J. (1995, May). *Congregational health services: A one year perspective.* Poster presented at the "Celebrating Science in Action" Third Annual Naurice M. Nesset Research Forum, Park Ridge, IL.

Solari-Twadell, P. A., Truty, L., & Ryan, J. A. (1994). *Congregational health services.* Park Ridge, IL: Lutheran General HealthSystem.

Solari-Twadell, A., Truty, L., & See, C. (1994, May). *Congregational health services: Age, gender and self-care issues.* Poster presented at the Second Annual Naurice M. Nesset Research Forum, Park Ridge, IL.

Truty, L., Solari-Twadell, A., Ludwig-Beymer, P., Yang, J. J., & Dunn, B. (1996, May). *Congregational health services database: Self-reported health using the health status questionnaire 2.0.* Poster presented at the "A Year of Discovery: Research Across Advocate" Fourth Annual Naurice M. Nesset Research Forum, Park Ridge, IL.

Ummel, S. L., Schaffner, J. W., Smith, B. D., & Ludwig-Beymer, P. (1995). Advancing the continuum of care: The Lutheran General HealthSystem experience. In S. S. Blancett & D. L. Flarey (Eds.), *Reengineering nursing and health care: The handbook for organizational transformation.* Gaithersburg, MD: Aspen.

Wylie, L. J. (1990). The mission of health and the congregation. In P. A. Solari-Twadell, A. M. Djupe, & M. A. McDermott (Eds.), *Parish nursing: The developing practice.* Park Ridge, IL: National Parish Nurse Resource Center.

14

Pastoral Reflections

Gerald Nelson

The voice on the other end of the phone said, "Our family needs spiritual comfort and direction. I called your congregation because we have heard you care."

An administrator of a junior high school called and said, "We have a young man who recently moved here. He is finding it difficult to adjust and he is acting out those difficulties. Is it possible for you or someone on your staff to meet this family and see if you can help?"

I recently participated in a panel that had been given the task of defining the unchurched and exploring how a congregation can reach out to those without a church home. One of the ways I noted was the importance of being known as a caring community. Our congregation has seen itself in that light, but it is quite true that 5 years after the advent of parish nurse in our congregation, others are now more likely to think of us as a parish who cares. Our own people can now quite easily say that their church home is a loving community.

Excerpts from a letter written by one of our members illustrates the image of a caring faith community:

My purpose in writing this letter is to comment for the record on the valuable service of Christian care recently given to our mom . . . and to us her children. Though I was serving as vice-president on the parish council at the time of the parish nurse education and implementation, I was not fully aware of just what this service could mean to a church member. One day in the midst of feeling inadequate in dealing with issues regarding Mom, and in prayer ("Oh, God, what more can I do?") the answer came, "Call Saralea Holstrom" (parish nurse). Saralea heard our story and called Mom the next day and became a dear friend to Marie, and a source of peace and support to us, her children. We are thankful for Saralea, her services, and who she is as a person. It is my intention that this letter be put on file as recommending the parish nurse as a valuable addition to the Parish Staff.

With the addition of a parish nurse to our staff, we have increased significantly our capacity for caregiving. That this is important is dramatized by how few institutions there are that really care. Although there are institutions and people who say "We care," what they care about are such things as our response, our business, or our vote. In most cases, it is unlikely that they will care deeply, if at all, if a loved one is ill, an income is lost, a child is struggling with self-esteem, substance abuse is destroying a life, or someone is desperately lonely. Congregations are concerned about such things! They believe there is a power in the community that gathers around the Word to help and bind up, to comfort and restore.

As our society becomes more and more fragmented, the congregation that seeks to carry out a healing ministry of caregiving is like a bright light in a dark place. We have a marvelous opportunity to bear witness to the love of God. The parish nurse program can move any congregation to a higher intensity of caregiving, for it helps to bridge the gap between concept and mission. Concept says we care. Mission is caring.

Our congregation has grown from 1,400 to over 3,100 baptized persons in the past 15 years. Much of that growth has happened because the congregation is seen as a caring community. All statistics indicate that over 75% of those who join congregations do so because of a friend. If members feel authentic caring in their church home, they will feel positive about sharing that church home with others.

I believe we must be able to link together the message that we are loved by God with the message that His grace frees us to be lovers ourselves. It is in that spirit that I relate that two of the most important decisions in our parish in the past 10 years were (a) to become a fully eucharistic community and (b) to add a parish nurse to our staff.

The first relates to the message that we are loved by God. By "fully eucharistic" I mean that we include the sacrament of Holy Communion at all four of our weekly worship services.

As the sacrament is shared, there is the powerful message of forgiveness, love, and new life. There is the opportunity for every person to be addressed with the Gospel. Then, too, as we give the bread, our pastors use the opportunity to touch each person. It might be a gentle touch or a squeeze of the hand. In that touch is communicated the message of love, that we are there for one another no matter how deep the hurt, worry, or concerns of the soul.

The second decision, that of adding a parish nurse to our staff, relates to our being a community in mission. A vital part of our healing mission is being available and competent in dealing with the hurts, needs, and concerns of people. One of the many touching moments connected to the healing aspect of our community occurred when a long-time member of our parish was seen in the sanctuary following worship. He was speaking with our parish nurse. What he said to her was, "I have cancer. I have been told I have only a short time to live."

He had received the eucharist. Now he was articulating the reality of human suffering and need. He was in conversation with someone who could understand the technical terms the medical profession had used to describe his illness. He asked for clarification, but mostly he practiced telling his story. As he told his story to our parish nurse in the sanctuary, he was strengthened by the eucharistic message received only moments before, that "because I live you shall live also." And healing, the healing of

Christ, was among them, and this beloved member of our congregation was able to add another crucial part to the telling of his story.

Let me raise again the claim I made earlier that the parish nurse program has not only enabled the image of a caring community but has indeed increased dramatically the caring we in fact accomplish. We stress that the parish nurse is available to our people on Sunday mornings. It is the weekly gathering time of the family. Each Sunday, she is surrounded by those who have discovered that she is a valuable resource, a confidante, an interpreter, an advocate, a source of referrals, a friend, one who can help identify options and sort through them. She is also available at other stated times during the week, but the Sunday coffee hours between services are a key time of availability. Her visible availability points up the message of the congregation being a caring place, a place of healing, a place that listens to one's needs and concerns.

It is very important to see the parish nurse as a part of the pastoral care team. Such a team might consist of the pastor or pastors on staff, the parish nurse, and lay volunteers. In our parish, it is our four pastors, parish nurse, and seminary intern. We meet early each week at a set time and review the parish needs and concerns. This has virtually eliminated those dreadful feelings that come to us when we are reminded that "Joe" came home from the hospital 2 weeks ago but no one has followed up on his progress or evaluated his needs.

We do follow up much, much better with a parish nurse on staff. One reason for this is that a nurse is a professional health care person. Nurses are accustomed to "checking in" on people. When we listen to a nurse in dialogue, we hear a steady pattern of conversation that is designed to draw out an articulation of "how are you doing?"

At each pastoral care staffing, we review those who have received care in the past several months and all who have been brought to our attention since the last time we met. We assess the need for follow-up and decide who will do it. Our parish nurse makes many of the follow-up contacts. Many can be made by phone. Her follow-up is valuable because a nurse is skilled at assessment and also because there are often questions of a medical nature.

We are sometimes asked if people accept the ministry of a parish nurse as easily as they receive a pastor's offer of care. The answer is yes. If there is hesitation, it is only prior to their having an opportunity to be helped by her ministry. Any hesitations quickly disappear when they have such issues as an aging parent, counseling relating to AIDS, depression in youth, sexual concerns among youth, chemical abuse questions, or the need for resources such as nursing homes, adult day care, and divorce or grief support groups.

A pastor has a great variety of responsibilities, such as being an administrator, preacher, teacher, worship leader, counselor, fund-raiser, and leader, but the parish nurse is able to be a specialist in the parish in the area of caring. Her focus is solely on caring. She demonstrates this caring through establishing support groups for caregivers, writing articles for the parish newsletter, arranging transportation for those who need outpatient treatment, and on and on.

This sense of specialty in caring is captured in a letter written by our parish nurse in which she was explaining her motivation and understanding of the program. She wrote,

I heard Granger speak about six years ago and was very interested in his vision of whole person health care based in the church. At the time, I was working as a Medicare staff nurse in a long-term care facility. My brother's wife had multiple sclerosis and I was caring for her on my day off. Several times I called her church encouraging a friendly visit, but this never took place. I felt their life could have been so different if they could have had a health advocate in their faith community. I have also seen numerous examples in my nursing experiences of how a patient with faith, a relationship with God and a faith community seemed to recover better from crisis and illness.

Out of her experience, she has helped us to realize as a congregation the powerful image we can have as a caring community of faith. We have had a surprising number of remarkable recoveries among the people of our parish. Although we do not pretend to understand the mysteries of God, we do understand that love and care can be essential to recovery from illness, injury, grief, and crisis of any kind. A caring parish can play a vital role in this process, and any parish increases its caring capacity when it has a care specialist on staff.

I am not saying that pastors are not caring persons. Quite the opposite is true. Pastors have such a wide range of responsibilities that we are seldom able to specialize in any area. When a parish nurse came on our staff, we began a new chapter of caring. We stepped it up. It took on new dimensions we had never known before. In my own heart I have always carried guilt and worry that I was not covering all the bases as I wanted. It was a heaviness that someone was forgotten or neglected, that opportunities were being lost. Once the parish nurse joined the caring team, there was a partner and specialist in caring. Several years ago, we had a young husband and father seriously injured in an automobile accident. Little hope was given for his survival. His parents, who lived out of state, came immediately to help with the children and to assist his wife in keeping the daily vigil at the hospital. In the days that followed, our pastoral care team, as we always do, talked together about how we could best give care to this hospitalized, comatose man and his family. Even though the hospital was 45 minutes away, we decided together that we would visit that man and his family every day. Our parish nurse was a part of that schedule. Every 5th day she visited, as we did not have a seminary intern at the time. She brought the same value of presence and prayer as did the pastors. She also brought the added dimension of being able to communicate with that family about medical procedures and concerns. She enabled dialogue and understanding that greatly aided the well-being of that patient and his family and helped them all in the healing process. It was a great day when that man returned to the sanctuary where so many prayers had been said on his behalf. As he embraced me after worship, he said, "Without the prayers and ministry of this People of God, I wouldn't be here!" And his eyes overflowed with tears of gratitude.

Another dimension of the caring by a parish nurse is in the way she draws others into the care arena. Not only does she draw volunteers from the parish who are recruited to do such things as provide transportation for outpatient needs, she draws all of us into the care arena through our contacts with her. A person who is modeling caregiving is one who gives others inspiration, motivation, and examples of how caring enriches life.

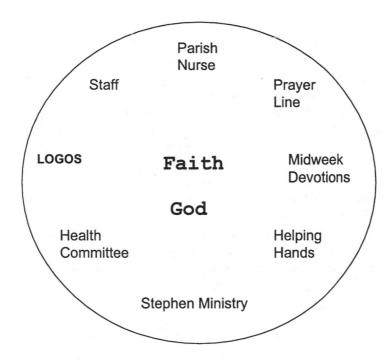

Figure 14.1. Caregiving in Our Saviour's Lutheran Church

Just recently, one of our members died following a brief illness. This person had always been very supportive to me and to the mission of our congregation. How can you not love a man who had been a supportive and articulate member of the stewardship committee for 33 successive years? After the funeral service, our parish nurse sought me out. She knew how hard his death was for me, not only because one pours one's self out in those times but because pastors, too, experience loss, even in the midst of the good news of eternal life. She reached out, this parish nurse, and put her arms around me, and all she said was "Oh pastor." That's all. Her view and her presence told me she understood. And, for that moment, I rested as a caregiver and received care and love from another. It makes a difference to have sensitive and caring people who league together in ministry either as volunteers or as part of a staff. Later, as I reflected on that moment, I was reminded again of how important it is to give to others that sense of how a parish nurse can draw others into the care arena through her contacts with them.

Figure 14.1 is not intended to be interpreted as an organizational model as much as an attempt to share some of the ways caregiving works in our parish. Each of the spokes of the wheel was initiated after the parish nurse program began or was revitalized or reshaped. My brief comments about the diagram are for the purpose of explaining the role of the parish nurse in some of these areas rather than a description of the program entity.

Prayer is a vital part of our faith life. We are all supported by the prayers of others. The Prayer Line is an encouragement for supportive prayers as well as intercessory petitions on behalf of those in need. The parish nurse recruits and meets with participants.

She is the one who gathers prayer concerns, doing so primarily through a prayer concern box, a form in each bulletin, telephone requests, and members of the pastoral care team.

The Wednesday morning midweek devotions are tied to the Prayer Line in that intercessory prayers are offered. The staff gives leadership to these 15- to 20-minute devotions held in the sanctuary. If you were to call the church office during this period of time, you would be greeted by a message that says, "The congregation is at prayer." The parish nurse is a part of these devotions, both as leader and participant. Her involvement models that one of the ways we maintain and guard our wholeness is through prayer and worship.

Stephen Ministry and LOGOS are both international programs available to all congregations. Stephen Ministry equips the laity for one-on-one caring. Our parish nurse relates to this program as a resource and as one who is alert to those in need of this personal caring. LOGOS is a youth and family ministry. As is true in many of our caring ministries, the emphasis is on enabling persons to develop in all the wholeness God intends. In this sense, we can speak of preventive medicine. LOGOS in our congregation embraces 6th- to 12th-grade youth and their families with the intent of giving spiritual nurture and direction, as well as building stronger ties to the church family. Our parish nurse serves as a table parent at the weekly meal and in so doing is present as a member of the faith family and available to staff and students as a resource person. By her presence she also experiences, firsthand, family concerns and needs.

Helping Hands is not an unusual group in any congregation, yet we find this deepened in that the parish nurse is often in a good position to assess the need for services the church family can offer, such as child care, meals, and transportation.

The Health Committee came into existence in connection with, and support for, the parish nurse program. The committee is focused on keeping health awareness before the congregation. It needs to be said that our parish nurse is a health educator. She leads adult and youth programs in all aspects of the stewardship of life. Her focus is often on children and youth. She gives leadership to church school units on human sexuality. We have two sessions of Vacation Bible School, and she is a part of each of those in her function as health educator.

In all aspects of the parish nurse program, and in our entire ministry of caring, it is our intention to articulate that the care given, the concern expressed, and the wholeness prayed for is done in the Name of our Lord who moved among the people as one who healed. In a letter received from one of our members, there were these words about our parish nurse: "Tell Saralea that when I get home I'm going to pin angel wings on her. What a marvelous caring person she is." What I want to emphasize here is that in the many letters we receive, the word "caring" is used over and over.

In the year when the stewardship theme of our church was "Signs of God's Gracious Love," one of our members gave a temple talk. He referred to the parish nurse program as one of those signs of gracious love:

> Without the parish nurse program some of us would be poorer in body and spirit. But with it here comes a feeling that God is near—that He comes and loves, that He heals and redeems. My wife and I have had various illnesses that seem to come with the aging process. We have been under the care of our parish nurse ever since this program was begun 5 years ago. We look forward to her visits because she comes on behalf of the

church, not only with medical knowledge and skill, but also with compassion and love that are uplifting and sustaining.

Returning to the thought of "angel wings," I am reminded of how after the temptation of Jesus in the wilderness, angels came and ministered to Him. I am grateful that God still sends angels to minister to His people. God calls out to all of us to be a part of the mighty group of caregivers—angels, as it were. And especially God calls His congregations to be people who are angels who minister in time of need.

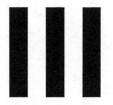

PARISH NURSING
Context for the Practice

15

Caring as a Context for the Practice

Patricia Benner

People are bound to one another through, among other things, love, sympathy, and solidarity. By love and friendship they are bound together in a spontaneous way, whereas in solidarity they are bound together more through cooperative endeavor and common circumstances. But whether these ties are formed spontaneously or socially, it is these ties that constitute a person's existence. The more intensely and comprehensively a person binds himself to other people spontaneously and socially, the more he will see that a selfish life lived at the expense of others is empty and unsuccessful and the more he will refrain from that kind of life (Logstrup, 1997, p. 126).

Parish nursing offers nursing a new opportunity to practice in a more whole and congruent way. Nursing has the opportunity to rediscover and extend the vision of what it means to care for one another as well as to promote health and well-being. Parish nursing brings to the faith community wisdom and know-how in health promotion, prevention of illness, coping with chronic illness, and being with the sick. Nurses have developed many fine arts of helping in our caring practices of (a) meeting and recognizing the other; (b) sustaining a sense of personhood and dignity through everyday practices of care and life; (c) bearing witness to life courage and travail, noticing and attentiveness; (d) comforting practices; (e) restoring trust; (f) caring for the dying; (g) preparing the family for birth; and many other well-developed caring practices not easily described except in concrete examples.

These are the strengths that parish nurses bring to churches. It is to be hoped that parish nurses will not bring familiar aspects of current market models of health care that break care down into procedural elements that can be sold at a fair market price. Turning the church into one more clinic will not be healing to the church or to society. The intent is that parish nursing does not assume the medicalization of life—that is, attending only to the technical repair of diseased parts and structures. Old, unseemly visions of the heroic helper who gains manipulative power over the other through "helping," or an unliberated view of the victimized, overburdened helping martyr are not to be rekindled and extended through the parish nurse role in the church.

Returning to communities of worship allows parish nurses to more freely link practices of meeting the other that is so central to nursing practice and to community life. Parish nurses use many metaphors and allegories for care that oppose control through efficiency, people processing, and other forms of disengaged care.

Society values high-status, highly paid, autonomous professionals who hold secret knowledge that has the capacity to solve problems. This ideal professional image overlooks the human care that renders such professional care safe. In a culture that values independence and self-sufficiency, care is overlooked and devalued. Helping, itself, can be a defense against feeling helpless and can cover over the helper's dependency. It is difficult to admit our mutual interdependence and need for care. When the helper seeks invulnerability through manipulation and control over the other, rather than meeting the other and helping out of a sense of solidarity and genuine concern for the other's well-being, the chances of doing harm are great. The chance of being open and responsive to the other's possibilities, constraints, and suffering are small. Either way, helping is relational. Despite the intents of the helper or quality of the help offered, the one being helped may potentiate and extend the help offered, whatever the quality, or he or she may refuse help and respond with fear as well as suspicion.

A technological understanding of the person views the person as a strategic agent engaged in rational calculation. This strategic view of the person is based upon assessing performance in line with strategic aims. It is essentially a technological view that calls for heroic actions and sweeping breakthroughs. Outcomes are highlighted. Such a technical view fits well with viewing the person as a consumer choosing commodities to foster health. Indeed, this market model of health care gives much of the impetus for seeking health and wholeness in religious communities, to restore an understanding of health for the whole person and decrease the commodification of helping relationships. Many technical cures would be rendered less necessary if we had a vision of health as daily care of the whole person within a family and a community.

From the perspective of the value of the ordinary life, the person, as created, is sacred and valued as intrinsically worthy. Strategic powers and performance criteria are not enough to characterize the human whose worth lies in his or her own worthiness as created and sacred. When we consider human concerns we encounter human forms of pride, shame, moral goodness, evil, dignity, suffering, human forms of love, and so on. Furthermore, these concerns determine the worth and approach to our strategic efforts towards reproduction, health maintenance, self-care, and so on. Outcome is no longer the only issue. Saving a life or prolonging dying become issues. Instrumental or means-ends strategic thinking can no longer be the only consideration. Maintaining ties, human connectedness and human concerns, responding to creation and to life as a gift are understood as constituting what it means to be a person. There are many examples of this from parish nurses who promote health and healing through assisting the patient in maintaining human ties and providing support that gives a patient the courage to weather illness and/or face death.

We are called to be healing communities, and faith does bring about healing, restoration, and recovery from the brokenness, alienation, and woundedness of illness, but such healing is not based on techniques that create unlimited control over outcomes or the precise specification of the means of our healing. As health professionals interested in providing whole-person care, we have to reassert the primacy of caring as a moral art and not as a mere science. Our science must be guided by our notion of health and the good life and by our notions of what it is to be a person.

Unfortunately, the implications of much of the research on the mind-body relationship is lost on us because we do not have good "scientific metaphors" to capture the way our bodies dwell in meanings in our everyday habits, postures, stances, fears, worries, joy, laughter, and tears. We end up with hopelessly simplistic views of radical freedom, that we can control the brain or the liver or our digestive organs with the mind, a mixture of New Age philosophy and technical rationality that seeks to directly control the body with the mind. This view ignores the ways our bodies are affected by our meanings, our faith, our concerns. Metaphors of the programmed computer, super-human willpower, mind over matter, or any of the other "control" metaphors do not capture the views of the created, finite "body as temple," responding and dwelling in a network of relationships and concerns. The problem with mind-over-matter control metaphors, other than their heretical stature, is that they cause us to blame the victim for not having the right thoughts, the right faith, the right kind of control over personal destiny.

Caring, ministering in specific ways to specific others, is a profoundly sacred, hopeful practice. Caring makes things, people, and events salient for us. What we care for and about constitutes what we experience as distressing and comfortable as well as creating possible responses. Caring determines what is accessible and whether it is experienced as helpful. Without caring relationships we would all perish. In the highly technical context of our current health care system, without careful coaching, interpretation, and care, which can make the various intrusive foreign interventions of highly technical medicine approachable and interpretable, people could be literally scared to death.

Moving Beyond the Ideal and Real Deficit View

Bonhoeffer (1954), in his book *Living Together,* introduces the radical notion that faith communities are communities of reality. They are not intended to be places for judging how far short everyone falls of certain standards. A healing community is a place of marvelous possibilities to be touched, healed, and redeemed in one's present circumstances. In such a reality-based community, one may be healed to more fully live in response to life as a sacred and unrepeatable gift. In moving toward health and wholeness, persons begin wherever they are and the movement is toward specific calls, specific concerns, and wholeness. In a "normal" technical view, the person has standards and ideals that are almost never actualized or achieved in reality. Thus, in a technical view of health, a gap is expected between the ideal and the real, and this tension is understood as the basis for striving, goal-oriented behavior. The same picture of reality is evident in psychological testing. People are measured against an ideal norm or standard unrelated to their particular context and are diagnosed in relation to that standard—how far they fall short of or exceed the standard. The move from viewing the person only in relation to prespecified standards to viewing the person in relation to their concerns, opportunities, and constraints can bring new possibilities of reconciliation and hope.

Shifting the parish nurse's perspective from that of a deficit view of the situation (i.e., assessing how deficient the real is compared to the ideal standard) to one of discovering the possibilities inherent in the situation opens up new options. Seeing only the deficits can block perceptions of the possible. The deficit view may also paralyze action if the emotional response is one of moral outrage or disappointment. Moral outrage helps only if we see alternative lines of action that bring justice and mercy in the situation. Moral outrage carries with it the danger that it may only produce cynicism and disillusionment and the person may cope by giving up the ideals altogether. Therefore a shift in perspective to what is possible in particular situations can open up new lines of action and empower the person through a decreasing sense of disappointment and powerlessness. Questions that open up possibility are: "What can be done now, in the meantime (before the ideal can be realized)?" "Is there another way to achieve the same end?" "Is the end in sight the most worthy?" Looking for the possibility inherent in the situation still requires a notion of what is good about what one is trying to achieve; however, decreasing the preconceived notions about how that good ought to be achieved or even the nature of the particular good can offer new points of departure and possibility.

Parish nurses have much to learn from the best and worst of caring practices. In the best practice we will discover selves of membership in common humanity that are given over or defined by specific concrete concerns and human relationships. Linking expertise and caring requires that we transform notions of expertise. Expert caring has nothing to do with possessing privileged information that increases one's control and domination over another; rather, expert caring unleashes the possibilities inherent in the self and other in the situation. Expert caring liberates and facilitates in such a way that the caring is enriched in the process. Instrumentalism, contract language, cost-benefit analysis, social exchange, enlightened self-interest, and all the language of autonomous selves of possession miss the relationship of the person that is constituted by concerns and human relationships (Taylor, 1989).

The self of membership and participation requires a language of commitment, meanings, skills, concerns, and aspirations. Meeting and understanding such human beings requires narrative and interpretation. Human capacities are best described in terms of possibilities and skilled practices, not just in terms of how well the person measures up to predetermined context-free criteria of performance (Benner & Wrubel, 1989). How do we take over our health care sciences so that they can do justice to our caring practices? In this age of scientism, ultimate authority is placed in science as a guide for living and for solving one's problems in contrast to drawing on science as one among many resources or sources of information. Science *is* our major authority and source of legitimization—how can we transform our science so that the definition of what it means to be a person is not always construed in advance as an unrelated, autonomous self of possession seeking strategic ends based only upon self-interest, enlightened or otherwise?

A revision of our understanding of the person will give new visions of healing relationships and coaching roles—our caring practices. These therapies already exist in the best of our healing communities, but we require a language that captures the nature and intent of these practices as they are carried out in real contexts and real relationships.

In lively communities, we gain a new respect over time for the concrete and specific, the courageous and meaningful. We will come to understand heroic action not only in terms of technological breakthroughs, but in terms of skillful comportment and excellence in the everyday demands of lives lived in relation to others, to nature, to the Eternal.

Typically, health policy experts do not worry about a society that does not care enough. Government officials do not at this time decry the negligence evident in a society that devalues caring and those who provide care. It is as if our health and social welfare policies are designed to hide our guilt about not caring enough. Faith congregations have lost many of their ties with the caring practices that constitute community. Indeed, many churches have unwittingly allowed unjust burdens of caregiving to be assumed by women and individual caregivers and not considered liberated caregiving practices for all members of the community. A societal preoccupation with the ends while ignoring the means is evident in the rational-technical model of the therapist, manager, salesperson, and consumer and typical in our technical, commercial age. Controlling can be confused with caring. The devaluation and confusion over caring and the elaboration of the view of the contractual, economic self has powerfully influenced our health care institutions, practices, and unjust patterns of caregiving.

A liberation from oppressive, domination/subordination-oriented, power-oriented views of caring. In returning to faith communities, we can discern the many ways we are called to love the other. In doing so, we can open up new opportunities to break free of psychologizing and temporizing about our relationships and responsibilities to each other. Freed of our former bureaucratic chains, we will have to face up to the ethical demands of whole-person care that meet the other in care rather than in domination and control. Bauman (1988/1998) points out the thin line between care and oppressive control that creates self-righteous practices of normalizing the other who is different:

> The Other is recast as my creation; acting on the best of impulses, I have stolen the Other's authority. It is I now who says *what* the command to love my neighbor commands. I have become the Other's plenipotentiary . . . and if I want to make sure that my responsibility has been exercised in full, that nothing has been left undone, overlooked or neglected, I will feel obliged to include in my responsibility also the duty to overcome what I can see as nothing else but her ignorance, or misinterpretation, of "her own best interest." If anything, my responsibility seems to be, gratifyingly, enhanced: naivety, imprudence, improvidence of the Other underlines my insight, prudence and circumspection.

The one caring feels more masterful in the face of another's weakness. Bauman (1988/1998) continues,

> Following its own logic, imperceptibly and surreptitiously, without fault of mine or ill will, care has turned into power. Responsibility has spawned oppression. Service rebounds as a contest of wills. Because I am responsible, and because I do not shirk my responsibility, I must force the Other to submit to what I, in my conscience, interpret as "her own good." There is no point in accusing me of greed or possessiveness, even of egotism: I still act for the Other's sake, I am still a moral self, unconcerned with self-interest, not counting costs, ready for sacrifice. There is really no other thing I am

to do, because I am responsible. So I will respond to the charges . . . there is no good solution in sight. If I do not act on my interpretation of the Other's welfare, am I not guilty of sinful indifference? And if I do, how far should I go in breaking the Other's resistance; how much of her autonomy may I take away? . . . There is but a thin line between care and oppression, and the trap of unconcern awaits those who know it, and proceed cautiously as they become aware of trespassing. . . . Post-modern ethics, suggests Marc-Alain Ouaknin, "is an ethics of caress, an allegory first used by Levinas for care in 1947. . . . The caressing hand, characteristically, remains open, never tightening into a grip, never 'getting hold of'; it touches without pressing, it moves obeying the shape of the caressed body." (pp. 91-92)

When we open ourselves up to our own woundedness and finitude and meet the other without trying to "fix" them and without omnipotent pretenses, we can begin to learn anew the healing power of love and the sufficiency of grace in the midst of the risks of life.

Mercy consists of an urge to free another human being from his sufferings. If it serves another goal, for example, the stabilization of society, it is replaced by an indifference towards the other person's sufferings. The ulterior motive transforms mercy into its opposite. (Logstrup, 1995, p. 380)

Cynicism and disillusionment over power and profit motives might tempt us to settle for benign benevolence for the sake of improving society, but removing the good in a particular relationship does not ensure benevolence in the larger society and diminishes a coherent understanding of health care practice for practitioner and patient alike. In faith communities and in outreach with health ministries, the goal is to meet the other face to face and reduce a measure of our cynicism. Faith communities have much to offer nursing through the enrichment and living out of caring practices. And nursing can gain a new, more open context to develop caring practices that foster well-being in the individual and community.

I offer a prayer and "Lamentation" that is an expanded and revised version published earlier in The *Journal of Christian Nursing* (Benner, 1992).

Give us a new vision and new dreams.
There are money changers in the temple.
Thirty-nine million are uninsured,
     meaning we cannot and will not give them access
     to our help, our potions.
Our language of healing has been replaced by economism,
     cost-benefit analysis, futility assessment and utilization reviews.
We offer managed care that focuses
     more on efficiency than reliability,
     more on curing than healing,
     more on controlling than caring.
Cost-saving formulas without considering what is worthwhile
     leave us impoverished.

People are assessed, diagnosed, found wanting and processed,
     and we do not notice that they are hungry,
     thirsty, and frightened.
World and care have broken down and we offer a sophisticated
     technical fix, glorying in our powers and prowess and
     covering over our powerlessness, our inattention, our arrogance.
We stand ready with our crash carts and emergency procedures,
     ignoring our environment, our poverty, our homelessness,
     the care of young mothers, our unhealthy workstyles.
Our "temples of healing" have become "Midas Muffler
     repair shops," specializing, breaking down into small parts,
     mastering, dominating, and controlling in ways that
     focus on the bottom line.
Our quality assurance focuses on complications,
     how far short we fell on our standards of control.
We pass over restoration, recovery, healing, thanksgiving,
     and celebration, forgetting to count what counts.
Our buildings and patient care rooms do not soothe us,
     our technology is jerryrigged. We have designed for
     techno-fix and medical specialization and have not
     created spaces for families, for communities,
     public spaces for healing.
We have desecrated sacred places for healing with noise,
     pollution, crowding, and neverending equipment.
Our "intensive care" units are frightening inhospitable places,
     where increasingly we restrain, paralyze,* and
     otherwise control bodies, failing to notice suffering
     participants and supplicants. Birth and death are no
     longer understood as meaningful human passages.
We long to have celebratory birthing rooms, but we do not
     find it economically attractive to cultivate the attentive,
     skilled know-how that prevents the need for excessive
     emergency surgical procedures.
Consequently, we have forgotten the ways of the body;
     we have failed to study and work with our embodied powers,
     preferring to substitute technical wizardry and quick
     technical fixes for daily care, nutrition, exercise, and love.
We have failed to notice that life is a gift filled with mystery,
     holy and worthy of our attentiveness and respect.
We need to create new lively traditions of justice
     and liberated caregiving.
A retreat to dead traditionalism and patterns of care based
     on inequality, domination, and subordination will not
     heal us. Returning to our sacred finite lives and
     diverse communities that celebrate and support life
     as creation is both a returning and a new beginning.

We overlook death as passage, destiny, tragedy, closure,
    epiphany. Our connections are broken. We seldom
    hold our loved ones as they die.
We do not know how to midwife our deaths.
Families and communities of memory are rushed in at
    the last minute after professional strangers have born
    witness to poignant human struggles and isolated suffering.
We are constantly in danger of being blinded by our desires
    to be heroic rescuers, preventing death at all costs, and
    we face the equal danger of not caring enough to notice
    the human possibilities of recovery and offering what
    we can in the midst of possible loss, possible "futility."
We have become invisible members of corporate systems of
    health as a commodity, commercial enterprises that
    encourage individuals to avoid diseases to minimize costs.
We have forgotten health as liveliness, blessing, gift,
    suppleness, as spirit and spiritedness.
Those that would bring healing and be healed have
    lost their place to stand.
We are wounded and wounding "healers," defining
    ourselves as codependents to people who have failed
    to manage their lives and their bodies so that they
    possess the precious commodity of health.
We are suspicious of the possibilities of mercy and
    generosity. After all, mercy, generosity, grace, and
    forgiveness would wreck our systems of control, of
    blame and shame, of inclusion and exclusion, our cost shifting.
Instead of standing alongside the wounded and suffering,
    admitting our common humanity, we try to fix the wounds,
    and failing that we blame the wounded for their attitude,
    their failed lifestyle, their lack of individual control.
We no longer understand our society, community, family,
    and our spirit as sources of healing.
We have a strange and estranged relationship with suffering.
We use it as a tool of pity, a source of blame, or experience
    it as a terrible embarrassment, a failure, a momentary
    breakdown of control—the technological promise.
We have colonized sickness and made it an industry
    of assessment, diagnosis, and deficit accounting;
    we give little attention to our healing arts.
We are like the man at the pool of Bethesda when asked
    by Jesus if he would be healed; we offer excuses
    and reasons why we cannot make it to the healing waters.
We prefer despair over freedom, understanding "freedom"
    as disconnectedness, disengagement, unencumberance:
    freedom *from* instead of freedom *to be* and to be with others.

We have made recovery a neverending project instead
    of an epiphany, a new beginning.
We do not understand how to be taught, healed,
    and comforted in our suffering.
Like ourselves, illness becomes a possession to be
    used instead of being a place of teaching,
    an occasion of courage and healing.
We make illness an altar of self-pity and secondary gains.
We have made "being healthy" a career and have
    forgotten its giftedness.
We have forgotten how to come together as communities
    of concern rather than competing individuals
    who forget that we all are needy at times.
We have covered over our embodied capacities and limitations.
We seek to transcend our bodies rather than respect and
    live within our bodily capacities and limitation.
We have lost our stories of healing.
We have lost our stories of suffering.
We have lost our stories that create us, sustain us,
    and bind us together as supplicants and celebrants.
We have colonized health and lost our ability
    to rejoice in it, protect it, and preserve it.
We need a new vision of health and well-being.
Give us new dreams and new vision.
Help us to hear your stories.

---

* Paralytic agents are increasingly being used in critical care units.

References

Bauman, Z. (1998). *Post-modern ethics.* Cambridge, MA: Blackwell. (Original work published 1988)

Benner, P. (1992). Lamentations. *Journal of Christian Nursing, 9*(3), 9-11.

Benner, P., & Wrubel, J. (1989). *The primacy of caring: Stress and coping in health and illness.* Redding, MA: Addison-Wesley.

Bonhoeffer, D. (1954). *Life together* (J. W. Doberstein, Trans.). New York: Harper.

Logstrup, K. E. (1995). *Metaphysics* (Vol. 2; R. L. Dees, Trans.). Milwaukee, WI: Marquette University Press.

Logstrup, K. E. (1997). *The ethical demand.* Notre Dame, IN: University of Notre Dame Press. (Original work published 1956)

Taylor, C. (1989). *Sources of the self.* Cambridge, MA: Harvard University Press.

16

Ethics as a
Context for the Practice

Marsha Fowler

Are the ethical issues encountered by the parish nurse different from those encountered by nurses in other areas of clinical practice? Will the ethical discussion within parish nursing practice sound the same as that within secular nursing contexts? What questions must we address as we begin an exploration of the ethical issues of parish nursing?

The fundamental issues that the parish nurse faces, particularly in relation to caring for members of the congregation, are much the same as those faced by other nurses. Issues of respect for the parishioner's wishes, of capacity to give consent or under-standing and informedness, of privacy and confidentiality, of end-of-life decisions including treatment cessation, of truthfulness and promise keeping, of advocacy and intercession, of equitableness and discrimination confront the nurse whether in the parish or not. These issues are a common ethical bond joining those who engage in the clinical practice of nursing, irrespective of the setting. No, the ethical issues that confront the parish nurse are not different from those that confront any other nurse.

But, yes, they are different. There are features of the parish setting that bring new meaning and emphases to ethical practice. For instance, the ethical duties of privacy and confidentiality, duties that we observe and preserve, are nonetheless exercised differ-ently in a prayer community where a more intimate involvement in the lives of others, a commitment to pray for one another, and a shared faith journey are norms from which moral action follows. The setting itself, that is, the nature of the community, may modify the way in which the parish nurse exercises her ethical responsibilities.

In addition, the discernment of right and wrong, good and evil (a task of ethics) is tied to the tradition's theology. That theology will shape and inform decisions. For instance, the notion that the body is intrinsically good and not to be despised or eschewed is rooted in the doctrines of creation ("God created . . . and God saw that it was very good," Gen 1:27-31) and the incarnation (Christ could not have become flesh if the flesh were evil). Questions such as assisted suicide, suicide, and euthanasia must be examined in the light of notions of stewardship, that is, that "life is a gift and a loan" and our lives and bodies are not our own—they belong to God. Questions of the allocation of social resources are informed not only by concerns for distributive justice (the fair distribution of costs, the emphasis of the current health care reform) but more by compensatory justice as a religious duty to benefit the least well off in society, those who were of old called "the lame, the halt, and the blind," "the widow, the orphan, and the stranger in your land."

The discernment of right and wrong, good and evil is also tied to a methodology that is somewhat different from that employed in the secular nursing context. Here, Scripture, prayer, reason, additional standards of a particular tradition (policy statements, social witness documents, creeds and confessions, responsa), pastoral counsel, church teaching, and so forth are essential to that discernment. Yet, even more important, the eternal, infinite, transcendent, and unchanging God is also the self-disclosing God, the one who leads, comforts, and sustains us. Within the Christian tradition, to which we turn in the discussion below, reliance upon the Holy Spirit is essential and imperative. In this, then, the moral discourse within parish nursing will sound different from that heard in the secular settings of nursing.

Ethics:
A Panoramic Snapshot

Ethics as Philosophy and Theology

Ethics, as a field, is related to philosophy as one of the five major divisions of philosophy: epistemology, logic, metaphysics (ontology and cosmology), aesthetics, and ethics. Ethics is the least well developed of the philosophical fields; philosophers have, in centuries past, generally been more interested in metaphysics than in ethics. In addition, of the three major divisions of ethical inquiry—metaethics, normative ethics, and descriptive ethics—philosophers have often been more interested in metaethics than in normative or applied normative ethics. Applied normative ethics has, however, always been a particular concern of religious bodies. Historically, religious leaders had the task of identifying acts for which the faithful should feel contrite and because of which they should be repentant, and the faithful depended upon religious leaders to help them discern right and wrong and good and evil when faced with the complexities of daily life. This was the case for individuals who sought the counsel of the priest or rabbi as well as for nations or communities that had gone astray only to suffer the scrutiny and furious condemnation of their prophets. Where ethics is seen as a part of theology, rather than philosophy, it is derived from Biblical or historical or constructive theology. Ethics within Biblical theology addresses those questions that are directly addressed by Scripture, questions such as right worship, usury, harmful speech, gluttony, and adultery. Ethical questions about recombinant DNA, nuclear warfare, or abortion cannot be addressed within Biblical theology per se, as Scripture does not mention these issues.

Instead, these and similar issues must be addressed through ethics in historical or constructive theology. Historical theology deals with what the church has believed and held to be the rule across centuries with regard to specific issues (e.g., priestly celibacy, nonmarital sex, usury, infanticide) and how those positions have developed. Constructive theology is concerned to bring Biblical and historical theology and philosophical-theological method to bear upon a wide range of questions, including those not directly addressed by Scripture (e.g., abortion, just war, national health insurance) but to which the observant believer must respond.[2]

There are some in philosophy who maintain that ethics is philosophical ethics and has no intercourse with theology. There are some in theology who maintain that ethics is theological ethics and is not informed by philosophy, or more specifically that religious ethics is ethics and that philosophy and theology do not meet. Between these poles, there are theologians and philosophers who fall all along the continuum. It is not our concern to debate this issue here. It is raised so that the reader will be aware of the variety of positions that exist and that exist even among Christian theologians. Where Christian theologians agree is on the point that there is no one ethics, no coherent system of ethics, to be found in Scripture itself; Scripture provides guidance (sometimes specific, sometimes general), but a coherent Christian ethic requires a constructive theological ethics. Here, some theologians will rely more and some less upon nonreligious philosophy, Scripture, reason, or revelation.

The Divisions of Ethics

Ethics is customarily separated into three main divisions (Frankena, 1973). Metaethics is the more speculative division of ethics and may be seen as theorizing about ethics. Its concerns include questions of meaning and justification (e.g., "Why be good?"), of logic, semantics ("What do we mean by *good* or *just*?"), and epistemology ("How do I know the good?"). The technical answers to metaethical questions fall into a domain that is principally of interest to professional ethicists. Descriptive ethics is concerned with examining what a given group or people believe or how they behave ethically. Descriptive ethics may fall within the field of ethics itself, particularly when its concerns lead to normative discussion, or may instead be a part of anthropology, sociology, or psychology, in which it would remain purely descriptive. Normative ethics is concerned with questions of right and wrong and good and evil. Where normative ethics is used to examine questions related to a specific context (e.g., profession, parish), it is usually termed *applied* normative ethics. Applied normative ethics, our chief concern here, is the domain of ethics that is the day-to-day concern of all those who seek to behave in a morally right manner in daily life and to be good persons besides.

Normative Ethics

Normative ethics is divided into two main approaches, under which a wide range of ethical theories fall (Fowler, 1987). *Norms of obligation* is that division of normative ethics that is concerned with right and wrong actions, with duties, that is with what we *do*. Its applied emphasis is on doing that which is right and refraining from doing that which is wrong. Norms of obligation fall into two main systems of theories of ethics:

teleological (e.g., Utilitarianism) and deontological (e.g., ethical formalism). Teleological and deontological theories determine an action to be right or wrong in different ways.
In teleological systems, an action is right or wrong depending upon the consequences it
produces as measured against a specific desired end. For instance, if the end that is sought
in a particular theory were "the golden mean," or moderation, then an action would be
right or wrong depending upon its consequences as they were measured against the end
of the golden mean or moderation. Deontological theories determine an action to be right
or wrong based upon something other than the consequences of the action, usually its
conformity to a moral rule. For instance, an action would be right or wrong depending
upon its conformity to a moral rule of truth telling, and not the consequences of having
told the truth. Consequences in this case are not irrelevant, but neither are they consti-
tutive of the right. Various theories of obligation (e.g., Utilitarianism, Kantian Formalism, Hedonism, Stoicism) determine what is right or wrong in different ways. What is
important for our purposes here is that contemporary bioethics, whether backed by a
teleological or deontological framework, predominantly focuses on the use of ethical
principles and rules in the determination of right or wrong. This is not, however, the only
way to proceed in ethics.

   Norms of value is that division of ethics that is concerned with good and evil in what
we are or in what we cherish or seek. Its applied emphasis is on being and seeking good
and not being or seeking evil. Thus, the ethical theories that arise from this approach to
ethics will focus on virtues, or what we are to *be,* and will also examine the *ends* that we
seek.[3] The dominant form of bioethical discourse in this country relies heavily, almost
exclusively, upon a norms-of-obligation perspective. It is indeed a smaller voice, but
often a religious one, that speaks of an ethics of virtue. Let us now look more closely at
these two approaches.

Principles in Bioethics

   Most clinical ethical discussion of cases or issues relies heavily upon the use of
principles and rules in its analysis. There are various lists of principles and rules, but
those most commonly and regularly used are the ones discussed in Beauchamp and
Childress's (1994) excellent work, *Principles of Biomedical Ethics.* Those principles are
justice, respect for autonomy, nonmaleficence, and beneficence. Rules derived from
these principles include the rules of informed consent, privacy, confidentiality, sanctity
of life, quality of life, and so forth. Rules differ from principles in that they are derived
from principles and, although abstract and still general, are nonetheless more specific
than principles. Rules and principles help us to understand what our moral duties are,
what is morally right to do. The "bedside" principles (those useful at the microlevel, in
individual cases) are respect for autonomy, nonmaleficence, and beneficence; justice
tends to enter the discussion at the broader institutional or societal level. The use of these
principles in case analysis has become almost formulaic. It has been my observation that
under most conditions, respect for autonomy receives about 60% of the weight in the
United States, with nonmaleficence and beneficence following behind, in that order.
Discussions of principles of community or solidarity, although frequent in the discourse
heard in other countries, are rare here. This is to say that when we embrace certain
principles, excluding a discussion of others, we reflect certain theoretical as well as

cultural perspectives, and we should be aware of this. With that caveat, the reader is referred to *Principles of Biomedical Ethics* as a starting point for an exploration of the nature of each of the principles above.

Ethical Decision Making

Using these principles, the steps of ethical decisions making are (a) identification and statement of the problem, (b) gathering the morally relevant facts, (c) analysis using principles, (d) evaluation of action alternatives, (e) action, and (f) evaluation. The statement of the problem should be a straightforward statement of the raw case conflict, couched in ordinary language (e.g., "The parishioner is receiving an unwanted treatment"). The collection of morally relevant facts includes clinical medical and nursing facts, facts about the individual's desires and her or his values, facts about the context, and so on. Parishioner values are important facts to collect. In this step, the parish nurse must resist the temptation to engage in endless fact finding, hoping that possession of enough facts will make the moral dilemma evaporate. It will not. Facts inform but will not resolve ethical questions that are questions of value. For instance, we can be factually certain that a certain person will die without a ventilator, but that still does not answer the value question of whether or not the person ought to be put on a ventilator. The step of analysis relies upon the various principles and rules of ethics and also upon the moral rules of the profession (nursing) and the community (church). Thus, additional moral documents, such as the *Code for Nurses* (American Nurses' Association, 1985), the Bible, and denominational creeds and confessions, will further inform the analysis and decision-making process. In the evaluation of possible actions, we measure those actions against the principles and rules that they affirm or violate and choose accordingly. Action follows choice and evaluation follows action. Here we must ask not only whether the outcome was as hoped, but whether the dilemma could have been prevented. The best ethics is preventive ethics.

If this process of decision making resembles the nursing process, it is not by accident. Although many have propounded various decision-making formats, decision trees, algorithms, and so on, there is no need to resort to a process that is different from that which is already embedded in nursing. Diagnostic decision making, whether medical or nursing or ethical or automotive, all takes place under conditions of uncertainty. For that reason, the steps of the processes must incorporate specific features that, in the end, make the processes essentially similar. It seems most reasonable not to forsake a process that is already fixed in nursing education and practice and is universal and serviceable. Rather, the process should simply be adapted to the ethical arena.

The principled approach is not the only approach to decision making. Depending upon the theoretician, it may be integrated with or supplanted by a virtue-based perspective.

Virtues and Excellences in Nursing's Ethics

Although ethical discourse has tended to focus on the use of principles and rules, nursing (and the Christian community) has always had an interest in an ethics of virtue. Indeed, an ethics of virtue dominated nursing's ethics until the 1970s, after which there was a shift toward an ethics of obligation. This shift took place in general society as well, but nursing's redirection took approximately 10 to 20 years longer, probably owing to the location of its education within relatively sequestered hospital-based schools (Fowler, 1985). These schools had many of the characteristics of Goffman's (1961) "total institution," where personal behavior was closely scrutinized and regulated. This early nursing ethics has often been characterized as an "ethics of etiquette," though this is to misunderstand and miscast it. Certainly questions of etiquette were addressed, but not as etiquette per se, rather as a piece of a larger ethics of virtue wherein no behavior (whether public, professional, or private) was seen as irrelevant to the character of the moral agent.

Virtues are habits of character that predispose a person to do what is right (i.e., the good person; Frankena, 1973). Excellences, a subset of virtue, are habits of character that predispose a person to do a specific task or job well (e.g., the good parish nurse; Youngblood, 1986). Virtues are universal and excellences are particular. In reviewing more than 100 years of nursing ethical literature in the United States, the following virtues and excellences thought to be important for the "good nurse" to possess were culled from the literature of approximately 700 articles and books. These virtues and excellences include:

> absolute accuracy, accepts criticism, adaptable, agreeable, alert, appreciative, calm, charitable, cheerful, Christian, clean, comforting, competent, conscientious, considerate, contented, controlled, cooperative, courageous, cultured, decisive, decorous, dependable, devoted, dignified, disciplined, discriminating, discreet, eager, economical, economizing, efficient, emotionally mature, enduring, enthusiastic, even tempered, ever ready, faithful, faithful to duty, fealty, finesse, firm, friendly, gentle, gentle words, gentler virtues, good breeding, good grammar, good memory, good posture, good reputation, gracious, healthful, healthy, helpmate, high thinking, honest, humanitarian, humble, humorous, impartial, industrious, inspires confidence, inspiring, intelligent, intuitive, joyful, kind, liberal of thought, likes people, long-suffering, loving, loyal, meek, mentally fit, morally pure, neat, noble, nonmalevolent, obedient, open minded, patient, patriotic, peaceable, perceptive, perfect woman, physically fit, plain living, pleasant personality, poised, praiseworthy, principled, protective, prudent, public spirited, punctual, pureheart, pure manner, pure speech, quickness, quiet, ready, reassuring, refined, reliable, reserved manner, resistant to infection, resourceful, respect for authority, responsible, restful, right living, righteous, satisfied, scientific attitude, seeks perfection, is self controlled, self respecting, self sacrificing, selfless, sense of fitness, sincere, skilled, smiling, soft hand, spiritual, spontaneous, stable, strong, studious, sweet, sympathetic, systematic, tactful, tasteful dress, teachable spirit, team worker, tender hearted, thorough, thoughtful, uncomplaining, unobtrusive, unselfish, unselfish soul, versatile, vigilant, virtuous, welcomes criticism, wholesomeness, womanliness. (Fowler, 1985)

When those "virtues" and "excellences" that are not really virtues or excellences are discarded, the list narrows to:

> benevolent, caring, compassionate, competent, courageous, devoted, faithful, integritous, just, kind, knowledgeable, loving, loyal, nonmalevolent, teachable, temperate, trustworthy, wise, understanding, veracitous.

These are, of course, the attributes of moral character that we would like to see in all nurses. The concern here is not to return to a scrutiny of the moral purity of the nurse but to ascertain the moral milieu that will best support and foster the development of such virtues among nurses in practice. Although it remains unexplored in the nursing ethical literature, there are excellences that are particular not simply to nursing in general, but to particular nursing specialties as well. For instance, the excellences that would make a good trauma nurse are not the same as might receive emphasis in the hospice nursing setting. As the clinical specialty develops, it would be fruitful to explore the particular excellences that would make a good parish nurse.

Clinical ethical discourse in the United States has emphasized the kinds of analysis and decision making that have relied heavily upon norms of obligation; that is, upon principled or rule-based reasoning. Early nursing ethics relied almost exclusively upon norms of value (that is, upon virtue ethics) to guide its practice. The presumption was that if the nurse possessed the proper moral character, that nurse would inevitably do what was right. Both approaches represent an overemphasis. It is not a situation of either/or but rather of both/and: principles and their subsidiary rules, without virtues, are impotent; virtue, without the principles and rules, is directionless (Frankena, 1973).

Ethics Within a Covenant Community

Parish Nursing as a Specialized Call and a Nursing Specialty

When we speak of ethics in parish nursing, we speak of nursing in a specific setting, one that shapes and informs practice. This specialty of nursing brings concepts of vocation and covenant community together with a specialized clinical nursing practice. Its identity is vocational, its intent is ministry, its instrument is nursing, and its involvement is covenantal.

Parish nursing's identity is vocational in the sense of vocation (from the Latin, *vocare,* "to call")[4] as a call or summons by God to "exercise a special function, especially of a spiritual nature," for which one has been gifted by God. It is a call to serve God, here, in a health ministry. It is a "special life work," a profession in the original sense (Latin, *professio,* a "public declaration") for which one has been given gifts, to which one has been called, and in which one finds self-identity.

Parish nursing's intent is ministry; that is, it serves a spiritual function, exercising spiritual gifts, to reclaim the fragmented parts of our lives, bringing them together in whole-person care that believes the spiritual to be the integrating and unifying force. Here, health is defined in terms of *shalom*[5] and also of reconciliation, healing, and incarnation rather than in terms of the World Health Organization's (1946) definition of health.[6]

Parish nursing's instrument is nursing, a concern for the person's "human responses" to actual or potential health problems, to the ends codefined by ministry and nursing goals. Here, at times, nursing may be subordinate to ministry.

Parish nursing's involvement is covenantal in that the nurse is a member of a community in which all members are bound to one another by God and seek faithfully to worship and serve God for God's glory, God's joy, and neighbor's good. Parish nursing, then, will be directed toward the community of faith itself *and* in outreach to the larger community surrounding it, sometimes toward society, and perhaps toward international missions as well.

Parish nursing is not public heath nursing with a change of venue. Parish nursing is not home health nursing with a change of venue. Because it is nursing, the values, relationships, aims, and ends of parish nursing share some commonalties with any other form of nursing, yet its practice is distinctive. Parish nursing is an emerging form of advanced nursing practice, an emerging specialty, that is chiefly defined by the spiritual and ministry values that undergird and drive its practice and by its concern for the spiritual aspects of care central to its existence and exercise. One's view of parish nursing is informed by nursing knowledge and practice but is also informed and shaped by the community of worship and fellowship, the sacred Scriptures, creeds and confessions, the canons of faith, prayer, and the spiritual disciplines. Nursing in a church that does not reflect this may be nursing in a church but it is not parish nursing; indeed, such nursing is to parish nursing as carob is to chocolate. There are certain similarities, but they are not interchangeable, and one is not a substitute for the other.

There are many other distinctive areas of parish nursing that make it radically different from other specialties in nursing, both in content and in patient population. Although space does not permit a detailed discussion here, two brief examples will suffice for substantiation. Parish nurses function intergenerationally. They function intergenerationally within the setting, as churches are inclusive of all age groups. However, parish nurses also function intergenerationally within any given family. In one church in which I served, I worked with families with four and five (and even six) generations of members in that church. In working with these families, individual members of the family were always "patients" in two senses: as individuals and as a family unit.

Another distinctive area of parish nursing is highlighted by what occurs when a parishioner dies. The parish nurse is a specialist in spiritual aspects of patient care. The parish nurse "walks" with the parishioner, often from before the time of symptom discovery or recognition through awareness of symptoms, diagnosis and treatment, to the "death vigil." When the person dies, the parish nurse bears the task of providing spiritual and bereavement support to the surviving spouse, to the family as a whole, and to the larger nonfamily relational community to which the person belonged. In some instances, this involves the parish-nurse-as-minister in conducting anointing, funeral, or memorial services and presiding at graveside burial or the scattering of ashes. Thus, other distinctive areas of parish nursing are the length of the involvement with an individual, the responsibility for assisting not just the patient and family to grieve during impending death and death but the community itself in mourning the loss of a member, and engagement in priestly functions. The parish nurse's patient is simultaneously (and longitudinally) the individual, the family, and the parish community. The patient is also simultaneously *patient* and *beloved member of the flock.*

A parish nurse is not, cannot be, and ought never to be reduced to "a nurse in a church." Parish nursing and nursing in a church are profoundly different. This fact has deep ethical implications.

Ethical Issues in Parish Nursing

There are a number of ethical issues that confront the parish nurse and are also encountered by nurses in other practice settings and specialties. For example, issues of privacy and confidentiality, of treatment at the end of life, of advocacy, and of the allocation of resources are not new to nursing. Yet, within the faith community, ethical dilemmas are shaped a bit differently and reflect some distinctive features in parish nursing. Intended as a basis for initiating discussion, a preliminary consideration of sample issues follows.

Privacy and Confidentiality

Issues of privacy and confidentiality are usually discussed in relation to their consideration as an aspect of the principle of respect for autonomy. Privacy refers to that sphere of personal experiences, including secrets, that one has a right to preserve and to have protected from discovery. Like a diary, these areas of life may not be entered by others without an invitation. It is a stringent (not an absolute) right, which is to say that compelling justification is necessary to override duties related to the protection of privacy or the maintenance of confidentiality. Confidentiality stems from a relationship of trust and mutual respect and refers to safeguarding information about others, information with which one has been entrusted or to which one has been allowed access. Such information is not to be passed on without permission of the person(s) involved. In the general arena of nursing practice, these concerns include the prohibition against unnecessary data collection and against disclosure of medical or nursing information without patient or family permission. These discussions provide general guidelines for all nurses, parish nurses included.

Yet the faith community within which a parish nurse labors possesses characteristics not common to other areas of nursing practice. First, there is a commitment to share one another's burdens, to walk with one another in the valley of the "dark shadow," and to pray for one another. This necessitates the disclosure of some of the darker moments of life—a child gone astray, chemical dependency, a haunting past—as well as public acknowledgment of life's more overt sorrows—spousal death, personal illness, increasing frailty. Second, faith communities are communities of confession, contrition, penitence, and repentance. We disclose not only our sorrows, but our sins, that we might be healed of them and renewed in faith and life. In this context, private as well as public disclosure may reach levels not encountered elsewhere in society. It is not unusual for the pastoral prayer during worship to include personal requests for health-related problems or for the "prayer chain" to be invoked for behaviors or conditions we would not openly discuss in other contexts. In some traditions, sins—not simply ones that have been or are about to be discovered—are openly confessed to the entire congregation and forgiveness is petitioned. These features of the faith community serve to relocate the lines of privacy and confidentiality as we understand them in general society, leaving the parish nurse in the quandary of discovering where those lines run in a particular congregation.

What then might be some guidelines for privacy and confidentiality? The sphere of individual privacy often narrows in the church community and even further in the pastoral relationship. Probing may be permitted in that relationship, beyond what is permitted elsewhere. Here both parishioners and pastoral caregivers enter into a relationship with sacred characteristics, one implicitly bound by a rule of silence and characterized by deep vulnerabilities. What is disclosed in these relationships, particularly where the parishioner understands them as sin, often calls for a specifically priestly response, one that may or may not fall within the authority of the parish nurse, depending upon the tradition involved. The power of those moments is profound, moving, and seductive. Parish nurses must bring to these encounters an awareness of their own needs for power and authority and must avoid, among other things, the temptation to seek private disclosure that is unrelated to the parish nursing role or beyond the authority or pastoral skill of the nurse. Uses of power and authority, or more specifically abuses of power or authority leading to the harm of others, are important ethical issues in themselves but beyond the scope of this article.

The simplest way to handle issues of confidentiality is to take the more stringent approach; that is, always to ask, never to presume, even in a community that is unusually open. Congregations are better served when the boundaries of privacy and confidentiality are made explicit. However, even in communities where secrets are openly shared and where the community understands them to be open secrets to which all have access, they are nonetheless open secrets *only* within that community and may not be shared beyond without permission. Permission to pass information to a church prayer chain or to include it in a pastoral prayer during worship is not permission to mention it at a diocesan (larger judicatory) meeting.

Treatment at the End of Life

Contemporary medical technology allows us to keep the lungs respiring, heart pumping, and cells metabolizing even in a dead body. This has profound implications for the choices that we make regarding the technological interventions available to us at the end of life. Where life can be sustained beyond all human dignity, some anticipatory consideration should be given to these choices. General bioethical guidelines for withholding or withdrawing life-sustaining treatment are fairly well-settled questions in the ethical literature. They are reflected by two statements that can be found in the President's Commission (1983) report *Deciding to Forego Life-Sustaining Treatment.* The first is that "neither criminal nor civil law—if properly interpreted and applied . . . forces patients to undergo procedures that will increase their suffering when they wish to avoid this by foregoing life-sustaining treatment" (p. 89). Patients do not have to accept treatment, even life-sustaining treatment, if, in their own estimation, it will increase or protract their suffering. In addition, the President's Commission notes that "the distinction between failing to initiate and stopping therapy—that is, withholding versus withdrawing treatment—is not itself of moral [or legal] importance. A justification that is adequate for not commencing a treatment is also sufficient for ceasing it" (p. 61). The adequate moral justifications for not commencing a treatment are (a) the patient does not want it (the principle of respect for autonomy), (b) it might harm the patient (the principle of nonmaleficence), or (c) it will not benefit the patient (the principle of beneficence). These three reasons are the same adequate moral reasons for ceasing treatment once it has begun—that is, for withdrawing treatment even if it is life sustaining.

The parish nurse is confronted with the issue of life-sustaining treatment in several ways. First, parish nurses often assist parishioners to complete advance directive forms (e.g., Durable Power of Attorney for Health Care, Living Will, Directive to Physicians) and must help sort out the issues in the light of their faith. Second, parish nurses are sometimes called upon to advocate for a parishioner who is receiving end-of-life treatment that is futile or that he or she does not want. The general ethical guidelines are clear and affirm those derived from Christian theological ethics, but the realities of hospital care often violate these guidelines and engage in *vitalism,* the preservation of human biological life at any or all costs.[7] It should be noted that as economic pressures on the health care delivery system increase, there may also be a tendency to withhold or withdraw treatment, perhaps on unacceptable moral grounds.

How does the Christian faith inform decisions about life-sustaining treatments? At the level of daily practice, ethical actions that are made in the secular or in the parish contexts may be indistinguishable from one another. Where they differ is in their ground of justification. The Christian and the non-Christian nurse may both agree that vitalism is morally wrong—but for different reasons. For example, the Nicene Creed states that "we believe in the Holy Spirit, the Lord and Giver of Life."[8] This reflects the Christian understanding that life is a gift of God and that all life belongs to God. Humankind is, consequently, not at liberty to take human life (one's own or that of another) except where allowed by God. Clearly, such a position would lead to discussions of capital punishment, warfare, abortion, suicide, and euthanasia. Our concern here is for the appreciation of life-sustaining treatment. If life is given by and belongs to God, it is, for us, a gift and a loan, and we are its stewards. The implications at their most basic are, first, that we may not choose death over life when there is a genuine choice within our power. Here, the life that is irretrievably moving toward death, or that entails unrelievable and unendurable suffering in the dying, does not present us with a genuine choice and preserving it may be seen as an idolatrous preservation of life or as an obstruction of God's will. The second implication is that we may not frivolously disregard life and health. Yet the lifestyles that many of us lead in the fast lanes of American society do, indeed, frivolously disregard health. In this brief chapter, it is impractical to draw out the nuances of this discussion. However, it is important to note that both implications relate to our understanding of the doctrines of God, creation, the incarnation, and stewardship and are profoundly informed by the Christian vision of life and its meaning.

Rendering Unto Caesar

There are ethical issues for parish nurses that extend beyond those of direct involvement with parishioners. For instance, a substantial number of ethical issues are raised when a parish nurse forms an alliance with a secular institution. One example might be when a parish nurse is formally the employee of a local hospital.

Although it is not a model that dominates in other parts of the country, California has many instances in which a hospital or HMO has hired a "parish nurse" as an employee. These organizations often are nonparochial—that is, explicitly nonreligious. Several issues arise here, not the least of which is the underlying motivation for creating this position. First, nurses are often lured with a substantial administrative-level salary (e.g., $60,000-$75,000). The effect of this is to bring applicants from all sectors of nursing, whether parish nurses or not; it is not unusual for the organization to hire the non-parish nurse (who may or may not have a faith commitment or an education or background in spiritual care) as a parish nurse. In addition, a salary of that amount, although perhaps warranted, engenders a loyalty to the institution that may subordinate the values of this emerging specialty or the community served.

In some instances, particularly where the institutions have been strongly secular, the spiritual care focal point of parish nursing is anathema to the organization. Parish nurses have been instructed either to set spiritual assessment and intervention aside or, worse, have been prohibited from such involvement. In other instances, it has been made clear that spiritual care is unwelcome but not prohibited. It must be conducted, however, on the nurse's own time, not the institution's. In situations such as these, the parish nurse runs the risk of being reduced to "a nurse in a church" and to having primary allegiance co-opted by salary.

Caesar can co-opt in another way. In one county, a health department held a free vaccination clinic and no one came. When the vaccines were given to a local church for their health fair clinic, the 500 vaccines were not enough to go around. Giving vaccines in a church-run health fair or clinic is not itself wrong. What is problematic is when the parish nurse who staffs the health fair is required to give the vaccines. Apart from the fact that parish nurses giving vaccines is not within the scope of their practice as it has been described in the literature, something is wrong when the labor costs of giving vaccines are borne not by the county health department but by the church. The church health fair needs to open its doors to county participation but not to do the work of the county.

Let us take this same example a bit farther. In the current health care context, society has been rightly concerned about cost cutting. What this has meant, however, has been shorter hospital stays, with patients emerging "quicker and sicker." The majority of these persons return to a home where, in most cases, a woman renders care. Cost cutting, then, has resulted in moving costs from third-party payors (who reimbursed a paid professional labor force) to an unpaid labor force of women in the home; this is cost shifting rather than cost cutting and raises serious ethical questions of the value and treatment of women in society. Similarly, in some public sector-church cooperation, there is a risk, again, of cost shifting, particularly through the use of women. As in the example above, when a local health department provides flu vaccine to a church and parish nurses, who are mostly women, administer the vaccine rather than facilitating the health department's access to parishioners, cost shifting to women may again be taking place. Cost shifting is not simply a matter of Caesar and the church; it is also a feminist issue. With regard to larger societal issues such as these, careful discussion of the role of the parish nurse (and women) and the relationship between the parish and society is essential.

Alliances with "Caesar" present ethical dilemmas for parish nurses, some of a subtle, and some of a not-so-subtle, nature. The parish nurse owes Caesar only that which is truly Caesar's. Parish nurses must be clear about identity, focus of practice, and primary allegiances and avoid the co-optation of the nurses or the church's labor.

One final word about ethics and labor. The church itself may use nurses wrongfully. Many persons donate their personal labor to the church; that is how a church functions.

For example, the deacons may divide the Sunday service flower arrangements and deliver flowers to shut-ins. Others may volunteer to teach the children of the congregation in Sunday School. Many professionals even donate their professional skills to the church; however, most do so only episodically or even just once rather than on an ongoing basis. For example, a congregant who is an architect may donate her or his professional skill to plan a classroom or nursery addition to the church facilities. Few professionals use or are called upon to use their professional skill by the church on an ongoing basis without compensation. Parish nurses who volunteer their professional skills must be careful that the church itself is not wrongfully taking advantage of professional, and usually female, labor.

Conclusion

Parish nurses face morally exciting times. Many of the most egregious moral failures of the health care delivery system can be addressed in new and more healing ways within the parish setting. The moral dilemmas that parish nurses face are similar to those faced by all nurses. Yet the faith community brings a different structure of values, a different understanding of life, a different understanding of our relationships with one another, and a different understanding of health and healing to bear upon these dilemmas. As parish nurses, insofar as we seek to use our gifts in the service of the living God, seeking "to do justice, to love kindness, and to walk humbly with God" (Micah 6:8), seeking to love God and neighbor as ourselves, we will find true healing and *shalom,* both for ourselves, for our parishioners, and for our neighbor.

Notes

1. I write from within the Western Christian tradition and endeavor to keep any remarks generally reflective of that tradition. Limitations of space prevent discussion of ethics as related to specific Western Christian traditions (e.g., Roman Eastern Christianity, or the Western traditions, or Eastern religions). Shul nursing is a term that I have coined to represent nurses in the synagogue with a Jewish faith commitment. It is my attempt to begin to widen the parish nursing lexicon to encompass and more accurately represent other non-Christian faith traditions as well. For instance, we need terms that will also be inclusive of the mosque. Note that the term "parish" is not a term used by all Christian denominations, although all would understand it. I do recognize the growing shul nurse movement in this country; I regret—deeply—that limitations of space permit me only to speak from within my own Christian tradition.

2. The doctrine of the Trinity, of God as a unity-in-trinity, is an example of an important doctrine that has chiefly been developed in constructive theology. Nowhere in scripture is the word *trinity* mentioned, and a theology of the Trinity is not developed in Scripture. The basics of the doctrine took almost 400 years to become established. Major disagreements continued for almost 12 centuries, and several remain with us today. This development and these questions would be addressed within historical theology. In some instances, constructive theology is seen to encompass historical theology.

3. In the interests of space, I will defer a discussion of nonmoral values (e.g., health, community, wholeness) here.

4. All definitions are taken from the *Oxford English Dictionary.*

5. The word *shalom* is customarily translated as *peace* in English, a translation that heartily fails to reflect the extraordinary richness and complexity of the concept. According to Youngblood (1986), the word shalom, "one of the most significant theological terms in Scripture, has a wide semantic range stressing various nuances of its basic meaning: totality or completeness. These nuances include fulfillment, completion, maturity,

soundness, wholeness (both individual and communal), community, harmony, tranquillity, security, well-being, welfare, friendship, agreement, success, and prosperity" (p. 732).

6. The World Health Organization (1946) has defined health as "a state of complete physical, mental, and social well-being, not just the absence of disease or infirmity."

7. *Vitalism* is a violation of the dignity of the person and is morally unacceptable. Sustaining biological life for the purpose of preserving organs for transplantation does not fall within the definition of vitalism.

8. The Nicene Creed, also called the Niceo-Constantinopolitan Creed, is regarded as one of the "universal creeds" affirmed by all of Christendom, East and West. It was written by the universal church council of Nicea and Constantinople and is credited to the Council of Constantinople of 381 A.D. (see Presbyterian Church, 1991).

References

American Nurses Association. (1985). *Code for nurses, with interpretive statements.* Kansas City, MO: Author.

Beauchamp, T., & Childress, J. (1994). *Principles of biomedical ethics* (4th ed.). New York: Oxford University Press.

Fowler, M. (1985). Nursing's ethics, 1898-1984. In A. Davis, M. Aroskar, J. Liaschenko, & T. Drought (Eds.), *Ethical dilemmas and nursing practice* (4th ed., pp. 17-34). Stamford, CT: Appleton & Lange.

Fowler, M. (1987). Introduction to ethics and ethical theory: A road map to the discipline. In M. Fowler & J. Levine-Ariff (Eds.), *Ethics at the bedside* (pp. 24-38). Philadelphia: C. V. Mosby.

Frankena, W. (1973). *Ethics* (2nd ed.). Englewood Cliffs, NJ: Prentice Hall.

Goffman, E. (1961). *Asylums.* New York: Anchor.

Presbyterian Church, (USA). (1991). "Nicene Creed," *Book of Confessions,* n.p., section 1.3.

President's Commission for the Study of Ethical Problems in Medicine and Biomedical and Behavioral Research. (1983, March). *Deciding to forego life-sustaining treatment.* Washington, DC: Government Printing Office.

World Health Organization. (1946). *Definition of health.* Geneva, Switzerland: Author.

Youngblood, R. F. (1986). Peace. In G. Bromily (Ed.), *The international standard Bible encyclopedia, Vol. 3* (Rev. ed.). Grand Rapids, MI: W. B. Eerdmans.

17

Parish Nursing
in Diverse Traditions

Mary Chase-Ziolek
Lawrence E. Holst

Introduction

Having begun in mainline Protestant and Catholic churches, parish nursing has grown to include increasingly diverse denominations and ethnic groups. For salaried parish nurses, this means there are more opportunities to work in congregations of faiths different from their own; the majority of unpaid parish nurses serve in their own congregations. For both, greater diversity in the field means an increased likelihood of participation in larger multicultural parish nursing groups of diverse faiths. For parish nurse coordinators, increasing diversity creates a challenge to create programs that are meaningfully interfaith and multiethnic.

The focus of this chapter will be on considerations for parish nurses and parish nurse coordinators who work with religious and ethnic traditions different from their own. The experience in this chapter reflects that of a long-standing, sizable, salaried parish nurse program and a newer, large, multiethnic, interfaith volunteer congregational health program.

Serving as a Parish Nurse in an
Unfamiliar Religious Tradition

Parish nurses who work in congregations with religious traditions different from their own will be required to become immersed in worship forms, doctrinal emphases, systems of governance, styles, nuances, and practices that may be unfamiliar. To be sensitive and responsive to these components of congregational culture is imperative if the nurse is to gain acceptance and respect and be integrated into the life of the faith community. Therefore, it is vital that nurses discuss these differences with the pastor or rabbi and be guided in appropriate background reading. Such reading should include historical overviews of a given faith's tradition, origins, founders, doctrinal emphases, and mission. In addition, nurses should become familiar with the history and current missions of the particular local congregation where they are employed because divergences exist as much within as between major faiths, owing to location, size, history, and lay and clergy leadership. For example, a small inner-city congregation may envision its mission and outreach quite differently than a large suburban congregation from the same denomination—which, likewise, may differ from a rural setting.

Although congregations of a major faith tradition will have much in common, there will always be unique local expressions. Some congregations are formal and ritualistic in their worship styles, others informal; some envision their missions as personal witnessing or evangelism, others as social activism; some may be doctrinally liberal, others conservative; some may be democratic in their polity, others authoritarian. These expressions are a reflection of the self-image of the congregation that shapes its way of being in the world (Dudley & Johnson, 1993). For nurses to move confidently through their assigned parishes, it is important that they have both national and local perspectives of their congregations and denominational affiliations.

The parish nurse needs to learn the culture of the congregation. One important component of the culture is language, which is a powerful social tool reflecting what is important to a given culture (Hall, 1976; Leininger, 1991). Attending to the words used to describe different components of congregational life helps to illuminate what is valued. Being sensitive to differences in terminology is also important in building relationships. For example, Catholic nurses working in Protestant churches would need to learn to refer to the Sunday morning service as a worship service rather than a mass and refer to the minister as a pastor rather than a priest. Another example of diverse terminology is the numerous descriptors and titles used for the ordained staff, such as pastor, minister, Reverend, Right Reverend, Very Right Reverend, Elder, Father, and Doctor. Pentecostal traditions often use the title Sister or Brother in reference to members, reflecting a sense of church as family. Table 17.1 provides questions to assist the parish nurse in beginning to learn the culture of the congregation.

Learning and using the appropriate language for a particular congregation is one way the parish nurse shows that she cares about what is important to the congregation and also that she belongs. The parish nurse should pay attention to frequently used terms and learn what they mean. Even with terms the nurse may be familiar with, such as *mission,* the nurse needs to learn what *mission* means for this particular congregation.

Parish nurses have been hired and worked effectively in congregations with traditions different than their own. That is, areas of conflict have been more theoretical than based on reality. For unpaid parish nurses, it can be difficult, although not impossible, to work in a congregation where they are not a member. One of the strengths of the unpaid parish nursing model, where the nurse typically serves in a congregation where she is a member, has been the ability of the nurse to build on existing knowledge of and commitment to relationships within a congregation. Volunteers are a mainstay of church and synagogue life, and it is not common for outsiders to volunteer for congregations.

TABLE 17.1 Questions for Parish Nurses to Consider When Working With Diverse Religious Traditions

1. What has the history of this congregation been?
2. How do they understand their mission or purpose?
3. How have they lived out this mission over time?
4. What historic, social, political, and economic factors have shaped this congregation?
5. How have health issues been addressed in the past?
6. What is happening in the congregation currently that promotes health and well-being?
7. What resources and materials are available from the denomination about parish nursing, health or health ministry?
8. How is the congregation organized?
9. What are the logical connections for parish nursing, including any groups with which the parish nurse should work?
10. What does the language of the congregation say about what is valued here?
11. What do any unfamiliar terms mean?
12. What documents are available that would help one gain an understanding of this congregation?

Why Have Conflicts Not Been Experienced?

This begs the question, Why have conflicts been minimal? The best that can be done is to summarize the experience of a long-standing salaried parish nurse program, with no claim that this experience is typical or even optimal. Paucity of conflict can mean there really is not much conflict, or it can mean that conflict is being denied. We can only hope that in this case, it is the former. The following reasons are cited as to why religious or doctrinal differences have not generated serious conflict between parish nurses and their employer congregations.

The Respective Partners

Parish nursing has tended to attract open-minded, curious, ecumenically oriented nurses who have easily adapted to unfamiliar religious practices. In fact, such differences have fostered creativity: Protestant nurses have come to appreciate the aesthetic beauty and structure of the Roman Catholics; Catholic nurses have had the opportunity to inaugurate services of healing in Protestant congregations. Tunnel vision has been overcome. It is also likely that any situation where religious differences would create a conflict are likely to be weeded out during the interview process. Congregations that would be uncomfortable with an interfaith program are not likely to even explore that option.

However, it should be noted that to date it has been predominantly mainline Protestant and Catholic churches that have caught the vision of parish nursing. In recent times, such traditions have become more cognizant of their common heritage and mission, fueled, no doubt, by religious pluralism, social mobility, and intermarriages. Such phenomena have tended to blur some denominational distinctions.

As one parish nurse, working in a congregation from a faith tradition different than her own, put it, "I was surprised to find so many parishioners who came out of my faith tradition."

The Spiritual Maturity of the Nurse

Much depends on the individual parish nurse and where she is on her spiritual journey. It would seem that personal confidence and spiritual maturity render one more open to newness and diversity, whereas a shallow, immature faith clings to rigid, restrictive patterns. Parish nursing, by virtue of its nontraditional nature, is likely to attract people who are open to new ideas.

None of the parish nurses interviewed related any major difficulties worshipping in the congregations where they work. They appreciated both the similarities and differences from the worship life they have known. Two practical problems did surface, however:

1. Because most nurses have Sunday morning responsibilities incumbent upon their positions, they are precluded from worshipping regularly with their own families, unless the families worship in the settings where the nurse is employed. When this does not occur, it is a real loss for the family. In the case of Catholic nurses working in Protestant settings, the issue may be somewhat minimized by the large selection of mass times available. In most cases, parish nurses are not required to be in their "employer churches" every Sunday, although there will be some interruption in the pattern of family worship practices.

2. When parish nurses worship in their assigned parish, sometimes they do not feel spiritually nourished—not because of doctrinal differences, but because they are always "working," even while worshipping. As one nurse put it, "It's hard for me to 'cool the motors': I catch myself looking around the worshipping congregation and identifying people I need to see that morning."

To worship where one is employed is not easy for any staff member; the distractions can be endemic. Of course, this problem would not be resolved even if the parish nurse were working in a congregation of her own faith tradition. It is an occupational hazard for employees of any church. Consequently, some parish nurses have had to seek spiritual nurture in other times and places, through spiritual advisers, small groups, or private meditation.

The Parish Nurse's Ministry Is Oriented to the Whole Person

The task of the parish nurse is to hear, assess, and respond to human needs by focusing on people in a broader faith context; she will rarely get involved in narrow doctrinal issues. As such, nurses are judged by their empathy, sensitivity, compassion, maturity, follow-through, and availability.

As hospital chaplains ministering to a spectrum of people have learned, hurts and needs are much the same the world over, and those common human denominators tend to pale religious, racial, or cultural differences. In fact, nurses say they have been surprised at how few in their congregation even knew the nurse's religious identity—and when they discovered it, it seemed to make little difference. As in other aspects of life, as relationships develop and trust grows, differences are easily absorbed.

No doubt it also helps that nurses are perceived as clinical persons, with specific and respected clinical skills. By tradition, they are perceived as helping, giving, nonthreatening persons. Although most parishioners are unaccustomed to seeing them in parish roles, most have encountered nurses in their lifetime and been helped by them.

The Mutual Respect Between Clergy and Parish Nurses

In most instances, parish nurses are considered part of the congregation's staff and are accountable to the clergy. Where it works—and it does in most cases—it is because clergy and nurse trust and respect one another. They are able to establish and live within parameters, meet with regularity, communicate openly, and adapt to each other's style. The strength of such a relationship can easily resolve conflicts over role, religion, competition, and/or personality. Trust allows feedback, which can head off problems. Troubles have more to do with the failure to trust and communicate than they have to do with denominational differences.

It also has been our experience that parish nurses working in a religious tradition different than their own pose problems less often then they create possibilities. In our judgment, this has been due to the mutual acceptance of the participating partners (congregations, pastors, and nurses), the nurse's and the congregation's spiritual maturity, the whole-person character of the nurse's ministry, and the mutual respect and communication capacities of the respective clergy and nurses.

Considerations for Parish Nurse Coordinators

From the perspective of a parish nurse coordinator, working with diverse religious groups presents unique challenges and opportunities. One challenge is to become familiar with the characteristics of different denominations as well as individual congregations. This begins with identifying denominational patterns that may affect the integration of parish nursing into congregations. Increasingly, denominations are developing materials on health, health ministry, and/or parish nursing. Any work done in these areas indicates a certain level of denominational awareness that may make individual congregations more receptive to the idea of parish nursing. Organizational patterns of denominations and individual congregations help to identify how parish nursing may fit into existing structures. That is, developing parish nursing is easier when there is a logical committee or area where it can fit within the culture of the congregation, such as a health and wellness board, ministry of care, nursing board, social concerns, or community outreach committee. The existence of pertinent committees can help to build a base of support for a parish nurse. In addition, it is important to help the congregation identify what health-related activities are already happening so the parish nurse can build on what exists rather than duplicating efforts.

Denominations all have a system of communication and regular meetings that can be used to expose multiple congregations to the concept of parish nursing. Asking to make presentations at these meetings or writing articles for denominational publications can be effective techniques for program development. When trying to include new religious groups in a program, the coordinator might try the useful approach of meeting with representative clergy and nurses from the group to talk about how a parish nursing program could fit into its denomination and congregations. These discussions may also reveal any pertinent language or programmatic considerations for incorporating parish nursing. Individual interviews or focus group techniques can accomplish this interchange.

Working with diverse religious groups also provides the opportunity to look at one's own faith and cultural assumptions. Often one is not cognizant of these assumptions until faced with someone who does not share them (Davis et al., 1992). Through becoming aware of their own assumptions about faith and culture, program coordinators will be better prepared to work with diverse groups without imposing their own values. Reflection, personally and with others doing similar work, is an effective way to gain insight into one's assumptions about religious and ethnic groups that are different from one's own. Having a willingness to learn about religious differences and similarities is an essential part of any coordinator's personal journey.

In addition, coordinators need a sincere desire to be inclusive in meaningful ways that go beyond simply transposing parish nursing from one setting to another. The seed of parish nursing is planted in each congregation and nurse, requiring room to grow in its own unique way. For individual congregations, this means not dictating what will happen but rather, through partnership, building on the unique interests, needs, and abilities of the congregation. For individual nurses, this means sensitive planning of orientation programs and support meetings that incorporate educational materials, devotions, and speakers reflective of the religious and ethnic groups of the participating parish nurses. One way to honor religious diversity within a parish nursing group is to have each nurse share something from her own faith perspective; a minority perspective cannot be successfully integrated if only the majority voice is heard.

Working With Synagogues

Examining efforts to include synagogues in parish nursing programs is a good example of issues that arise in working with diverse religious traditions. Parish nursing has developed almost exclusively within Christian churches, fitting well with the tradition of the healing ministry of Jesus. As parish nursing programs have grown, one logical question has been, how will this concept fit into other religious traditions, such as Judaism? Through working with synagogues to develop an interfaith volunteer congregational health program, a base of shared values was observed, as well as some significant differences. The values that Christians and Jews share include the Judeo-Christian tradition, reverence for life, concern for human welfare, shalom (see chapter 16), justice, wholeness, and the Hebrew Bible. Some significant differences between Christians and Jews include religious observances, cultural heritage, patterns of gathering, language, and Jewish law. The shared values provide an opportunity for building bridges from the parish nursing community to synagogues. The significant differences identify areas to be understood in making parish nursing relevant to the synagogue.

Many elements of Judaism support the role of health and healing within the congregation, including the essential emphasis on the sanctity of human life represented by the fact that preserving life is a *mitzvah* (commandment or obligation) that takes precedence over all others. There is also a religious imperative for keeping the body and soul healthy, reflected in the principle of *pikkuach nefesh*. Historically, the *kohanim* (priests) were responsible for the public health of the community, which reflected an interrelationship between religion and health. Likewise, Judaism has esteemed medicine, as it seeks to preserve life (Feldman, 1986).

There are theological roots that support the synagogue as a healing place, but functional differences between churches and synagogues do affect the introduction of parish nursing into the synagogue. Synagogues function in patterns that differ from those of many churches. For example, in urban areas, the provision of needed services has typically been organized through the larger Jewish community by the Jewish Federation. Services are provided for all Jews, regardless of synagogue affiliation, and in fact many Jews are not affiliated with a synagogue (Council of Jewish Federations, 1991). In Chicago, agencies such as the Council for Jewish Elderly, Jewish Children and Family Services, Jewish Vocational Services, and Jewish Community Centers provide services to the wider Jewish community, meaning that there are many organizations within Judaism other than the synagogue where needs are being identified and met.

The nature of Judaism (both a culture and a religion) is reflected in the pattern of organizing services for the broader community regardless of synagogue affiliation. In a survey of American Jews (Council of Jewish Federations, 1991), the majority (90%) saw Judaism as an ethnic or cultural identity, although 5% saw Judaism only as a religion. This interrelationship between culture and religion marks one of the differences between synagogues and many churches. An understanding of both Jewish culture and Judaism as a religion is needed to identify how parish nursing can be implemented in the Jewish community.

Currently, there is a growing interest in health and healing within the Jewish community, as demonstrated in the growth of Jewish healing centers (Flam, 1994). Synagogues are becoming increasingly involved in issues of health and healing. Several synagogues in the Chicago area have a congregation nurse. Others have regular healing services (Greene, 1994). One synagogue has had a support group for people who are chronically ill. Another synagogue has a health cabinet that addresses the health needs of the congregants (Ostrovsky, 1985).

In working to include synagogues in volunteer congregational health programming, those involved have raised such issues as language, the availability of Jewish nurses as potential volunteers within synagogue membership (it was felt that it would be much easier to find doctors and social workers), how the role of the nurse would fit within the congregation, and how this program would relate to (or compete with) other services within the Jewish community of services. Language differences were addressed by several rabbis during the development of the program. The language of parish nursing has developed from a Christian paradigm that, although it shares much with Judaism, does have distinct differences. *Parish* is a distinctly Christian term, as is *ministry*. Terms that some rabbis have identified as being more appropriate are *kallilah* (community) nurses or *congregation* nurses, and the concept of *mitzvah* is seen as more acceptable than *ministry*. Marsha Fowler elaborates on the term "shul nursing" in her notes to chapter 16 in this book. The concept of ministry also comes from a Christian perspective and is not shared by all world religions. The term *congregational health* rather than *parish nursing* was chosen for the interfaith volunteer program, to show sensitivity to these linguistic differences. *Congregation* is a more inclusive term that can be used for Christians and Jews. However, in Catholicism, congregation generally refers to religious communities.

In building bridges to synagogues, there are other Hebrew concepts that can be used to relate to congregational health. In addition to mitzvah, there is *bikkur cholim,* which is visiting the sick, and *pikkuach nefesh,* which is a religious obligation to protect health (Feldman, 1986). These are just a few examples that reflect the challenge of developing a language for parish nursing that will be sufficiently broad to comfortably include Christians, Jews, Muslims, and Buddhists and yet also be specific enough to be meaningful.

There are a small number of nurses working with synagogues in a parish nurse role; they are more commonly referred to there as congregation nurses. Although Judaism is well represented in medicine, nursing has not been a common profession. The common presence of nurses in churches (Westberg, 1990) is not duplicated in synagogues. For the nurses in the interfaith volunteer program who worked with synagogues, there were challenges in getting people to think of a nurse in the synagogue as being useful. This, in addition to the fact that the majority of members in their synagogues were very well connected to medical services, made a volunteer congregational health program a difficult concept to integrate into congregational life. However, salaried congregation nurses in various other programs have had more success.

In looking at the Jewish community in Chicago, it can be observed that the synagogue has not been the focal point for providing for social service or health needs. This has been done through the wider Jewish community. There have been rabbis who were very interested in the idea of a congregation nurse; however, one rabbi suggested that the Jewish Community Centers, instead of synagogues, might be a more appropriate way to address health needs in the Jewish community.

For what has been called parish nursing to fit within synagogues, new language and images, as well as flexibility, will be required. More people within the Jewish community asking the question of how this role fits into synagogue life will also be needed. This will take time and persistence. Typically in the Jewish community, when there has been a need identified, there has been excellent response in mobilizing resources to address that need. It is possible this will happen with a nurse within the congregation, if this is seen as a way to respond to an identified need within the broader community. It is also possible that, because of the unique tradition of the Jewish community, synagogues will develop a unique way of being a health place that may or may not use a nursing model.

Parish Nursing in African American Churches

The African American church is a good example of the importance of building on existing cultural and religious traditions when developing parish nursing programs. African American churches include many different denominational backgrounds but share similar historical and cultural roots. In African American culture, the church has been a focal point of community life, and as such, has been and is a very logical place to address health concerns (Armmer & Humbles, 1995). One of the frequently heard comments in speaking with African American clergy is the whole-person nature of their church's ministry, which means that anything of concern to the congregation is an appropriate arena for ministry. The relevance of health concerns to the life of the church is reflected in the multiple research studies that have used African American churches as a site for specific health programs, including hypertension screening (Saunders & Kong, 1983; Smith, 1989), weight reduction (Kumanyika & Charleston, 1992), smoking (Stillman, Bone, Rand, Levine, & Becker, 1993), and other health issues.

In some African American churches, there has been a tradition of a nursing board or church nurses who serve a first-aid and/or social function and may also be involved in larger health issues (Johnson, 1988). The members of these boards are not required to be licensed nurses, and they serve in a lay capacity. In working with churches who have a nursing board, parish nurses may find that such groups can be an important network. In some cases, the nursing board may also function as a health and wellness committee. When introducing a program that is called parish nursing into a church that already has a program called "nursing," it is important to build bridges so the two concepts will complement each other rather than compete. The advantage of having an identified nursing group is that it can provide a base of support for the parish nurse. In the Interfaith Volunteer Congregational Health Program, which had a very good response from African American churches, several nurses are also the president of their church's nursing boards and see the role of parish nurse as a way to enhance the work of the nursing board. This kind of bridge building between what already exists and what could exist is important in developing parish nursing in diverse congregations.

Conclusion

Looking to the future development of parish nursing, it is reasonable to expect increasingly diverse configurations and affiliations. This diversity will increase the richness of the parish nursing community. As bridges are built and new partners created, parish nurses need to be mindful of the unique contribution that each denomination, congregation, and nurse can make to what is known as parish nursing. The role of religions in health and healing may be universal, but how that role is acted out will be distinctly unique.

References

Armmer, F. A., & Humbles, P. (1995). Extending health care to urban African-Americans. *Nursing & Health Care, 16*(2), 65-68.

Council of Jewish Federations. (1991). *Highlights of the CJF 1990 national Jewish population survey.* New York: Author.

Davis, L., Dumas, R., Ferketich, S., Flaherty, M. J., Isenberg, M., Koerner, J. E., Lacey, B., Stern, P., Valente, S., & Meleis, A. (1992). AAN expert panel report: Culturally competent health care. *Nursing Outlook, 40*(6), 277-283.

Dudley, C. S., & Johnson, S. A. (1993). *Energizing the congregation.* Louisville, KY: Westminster.

Feldman, D. M. (1986). *Health and medicine in the Jewish tradition.* New York: Crossroads.

Flam, N. (1994). The Jewish way of healing. *Reform Judaism, 22*(4), 35-39.

Greene, A. (1994, Winter). The spiritual dimension. *Faith & Health, 6.*

Hall, E. T. (1976). *Beyond culture.* New York: Doubleday.

Johnson, M. (1988). *Johnson's manual for church nurses.* Cleveland, OH: B.J.W. Art & Printing.

Kumanyika, S. K., & Charleston, J. B. (1992). Lose weight and win: A church-based weight loss program for blood pressure control among Black women. *Patient Education and Counseling, 19,* 19-32.

Leininger, M. (1991). *Culture care diversity & universality: A theory of nursing.* New York: National League for Nursing.

Ostrovsky, R. (1985). Renewal in a congregation: Establishing a health cabinet. *Conservative Judaism, 38*(1), 62-70.

Saunders, E., & Kong, B. W. (1983). A role for churches in hypertension management. *Urban Health, 12,* 49-51, 55.

Smith, E. D. (1989). The role of Black churches in supporting compliance with antihypertension regimens. *Public Health Nursing, 6*(4), 212-217.

Stillman, F. A., Bone, L. R., Rand, C., Levine, D. M., & Becker, D. M. (1993). Heart, body and soul: A church-based smoking cessation program for urban African Americans. *Preventive Medicine, 22,* 335-349.

Westberg, G. (1990). A historial perspective: Wholistic health and the parish nurse. In A. Solari-Twadell, A. M. Djupe, & M. A. McDermott (Eds.), *Parish nursing: The developing practice* (pp. 37-39). Park Ridge, IL: Lutheran General Health Care System.

18

Translating Nursing Conceptual Frameworks and Theory for Nursing Practice

Sandra Schmidt Bunkers

Introduction

Nursing conceptual frameworks and nursing theory-based practice models can serve as a guide for the evolution of parish nursing. "The challenge for nursing in the 21st century is to ground nursing practice in nursing science. Such grounding means that the philosophical foundation and belief system guiding nursing practice is based on nursing theory" (Bunkers, Allchin-Petardi, Pilkington, & Walls, 1996, p. 33). Presented in this chapter are explicit models of (a) a nursing theory-based conceptual framework created to guide the development of a curriculum through which to teach nursing theory-based practice and (b) a theory-based parish nursing practice model developed to address health and quality-of-life issues in a faith community. Health as the process of living one's life and quality of life from the person's and community's perspective emerge as the cornerstones for developing these new and innovative nursing practice models.

The Parish Community: Living in Relationship

A parish community consists of living in relationship. This living in relationship is composed of an interconnectedness of persons, ideas, hopes, and dreams. Nurse theorist Rosemarie Rizzo Parse (1996a) suggests that community "refers to the universe, the galaxy of human connectedness" (p. 4). In being part of this human connectedness, the parish nurse addresses lived experiences of health "of people in intentional communities or communities of faith located in the places where people live, work, and worship"

AUTHOR'S NOTE: The author wishes to acknowledge the following nursing faculty who cocreated this conceptual framework: Mary Auterman, Mary Brendtro, Sandra Bunkers, Karen Dorn, Karen Fritz, Jacquelyn Howell, Lois Kelley, Cheryl Leuning, Joyce Nelson, and Margot Nelson.

(Magilvy & Brown, 1997, p. 71). A parish nurse brings to this human encounter of living, working, and worshiping together a belief system about persons, health, quality of life, and professional nursing. The nurse's belief system, whether articulated explicitly or not, is manifested in how the nurse lives her nursing practice in relationship with others in the parish. Thus the development of conceptual frameworks and theory-based practice models that delineate a belief system concerning nursing can serve as signposts in the creating of future parish nursing practices.

The Nursing Conceptual Framework: A Guide

The faculty of nursing at Augustana College in Sioux Falls, South Dakota, developed a conceptual framework to guide the teaching of nursing theory-based practice at both an undergraduate and graduate level (see Figure 18.1). This conceptual framework consists of selected core concepts deemed important to the profession of nursing and a set of accompanying assumptions linking these concepts in an organized expression of meaning for the profession. The conceptual framework provides the foundation for a philosophy of nursing and the development of course content.

Core Concepts Concerning Person, Health, Quality of Life, and Nursing

The interrelated core concepts of Augustana's conceptual model, linked with the assumption that the focus of nursing practice is the health of the community, include person, health, quality of life from the person's perspective (Parse, 1994), caring in the human health experience (Newman, Sime, & Corcoran-Perry, 1991), the nurse-person process, environment, valuing, caring, and knowing. These core concepts are grounded in nursing theory that has evolved from theory-based research; they support nursing theory-based practice models. The nursing theorists informing the creation of this conceptual framework include Drs. Margaret Newman, Rosemarie Rizzo Parse, and Jean Watson.

According to Augustana's conceptual model, *person* can be viewed as an individual, as a family, or as a community or country. The person is a unitary, indivisible whole and interrelates with others in the environment while experiencing the past, present, and future all at once. At an abstract level, person denotes humankind.

A nurse practicing in a parish, understanding that person includes this interconnectedness of others with past, present, and future, will appreciate the history that individuals, groups, or a community bring to a present encounter while knowing that the future is being cocreated in that moment. The nurse knows that people coauthor their own health and are characterized by patterns of relating. The nurse appreciates the primacy of the nurse-person relationship in working together in matters of health and quality of life.

Health is viewed as a personal commitment to a lived value system (Parse, 1992); the pattern of the whole of one's life (Newman, 1986, 1994). Health is living that which is important to a person and can only be described by that person.

A parish nurse, practicing from the perspective that health is the way one lives life, will focus on many health and human issues important to the person and community and

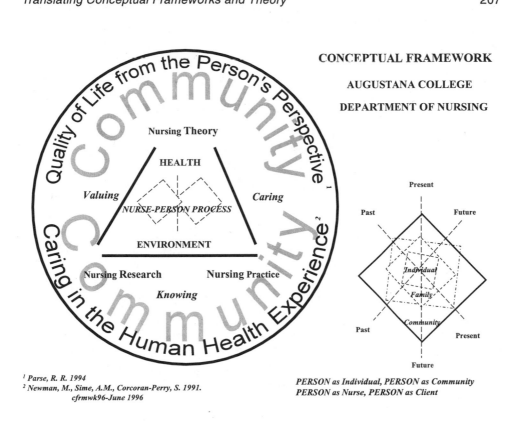

[1] Parse, R. R. 1994
[2] Newman, M., Sime, A.M., Corcoran-Perry, S. 1991.
          cfrmwk96-June 1996

PERSON as Individual, PERSON as Community
PERSON as Nurse, PERSON as Client

Figure 18.1. Nursing Conceptual Framework Developed by the Augustana College Department of Nursing, Sioux Falls, South Dakota

will not limit nursing practice to addressing illness and disease. With today's increasing emphasis on a person's responsibility for his or her own health, the parish community's concern for health and human well-being can make possible abundant parish resources to create desired programming that makes it possible for individuals and groups in the parish to choose to change their health patterns.

Quality of life from the person's perspective (Parse, 1994) is seen as the essence of nursing, according to Augustana's conceptual framework. Quality of life is the way one lives one's health, the "whatness" of one's life. It can only be described by the person living that life. Nurses practicing with this view respect the meaning of lived experiences of health as described by persons themselves, and they value others' human dignity and freedom to choose within situations. "People and communities will identify what is important to them and what is desired for quality of life" (Bunkers, Michaels, & Ethridge, 1997, p. 80).

Believing that the person (or community) is the expert in his or her health calls forth a very different type of nursing practice than the type of nursing that views the nurse as the expert in another's health. This alternative model of nursing practice is not based on the traditional nursing process and nursing diagnosis; it is based on what emerges in the nurse-person process. The nurse-person process involves being present and attentive to others, with receptivity and openness in responding to differing values and worldviews.

For example, Parse (1992) identifies true presence with others as "a special way of 'being with' in which the nurse bears witness to another's living of value priorities" (p. 40). Bunkers et al. (1997) suggest that there is a "nurse-person-community-health process characterized by the nurse living presence with others" (p. 80). Such presence depicts a valuing and acknowledging of the person's or community's value choices in living health. "The nurse, in being present, will work with them and walk with them as they identify struggles and concerns as well as joys in living their health" (Bunkers et al., 1997, pp. 80-81).

The nurse's presence, from the perspective of Augustana's conceptual framework, involves caring in the human health experience (Newman et al., 1991, p. 2). Watson (1997) suggests that "caring calls forth an authenticity of being and becoming, an ability to be present, to be reflective" (p. 50). Parish nurses living presence with others will concern themselves with persons' meanings of lived experiences and will be with them in an open, caring manner.

Weaving Nursing Theory Into Education, Practice, and Research

Augustana College's Department of Nursing's conceptual framework serves as an example of how nurses can be educated using a nursing science foundation. The discipline of nursing is evolving its own science, and with that evolution, more than one worldview is surfacing concerning the focus of nursing. These differing paradigms are a sign of a developing discipline and a developing nursing science. Margaret Newman (1995, p. xiii) refers to this development of nursing science as a progression of "the seamless whole of TheoryResearchPractice." Rosemarie Rizzo Parse (1996b) writes,

> As the 21st century approaches, it will be increasingly important for nurses to foster use of nursing theories and to continue to carve out an original path, so that nursing's presence in the health care system is recognized as contributing a unique perspective. (p. 85)

Parish nurses who choose to base their practice on the science of nursing instead of science borrowed from other disciplines will advance the practice of nursing as an independent profession, with its own unique knowledge base. The definitions and meanings of core concepts important to the knowledge base of the profession can be expanded through the creation of theory-based conceptual frameworks; nursing theory-based research; and original, theory-based practice models. Such an original practice model has been created at First Presbyterian Church in Sioux Falls, South Dakota, with the development of a parish nursing practice based on Parse's nursing theory of human becoming paralleled with the Eight Beatitudes. This parish nursing practice model serves as an example of the possibilities present for cocreating transformation in nursing. "Theory for nursing practice is more than the application of single-dimension theories in specific practice situations. It is a matter of the nurse's being transformed by the theory and thereby becoming a transforming partner in interaction with clients" (Newman, 1995, pp. 282-283).

Transforming:
A Nursing Theory-Based Health Ministry

The development of a nursing theory-based health ministry at First Presbyterian Church in Sioux Falls, South Dakota, based on Parse's theory of human becoming, occurred through months of study and dialogue. The central focus of this nursing theory-based health model is quality of life in the parish community. Health is viewed as a personal commitment to a lived value system: a process of human becoming (Parse, 1990). Central to parish nursing practice is living true presence with those in the parish. A graphic model was created (see Figure 18.2) to depict the belief system guiding nursing practice in the parish. Paralleled with the concepts of the human becoming theory are the Eight Beatitudes. Concepts of nursing theory, when interwoven with beliefs fundamental to the parish community's culture, brought together shared values concerning health and faith.

The Eight Beatitudes and Parse's Theory of Human Becoming

"Blessed are the poor in spirit, for theirs is the kingdom of heaven" recognizes that individuals coexist with one another and a great Wisdom (Ward, 1972). Simon Tugwell (1980), in his book *The Beatitudes,* suggests that this beatitude is also about risk taking. Tugwell writes,

> The Lord calls us to the poverty of being always ready to relinquish everything that is given to us, so that it can be given back to us enhanced and multiplied. Unless we are prepared to play the game of time like this, and risk losing everything, even what we thought we had will be taken away from us sooner or later. (p. 23)

The theory of human becoming posits that humans are in a process of cotranscending with all possibilities. "The theory is grounded in the belief that humans coauthor their becoming in mutual process with the universe, cocreating distinguishable patterns that specify the uniqueness of both humans and the universe" (Parse, 1995, p. 5). Thus, the process of cotranscending with possibilities involves unpredictability and a spirit of risk taking in living one's values. The parish nurse, practicing from the human becoming perspective, supports others as they live with risks in moving with their hopes and dreams.

"Blessed are those who mourn, for they will be comforted" presents the notion of deep sensitivity to the life experiences of others (Ward, 1972). This beatitude concerns itself with the interconnectedness of human beings in suffering and in uniting that suffering with Christ. "Uniting our suffering with that of Christ does not, in some mysterious way, change the actual quality of our suffering. It gives it a different perspective, which may make it more possible for us to live with it" (Tugwell, 1980, p. 63).

From a human becoming perspective, the nurse, in true presence, respects the person as one who knows the way, a chosen personal way of being with life experiences. A person's reality is viewed as a symphony of becoming. "True person-focused care from

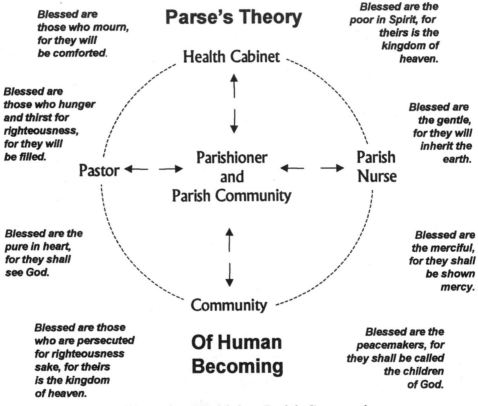

Figure 18.2. Congregational Health Model, First Presbyterian Church, Sioux Falls, South Dakota
SOURCE: Bunkers and Putnam (1995). Used by permission.

the human becoming view requires the health care provider to join the song as a presence, therewith attending to the meaning being shared by the person without judging or labeling" (Parse, 1996c, p. 182). The parish nurse, in joining with another's song of pain, struggle, and feelings of ambiguity about the future, participates with the other in exploring new ways of living.

"Blessed are the gentle, for they will inherit the earth" depicts the idea of an openness to the learning of new truths and new ways of being (Ward, 1972). This beatitude suggests that we act "with detachment from the results of action. What is important is what we are doing, not what we are trying to do" (Tugwell, 1980, p. 41).

The theory of human becoming emphasizes openness to new ways of evolving. People change moment to moment as they live their value priorities. The nurse does not try to change the other person. The nurse understands that what is important is participating in the *now* with the other as that other changes and grows depending on how he or she chooses to live health. "Humans change moment-to-moment as they actualize dreams and hopes through inventing new ways to propel beyond what is to what is not-yet" (Parse, 1995, p. 8).

"Blessed are those who hunger and thirst for righteousness, for they will be filled" expresses the desire for a deep, loving relationship with people and with God (Ward, 1972). This beatitude suggests that humans hunger for fulfillment and this fulfillment will be with God. "The gift which God makes of himself in this life is known chiefly in the increase of our desire for him. And that desire, being love, is infinite, and so stretches our mortal life to its limits" (Tugwell, 1980, p. 81).

True presence, in the human becoming tradition, is a loving intent to be with a person and honor his or her uniqueness. In true presence, the nurse flows with the person's rhythms of illuminating meaning (making explicit what is) and synchronizing rhythms (dwelling with the ups and downs of connecting-separating with others) while mobilizing transcendence (moving beyond). Parse (1997) writes regarding true presence,

> The person at all realms of his or her universe experiences the intent of the nurse, which is to bear witness to changing health patterns. The intent of the nurse is languaged in his or her whole being, in the subtle knowings of the messages given and taken at all realms of the universe, so words are not necessary to live true presence in the nurse-person process. (p. 35)

The nurse, in living true presence with a parish community, intentionally contributes to a valuing of love, faith, and health in quality of life.

"Blessed are the merciful, for they will be shown mercy" encourages activities of care for the wounds and hardships of broken lives (Ward, 1972). This beatitude encompasses the idea of forgiveness. "Forgiveness. . . . It is the dogged refusal to settle down in such a world of discord. Forgiveness is the hunger and thirst for total rightness" (Tugwell, 1980, p. 90).

When a person indicates suffering and a desire for mercy, the nurse practicing from a human becoming perspective bears witness to such suffering and is with the person in ethically appropriate ways. Daly (1995) suggests that from a Parsean perspective one "highlights the need to explore the meaning of the context for the individual sufferer" (p. 58). Thus, the parish nurse realizes that a person's request for mercy, forgiveness, and care is unique and individual, depending on the person's assigned meaning of what is occurring in his or her life.

"Blessed are the pure in heart, for they will see God" describes a singleness of purpose for living an ethic of love and care for others (Ward, 1972). This beatitude alludes to the mystery of being. Tugwell (1980) writes,

> To have a pure heart is to have a life which wells up in us from a source too deep for us to plumb. To have a pure heart is to have a heart that is not just created by God and then abandoned to us for us to make the most of it; it is to have a heart which is constantly being created and sustained by the newness of the life of God. . . . If purity of heart means recognizing a mystery within ourselves, it leads us also to confront the related mystery that there is in all other created things. (pp. 97, 99)

The nurse, practicing from a human becoming perspective, lives an ethic of love and care that honors the mystery of human freedom. The mystery of human freedom is central to the human becoming theory. Health and human freedom are interconnected in the process of evolving and changing. Mitchell (1995) suggests,

> To honor and respect others' freedom to choose their own way is one of the most challenging aspects of Parse's theory, perhaps the most challenging. . . . In a moment of silence people will indicate where they want to go and how they want to be. Quite often, the person's creations of meaning and possibilities far surpass what the nurse might be able to offer. (pp. 38-39)

The nurse, living these beliefs in parish nursing practice, will coparticipate in the unfolding mystery of life in the parish.

"Blessed are the peacemakers, for they will be called children of God" suggests a focus on reconciliation of the hostile and estranged in the world (Ward, 1972). This beatitude also concerns itself with truth leading to inner peace. Tugwell (1980) suggests,

> The way to peace is the acceptance of truth. Any bit of us we refuse to accept will be our enemy. . . . It is in Christ that our broken humanity is united with divine whole-ness. . . . The peace that we seek is a wholeness that does not exist simply in ourselves, it is in Christ. (pp. 112-113)

Acceptance and valuing of others and self is inherent in the practice of nursing based on the human becoming theory. People are viewed as whole: "Nursing's phenomenon of concern is the unitary human-universe-health process, and nursing's uniqueness is in its unitary focus" (Parse, 1996c, p. 183). The nurse honors how others choose to create their world and seeks to know and understand the wholeness of their lived experiences of faith and health.

"Blessed are those who are persecuted because of righteousness, for theirs is the kingdom of heaven" denotes an understanding that choosing to live a certain ethic may

mean adversity. But it also denotes a sense of happiness or good fortune when one chooses one's own way (Ward, 1972). This beatitude focuses on an ethic of love and compassion. Tugwell (1980) points out,

> It is surely no accident that the people who do get martyred are often precisely the people who have shown most love. . . . Could it not be that it is precisely their devoted service which draws martyrdom towards them? Because they have been seen to love, they give confidence to those who are unsure of love; but this confidence eventually becomes a need to probe further. (pp. 132-133)

The nurse, practicing from a human becoming perspective, chooses an ethic of reflective love in true presence that includes honoring human freedom. In living this ethic in the parish, the nurse respects choices persons make concerning living with good fortune and adversity. The nurse listens at all levels of her being as others give voice to their cares, to their hopes, and to their dreams. The nurse walks with others in the parish as they move with the certainty-uncertainty of creating their lives in hope and faith. Parse (1990) writes,

> Health is how I live my life—my own personal commitment to being the who that I am becoming. . . . Listen to me nurse, when I tell you how I am, and what I will do—since that is how I am going to be me. (p. 140)

The nurse, in honoring a person's and a parish's own way, can transform nursing practice in a parish. "A clarity of purpose of the First Presbyterian Congregational Health Model has been established by using constructs from theology and Parse's theory of human becoming to guide model development and nursing practice in the parish" (Bunkers & Putnam, 1995, p. 210). This clarity of purpose originates in clearly articulating the beliefs surrounding person, health, quality of life, and faith that guide nursing practice in the parish.

Conclusion

Transformation in nursing, which can occur with theory-based nursing education and practice models, is the promise of this generation in nursing. Living such a promise encompasses the study of the different nursing paradigms and theories and the choice of delving deeper into knowing and understanding nursing science. A nursing theory-based guided practice offers the richness of interweaving nursing beliefs and values and the faith values of a parish community. This richness of creating new meaning and understanding of the interrelationship of faith and health can unfold endless possibilities for quality of life.

References

Bunkers, S. S., Allchin-Petardi, L., Pilkington, F. B., & Walls, P. (1996). Challenging the myths surrounding qualitative research in nursing. *Nursing Science Quarterly, 9,* 33-37.

Bunkers, S. S., Michaels, C., & Ethridge, P. (1997). Advanced practice nursing in community: Nursing's opportunity. *Advanced Practice Nursing Quarterly, 2*(4), 79-84.

Bunkers, S. S., & Putnam, V. J. (1995). A nursing theory based model of health ministry: Living Parse's theory of human becoming in parish nursing. In *Ninth Annual Westberg Parish Nurse Symposium: Parish Nursing: Ministering Through the Arts* (pp. 197-212). Northbrook: Advocate Health Care.

Daly, J. (1995). The view of suffering within the human becoming theory. In R. R. Parse (Ed.), *Illuminations: The human becoming theory in practice and research* (pp. 45-58). New York: National League for Nursing.

Magilvy, J., & Brown, N. (1997). Parish nursing: Advanced practice nursing model for healthier communities. *Advanced Practice Nursing Quarterly, 2*(4), 67-72.

Mitchell, G. J. (1995). The view of freedom within the human becoming theory. In R. R. Parse (Ed.), *Illuminations: The human becoming theory in practice and research* (pp. 27-43). New York: National League for Nursing.

Newman, M. (1986). *Health as expanding consciousness.* New York: C. V. Mosby.

Newman, M. (1994). *Health as expanding consciousness* (2nd ed.). New York: National League for Nursing.

Newman, M., Sime, A. M., & Corcoran-Perry, S. A. (1991). The focus of discipline of nursing. *Advances in Nursing Science, 14*(1), 1-6.

Newman, M. A. (1995). *A developing discipline.* New York: National League for Nursing.

Parse, R. R. (1990). Health: A personal commitment. *Nursing Science Quarterly, 3,* 136-140.

Parse, R. R. (1992). Human becoming: Parse's theory of nursing. *Nursing Science Quarterly, 5,* 35-41.

Parse, R. R. (1994). Quality of life: Sciencing and living the art of human becoming. *Nursing Science Quarterly, 7,* 16-20.

Parse, R. R. (1995). The human becoming theory. In R. R. Parse (Ed.), *Illuminations: The human becoming theory in practice and research* (pp. 5-8). New York: National League for Nursing.

Parse, R. R. (1996a). Community: A human becoming perspective. *Illuminations: The Newsletter of the International Consortium of Parse Scholars, 5*(1), 4.

Parse, R. R. (1996b). Nursing theories: An original path. *Nursing Science Quarterly, 9,* 85.

Parse, R. R. (1996c). Reality: A seamless symphony of becoming. *Nursing Science Quarterly, 9,* 181-184.

Parse, R. R. (1997). The human becoming theory: The was, is, and will be. *Nursing Science Quarterly, 10,* 32-38.

Tugwell, S. (1980). *The beatitudes: Soundings in Christian tradition.* Springfield, MO: Templegate.

Ward, W. (1972). Matthew. In H. Paschall & H. Hobbs (Eds.), *The teacher's Bible commentary* (pp. 586-616). Nashville, TN: Broadman.

Watson, J. (1997). The theory of human caring: Retrospective and prospective. *Nursing Science Quarterly, 10,* 49-52.

19

Parish Nursing and the Nursing Process

Phyllis B. Heffron
Jean King

Introduction

The parish nurse has an excellent tool available that provides a framework for the delivery of nursing care: the *nursing process*. It is based on the scientific method of problem solving and is designed to assist all nurses as they work with individual clients, groups, or special populations. More specifically, the nursing process is a set of directions or steps that enables the nurse to gather and organize facts, to analyze and label those facts, and to make clinical decisions based on nursing knowledge as applied to those facts. The process is flexible and open, and it encourages the nurse to confirm and evaluate nursing care decisions and modify or change them as necessary. Figure 19.1 lists and describes the five steps of the nursing process.

Nursing knowledge is often complex in nature, and nursing care is delivered in a wide variety of settings. Given that human beings are also complex, as well as highly individual and dynamic, it is crucial that nursing knowledge is applied deliberately, carefully, and systematically. Parish nurses reflect these facts in their philosophy of adhering strongly to the model of whole-person health. In their practice, nurses strive to include the client's cultural, religious, spiritual, socioeconomic, educational, psychological, and physical dimensions as they make assessments and plan care. The purpose of the nursing process is to guide the nurse in thinking critically about the client as a whole person and to expedite an orderly process for making nursing diagnoses and for planning, evaluating, and implementing high-quality nursing care.

Historically, the nursing process has been in use for nearly 30 years. Major credit has been given to Helen Yura and Mary B. Walsh (1967), who wrote the first comprehensive textbook addressing the nursing process. Over the years, the concept and use of

1.	Assessment	Assessment is the systematic collection of relevant data about the client for the purposes of identifying nursing diagnoses and planning nursing care. During this phase, the nurse obtains facts and pieces of information, organizes and sorts them, and documents them in the form of a database.
2.	Nursing Diagnosis	A nursing diagnosis is a proposed statement about the client's health care need or problem that describes a healthy, unhealthy, or potentially unhealthy response to an illness, injury, or environmental situation. A nursing diagnosis includes possible causes of or factors related to the identified need. The nursing diagnosis is derived through clinical decision making based on the analysis of data collected during assessment.
3.	Planning	Planning involves the development of a nursing care plan that will direct how the client's care will evolve and, specifically, how the nursing diagnoses will be resolved. Priorities are established, along with goals, objectives and outcome criteria, to measure effectiveness of the actions.
4.	Intervention/ Implementation	This is the action phase of the nursing process, during which the nurse carries out activities and treatments aimed at resolving the nursing diagnosis. Nursing interventions are initiated according to the plan of care and may include self-care actions carried out by the client and actions carried out by others. Written or electronic documentation of the nursing actions is an important part of this phase.
5.	Evaluation	Evaluation is an ongoing and intentional activity for the purpose of determining how well the client is progressing toward meeting the care goals and resolving stated nursing diagnoses. Evaluation involves judgment on the part of the nurse, as she compares the outcome criteria statement to what is actually happening to the client. If the goals of care have not been met or have been only partially met, it may be nec-essary to reevaluate by reentering the assessment phase and going through the steps of the nursing process again.

Figure 19.1. Steps of the Nursing Process

the nursing process have evolved in importance to provide a framework for legal and professional accountability in practice and to assist health care agencies and nursing organizations express their standards of care (Heffron, 1997). Parish nurses, for example, practice in diverse roles and care for clients in nontraditional settings. In their care for individuals and families in faith communities, they have a unique opportunity to focus on spirituality and spiritual care and on how these concepts affect healing and health care. The nursing process can be used effectively at different levels of care—whether the extent of care is confined to an hour of therapeutic listening or the management of a client who collapses with chest pain during a worship service. The nursing process can also be important to nursing research by providing a uniform way to express and document all of the phases of nursing care. Current and ongoing nursing research on nursing classifications and nursing outcomes provide a good example of this importance (McCloskey, 1995). The nursing process goes into effect any time there is contact between a nurse and a client or between a nurse and another source of information about that client. The process always begins with assessment, the first step of the nursing process.

Assessment

The assessment step develops the *client database,* which can be defined as an organized pool of comprehensive information about the client that is systematically gathered from many sources. An important source for parish nurses is other members of the ministerial team of the congregation. Assessment is done for the purpose of identifying and obtaining data that affirms the person's state of health and wellness. From a nursing perspective, the health assessment implies a broad focus, incorporating data from all dimensions of the person. This emphasis on the whole person ensures that the physiological, psychological, sociocultural, and spiritual components of the person's life will be addressed. Assessment is done in accordance with the reality of the nurse-client encounter and can take place in a complete and orderly fashion or, over time, in segments. Assessment also varies according to the setting (hospital or home), the acuity of the client (semiconscious or ambulatory and alert), the cognitive and sensory abilities of the client, and other environmental or institutional differences. This chapter will present assessment as it would be done in an ideal situation, with the client cooperative and able to participate in the process. Traditionally, the two major components of a comprehensive assessment are the *health history* and the *physical examination.* The health history is obtained through an interview process. The physical examination includes using the skills of inspection, palpation, percussion, and auscultation. This depth of physical examination is not within the scope of parish nursing and thus is not addressed in depth in this chapter.

The health history is an extremely important part of the health assessment for several reasons. First of all, it is the beginning of the process when the nurse and client are forming impressions of one another and establishing the groundwork for a relationship marked by friendliness, openness, and trust. It is the time when the nurse asks the client to explain in his own words the primary reason for seeking care. The nature of the reasons can guide the nurse throughout the assessment as she asks further questions and pays particular attention to relevant areas. The information contained in the health history needs to reflect the client as a whole person and includes past as well as present health considerations. In addition to problems, weaknesses, and dysfunctions, the health history includes client strengths and positive health behaviors that can be used therapeutically.

Assessment data are classified as *subjective* and *objective* data. The health history contains subjective data, which is information based on what the client tells the nurse. Subjective data cannot be measured directly and are only what the client experiences, perceives, and verbally reports. Objective data, on the other hand, are measurable data that the nurse collects through the skills of listening, observing, feeling, smelling, or manipulating through the use of an instrument such as a thermometer. Examples of these two kinds of data are as follows:

Subjective: sensations of nausea or pain; feelings of sadness, grief, or depression; report of falling

Objective: blood pressure, body temperature, description of a skin lesion, description of behaviors indicating anxiety, physical or spiritual distress

The health history information is elicited both formally and informally. Most nurses find it helpful to have a written health history outline or form to fill in. This helps to guide the interview and to assure that all important areas are addressed. It also serves as a documentation mechanism. Formalized health history guides can be as numerous as practitioners, organizations, and health care institutions. For example, parish nurses may use a spiritual assessment tool in addition to a more generic health history form. Formats can be based on theories or models or on a combination of these. Physicians typically use a format known aptly as the *medical model*. This model uses the physiologic systems of the body as a basis (e.g., the gastrointestinal system or the neurological system) and may include selected areas of inquiry on socioeconomic and psychosocial factors. All formats will have some type of biographical and demographic data area, but these will vary in depth and detail. Figure 19.2 lists components of a typical nursing history and examples of areas of inquiry using Gordon's (1997) Functional Health Patterns.

Many nurses incorporate the *review of systems* into the health history. The review of systems is borrowed from the medical model and serves as a way to double-check the past and present status of all the major anatomical areas of the body. There are conventional questions that can be asked in relation to each area of the body, such as for the eye: "Have you ever experienced blurred vision?"

The physical examination is also carried out in an organized way, using some type of written format as a guide. As with the history interview, the format design will vary from nurse to nurse and from institution to institution. It doesn't really matter whether the format is theory based, anatomically based or sequentially based (from head to toe). What matters is that it is done methodically, thoroughly, and in a context that fits the client situation.

Documentation of the findings of a health history establish a permanent means of communication for the initiation or continuation of the legal medical record. Parish nurses keep records not only for their own use and reference, but for professional accountability and to assist in making referrals to other health practitioners. The importance of clear, accurate, and complete documentation cannot be overemphasized.

Nursing Diagnosis

The second step of the nursing process is formulating the *nursing diagnosis*. A nursing diagnosis is defined as a clinical judgment about a client, a family, or a community response to an actual or potential health problem or life process (North American Nursing Diagnosis Association, 1992). Nursing diagnoses provide the basis for choosing nursing interventions to achieve outcomes for which the nurse is accountable. It is important to understand the difference between a *medical diagnosis* and a nursing diagnosis. A medical diagnosis is made by a physician and is an illness or condition that reflects an alteration of the structure or function of organs or body systems. Medical diagnoses do not usually change and can be verified by various medical diagnostic measurements. Nursing diagnoses differ in that they reflect the client's *response* to the medical diagnosis or to whatever health problem may be present. Nursing diagnoses change as the client's response changes; that is, as healing and other developments occur, the nurse adjusts the nursing diagnosis accordingly. Nursing diagnoses are

PATTERNS	EXAMPLES OF HISTORY QUESTION AREAS
Biographical data	Name, address, other identifying data, age, birth date, sex, marital status, race/ethnicity, religious preference, educational background, current and past occupations
Health perception and health management	
Current health	Reason for visit, allergies, blood type, prescription and OTC (over the counter) drugs
Past health	Childhood illnesses, hospitalizations, surgeries, major illnesses, medication history
Health habits	Smoking, substance abuse, caffeine use
Economics	Amount and source of income, insurance
Environment	Home, community, and work environment
Health behaviors	Immunizations, frequency of physicals, routine lab and X-ray exams
Family history	History of familial diseases (e.g., diabetes)
Cognition and perception	
Sensory	Eyes and vision, ears and hearing, touch
Mental status	Memory, decision-making ability, learning disabilities, ability to express self, past treatment by a psychiatrist
Motor	Headaches, fainting, seizures, tremors, gait difficulties, head injuries
Coping and stress tolerance	Current and past stressors, measures used to relieve stress, effectiveness of coping strategies, understanding of effects of stress
Nutrition and metabolism	Weight, height, appetite, usual diet, dietary supplements, appetite suppressants, 24-hour recall of food and fluids, religious and cultural influences on diet, knowledge of nutrition, daily activity level, history of eating disorders, hormone use, personal hygiene, medication affecting appetite
Elimination	
Urinary system	Review any kidney or bladder problems, past surgeries or injuries to kidneys
Lower GI (gastro-intestinal) system	Usual bowel patterns, constipation, diarrhea, bowel or rectal surgery, GI diseases
Sleep and rest	Usual sleep pattern, snoring, sleep apnea, sleepwalking, periods of frequent wakefulness during night, morning headaches, teeth grinding, falling asleep during the daytime, usual rest patterns
Activity and exercise	Describe ability to carry out activities of daily living in terms of being independent, partially dependent, needing assistance, or dependent
Roles and relationships	Types of family relationships and frequency of contact with family, friendships—number of and frequency of contact, who the client turns to in time of crisis, social activities, job-related friendships and relationships, role of religion in daily life, relationship to God

Figure 19.2. Components of a Health History Based on Functional Health Patterns
SOURCE: Adapted from Gordon (1997).

inclined to reflect the whole person orientation of nursing and the relationship between psychosocial and physiological entities. They cover a wide variety of patient responses, such as activities of daily living, behaviors and feelings, coping mechanisms, and role functioning.

In regard to the nursing process, the nursing diagnosis is somewhat of a newcomer. Nursing diagnosis was developed as a model after the establishment of and subsequent influence of the North American Nursing Diagnosis Association (NANDA). NANDA was established in 1973 as an organization devoted to the continued development and maintenance of a taxonomy of nursing diagnoses. In 1980, the American Nurses' Association formally accepted the term *nursing diagnosis,* and soon after, it became accepted as the second step of a five-step nursing process.

Nursing diagnosis is a process within itself. The diagnostic process starts with analysis of the data at hand. Even during the assessment phase, as data are being collected, the nurse is beginning to sort them out and make interpretations about what is significant and which data can be clustered together. As the data are organized further, patterns may begin to emerge and data can be validated and compared to norms and standards. The nurse uses knowledge of past clinical experiences with clients, collaborates with others on the health team, and listens to her own intuition to complete the process.

The next step in the diagnostic process is to attach a label to the identified focus area or problem for which the nurse believes nursing care is warranted. NANDA (1997) has developed the most extensive terminology for nursing diagnosis, called the NANDA Taxonomy. The framework for this taxonomy is a listing of nine human response patterns, as follows:

1. Exchanging: mutual giving and receiving, such as fluid exchange
2. Communicating: sending verbal or written messages
3. Relating: establishing bonds, social exchanges, roles, relationships
4. Valuing: ascribing worth, belief patterns, spirituality
5. Choosing: selecting alternatives, coping mechanisms, decision making
6. Moving: activity, mobility, exercise, daily activities
7. Perceiving: receiving and comprehending information, self-concept
8. Knowing: comprehending knowledge, exhibiting understanding
9. Feeling: subjective awareness of information such as pain, depression

NANDA continually updates its taxonomy of nursing diagnoses, and as each new listing is published, the diagnoses are grouped under each of these nine areas. Each nursing diagnosis is formulated using the taxonomy and appears as two statements joined by the word "related to." The first statement reflects a human response, such as verbalization of a feeling of pain, anxiety, or depression (Pattern 9) and the second statement reflects contributing factors related to the response, such as a diagnosis of cancer, death of a loved one, surgery, or other major life event. One example of a nursing diagnosis using the above terms might be *anxiety related to cancer surgery.* By adding more specific assessment information to this situation, a second more accurate diagnosis may result. For example, the client may discuss fears of dying and the meaning of life in relation to her surgery. She may communicate in generalities or very specifically (i.e., "I wonder if God is punishing me!"). This information raises a flag for the nurse to consider the category of *spiritual distress* (Pattern 4, Valuing) as the human response portion of the nursing diagnosis.

Another popular method used to guide nursing diagnosis formulation is known as PES: P = problem, E = etiology, and S = signs and symptoms. The problem is a clear description of the client's actual or potential health status or problem. It is a description of the client's condition and determines the diagnostic category. The etiology of the problem identifies any environmental, sociological, spiritual, psychological, or physiological factors that are related to or are the probable cause. The signs and symptoms include those objective and subjective factors that define characteristics of the problem or provide evidence that a pattern exists. When writing a nursing diagnosis using this format, the problem is stated first, then connected to the etiology by the phrase "related to," followed by any signs and symptoms for credibility. The following is an example of preparing a nursing diagnosis using the PES format.

(P) = the client has received the diagnosis of uterine cancer

(E) = the client verbalizes anxiety about dying and wonders if God is punishing her

(S) = the client exhibits hand-wringing behavior, prays frequently, and cries spontaneously

Spiritual distress, moderate, related to medical diagnoses as evidenced by verbal reports and anxious behavior would be a correct format for the nursing diagnosis for the above example.

Planning

The planning phase, the third step of the nursing process, is characterized by organization of the nursing diagnoses by priority, determining goals and objectives, establishing outcome criteria for each diagnosis, and writing the nursing care plan. The focus is toward choosing those nursing interventions or actions that would be most appropriate to effectively address the client's needs and problems. Inclusion of the client in the steps of the nursing process is important overall, but it is especially crucial in the planning process. If the client does not believe that a problem exists and there is little or no commitment to intervention, the chances are slim for a positive outcome.

There are a number of criteria that can be used when setting priorities among multiple diagnoses. First and foremost is usually the acuity of the situation. Anything life threatening such as suicidal or other acute self-destructive behaviors, excessive bleeding, breathing difficulties, and so forth would obviously be candidates for the top of the list. Maslow's (1970) hierarchy of needs, known to most nurses, provides an excellent theoretical basis for this kind of priority setting. Temporal, human, and material resources also play a part in this process. The nurse must look at the time she has allotted to work with the client, the client's financial resources (in some cases), and general resources available in the community. Priorities can also change as the client's health care status changes.

The next step in the planning phase is to establish client goals and objectives related to each nursing diagnosis. Short- and long-term goals are broad guidelines that direct nursing interventions and communicate the purpose of the plan. They also establish the pace of care activities for the client. An example of a short-term goal would be *client will make a dental appointment within 1 week.* Long-term goals are broader and direct nursing care over time. An example of a long-term goal a parish nurse might write for a spiritually stressed geriatric client who is "angry that God has allowed her to keep on living" might be *client will arrange for and attend weekly scheduled counseling sessions with her parish priest and/or parish counselor for the next 3 months.*

After arriving at a minimum of one goal for each diagnosis, the next step in planning care is to write *behavioral objectives* for each goal. A behavioral objective is a statement that measures the client's progress in terms of behavioral language. In the case above, where the client is advised to maintain attendance at counseling sessions, the behavioral objectives under the goal might be as follows: "The client says that she has contacted the parish counselor and set up weekly appointments for discussing her spiritual concerns. The client has also made plans to visit with the parish nurse to discuss her progress on a monthly basis for the next 3 months." The last example, which gives a specific time frame, is known as an *outcome criterion.* Outcome criteria are very similar to behavioral objectives, the difference being the added specificity of a time frame. Many nurses progress to writing outcome criteria directly after writing the goal.

At this point, writing of the *nursing care plan* is usually started. This document is like a blueprint that guides the nurse as she goes about giving nursing care. It is part of the client's health record and may be in computerized form or in hard copy. The final task is to choose *nursing interventions.* Nursing interventions are those specific strategies or actions designed to assist the client in achieving the outcomes related to each nursing diagnosis. Deciding upon the appropriate nursing interventions is a critical responsibility of the professional parish nurse and must be individualized and balanced between numerous factors. A good starting point for this task and a dependable resource is to consult the latest Nursing Interventions Classification (NIC) publication (McCloskey & Bulechek, 1996). NIC is a comprehensive taxonomy of standardized nursing interventions developed and researched by faculty from the University of Iowa College of Nursing. NIC interventions are classified under six general domain headings and include physiological and psychosocial nursing actions as well as illness treatment and prevention and health promotion behaviors. Each NIC entry has three parts: a label, a definition of the concept, and a summary of the actions recommended for implementation. A reference list is also provided for each NIC intervention.

NIC provides the nurse with a list of options to consider for determining which interventions to include on the nursing care plan. As these options are pondered, there are other influences to factor into the decision. Examples of some of these factors are listed below:

- Consult with the client and possibly with family members
- Consult the current literature for new advances
- Consult nursing standards
- Consider factors such as age, sex, maturity, education, sociocultural background, and spiritual and religious practices

- Consider safety and comfort factors
- Consider the fit between outcome criteria and the chosen intervention
- Consider the fit between the intervention and the ability and availability of staff and equipment

The parish nurse will use the completed care plan for her own reference as she interacts with clients and as she consults with others on the ministerial team. Nursing care plans are meant to be shared and are a valuable source of communication in settings where many health care professionals come into contact with one client. The care plan is updated periodically as nursing diagnoses are resolved and/or other changes need to be made.

Implementation

Implementation is the fourth step of the nursing process; its purpose is to put the nursing care plan into action. The performing of nursing interventions can begin as soon as the care plan is completed. Just as the nursing diagnoses are prioritized, if there are several interventions listed, the nurse may need to reorder these to suit the individual situation. The ability and condition of the client and the nature of the action will help guide this process. For example, in a counseling situation, the intervention may be to listen and give guidance as necessary. In this instance, the nurse is likely to focus on reviewing the goals and objectives rather than looking at the designated intervention. Therapeutic counseling is an advanced nursing skill, and nurses experienced in this specialty often need to be especially flexible and innovative in their approach to intervention.

In implementing care in certain nursing situations, it may be useful to distinguish between *client-focused* activities and *nurse-focused* activities. Nurse-focused activities are those in which the nurse is directing and providing the care. Clients may be unable to do for themselves, may not want to do the activity, or may not be competent. Client-focused interventions are those activities clients do by themselves, with or without supervision. A parish nurse may, for example, assist a client to initiate and maintain a weight loss program. The client would be encouraged and counseled to do certain activities on his or her own, such as keeping a written progress record, following a dietary plan, increasing water intake, exercising on a daily basis, and so forth.

Documentation of nursing actions is done in accordance with the outcome criteria. For the sake of accountability and clear communication, the documentation language should adhere to and complement the language used in the nursing care plan. Documentation also represents the individuality the nurse has exercised in providing care; it also serves as a basis for evaluating the care.

Evaluation

The final step of the nursing process is evaluation, and its purpose is to determine whether desired outcomes have been met. The client's response to the care given is evaluated generally and specifically according to each outcome criterion on the care plan. The evaluation plan is built into the process when the nursing care plan is completed; the actual evaluation is done by comparing the outcome criteria to the reality of what is happening to the client. Periodically, the outcome criteria are reviewed and labeled as met, unmet, or partially met. This action is a basic and intentional way to begin the evaluation process. Those criteria that are unmet or partially met need to be further scrutinized if the time period for resolution has passed.

Evaluation is also a continuous process that arises any time there is a change in the client's health status or an event that triggers the need for reassessment. Reassessment is done routinely during care giving and the monitoring of patient responses. As new data is collected during the implementation of the care plan, evaluation or reassessment determines the following (Doenges, Moorhouse, & Burley, 1995):

- Appropriateness of the nursing actions
- The need to revise the interventions
- Development of new client problems and needs
- The need for referral to other resources
- The need to rearrange priorities to meet the changing care needs

Outcomes can be evaluated using various methods: direct observation, talking with the client, talking with other members of the ministerial team, and reviewing various parts of the health record. Parish nurses may choose more formal methods of evaluation that can be used when working with groups in the faith community or other specialized populations involving more than a few individuals. Surveys, focus groups, and questionnaires would fall into this category.

One again, it should be emphasized that evaluation enhances credibility and attention to documentation. Notations about the evaluation of care are sometimes placed directly into the care plan or in another part of the health record. The documentation needs to clearly indicate whether the goals were met, unmet, or partially met and provide appropriate explanations if they were not fully met.

Evaluation in itself is not the end of the nursing process. As long as there is a nurse-client relationship, the nursing process is cyclical, and ongoing assessment starts up new cycles of care. When the client terminates from nursing care, either through discharge, mutual understanding between the nurse and the client, geographic relocation, or death, the nursing process comes to an end. If the client is discharged from the nurse's care and reenters care at a later date, the nursing process is simply reactivated and can be picked up where the situation last left off.

Summary

The nursing process is described as the central core of nursing care. A major advantage of the nursing process is its ability to be used as a framework in any nursing setting and with any type of client, whether that client is a single individual, a family, or a special population such as a faith community. The nursing process begins when the client first meets with the nurse and continues throughout the care period.

The organization and consistency provided by the nursing process allow for the maintenance of professional accountability and for the retrieval of nursing care documentation. For parish nurses, who usually work as solo practitioners, the nursing process assists them in meeting each client with a manner that reflects credibility, purposeful activities, and a planned course of action. Parish nursing, along with all areas of nursing practice, is continually strengthening its professional base. As parish nursing strives to meet the ever-changing needs of the faith community and respond to the dynamics of the health care system enterprise, the nursing process will remain as a steady and unifying guidepost.

References

Doenges, M. E., Moorhouse, M. F., & Burley, J. T. (1995). *Application of nursing process and nursing diagnosis: An interactive text for diagnostic reasoning* (3rd ed.). Philadelphia: F. A. Davis.

Gordon, M. (1997). *Manual of nursing diagnosis, 1997–1998.* St. Louis, MO: Mosby-Yearbook.

Heffron, P. B. (1997). *Nursing process.* In R. Kearney-Nunnery (Ed.), *Advancing your career: Concepts of professional nursing* (chap. 14, p. 231). Philadelphia, PA: F. A. Davis.

Maslow, A. (1970). *Motivation and personality* (2nd ed.). New York: Harper & Row.

McCloskey, J. C. (1995). Help to make nursing visible. *IMAGE: The Journal of Nursing Scholarship, 27*(3), 170.

McCloskey, J. C., & Bulechek, G. M. (Eds.). (1996). *Nursing interventions classification (NIC)* (2nd ed.). St. Louis, MO: Mosby-Yearbook.

North American Nursing Diagnosis Association. (1997). *NANDA nursing diagnoses: Definition and classification, 1997–1998.* Philadelphia: Author.

Yura, H., & Walsh, M. (1967). *The nursing process.* Norwalk, CT: Appleton-Century-Crofts.

Additional Reading

Barkauskas, V. H., Stoltenberg-Allen, K., Baumann, L. C., & Darling-Fisher, C. (1994). *Health and physical assessment.* St. Louis, MO: Mosby-Yearbook.

Bates, B., Bickley, L. S., & Hoekelman, R. A. (1995). *A guide to physical examination and history taking* (6th ed.). Philadelphia: Lippincott-Raven.

Carpenito, L. J. (1997). *Handbook of nursing diagnosis* (7th ed.). Philadelphia: Lippincott-Raven.

Carson, V. B. (1989). *Spiritual dimensions of nursing practice.* Philadelphia: W. B. Saunders.

Cox, H. C., Hinz, M. D., Lubno, M. A., Newfield, S. A., Ridenour, N. A., Slater, M. M., & Sridaromont, K. L. (1997). *Clinical applications of nursing diagnosis.* Philadelphia: F. A. Davis.

Hogstel, M. O., & Keen-Payne, R. (1996). *Practical guide to health assessment through the lifespan* (2nd ed.). Philadelphia, PA: F. A. Davis.

Iyer, P. W., Taptich, B. J., & Bernocchi-Losey, D. (1995). *Nursing process and nursing diagnosis* (3rd ed.). Philadelphia: W. B. Saunders.

20

Accountability and Rationale

Mary Ann McDermott

Overview

What first comes to your mind and heart when you hear the term *accountability?* How have you been accountable up to this point in your nursing career? If we consider professional nursing as a covenant with patients, what are the terms of the covenant we have with the members of the congregation, and what is our accountability in the parish nurse role? Dictionary definitions hint at accountability as a reckoning, a valuing, a narration, an explanation—which is why we often move right into the subject of documentation and specifically charting.

I ask you to think initially about accountability in a broader sense. Terms related to accountability may come to mind: authority, responsibility, legality, liability, and concepts such as professionalism and ethical or moral codes of conduct. I believe there are no distinctions in accountability for persons who take on the parish nurse role in either the paid or the unpaid model. Others might wish to disagree. A position description for the parish nurse, in the initial negotiation for assuming this role, *must* address the matter of accountability: for what, of what, to whom, and the manner in which the nurse will be accountable. I offer several definitions for your consideration:

> Accountability . . . means that an agent, public or private, entering into a contractual agreement to perform a service will be held answerable for performing according to agreed-upon terms, within an established time period, and with stipulated use of resources and performance standards. This definition of accountability requires that the parties to the contract keep clear and complete records and that this information will be available for outside review. It also suggests penalties and rewards; accountability without redress or incentive is mere rhetoric. (Lieberman, 1972, p. 2)

> Accountability is the fulfillment of a formal obligation to periodically disclose in adequate detail and consistent form to all directly and indirectly responsible or properly interested parties the (1) purposes, (2) principles, (3) procedures, (4) relationships, (5)

results, (6) incomes and expenditures involved in any activity, enterprise, or assignment, so that evaluations and decisions can be made. (Matek, 1977, p. 4)

Accountability denotes liability and is defined as the liability for task performance. It is created by the assignment of responsibility and the grant of authority. It means that the subordinates are answerable and liable to the superior for the quality and quantity of the assigned task. Accountability flows upward. It is the concept of "the buck stops here." Accountability is a retrospective analysis of what occurred to determine if what occurred was appropriate in the situation. (Multiple sources, as abstracted by Huber, 1996, p. 233)

Given these definitions of accountability, certain elements of accountability emerge as it applies to the parish nursing role. Promise fulfillment as an element springs from the contractual (I prefer the terms *covenantal* and *relational*) nature of the position. A certain amount of formality in the arrangement is implied. An accounting must first and foremost be appropriate for the endeavor. It would appear that this needs to be done efficiently, effectively, in adequate detail, periodically, and on a consistent basis. There is an obvious relationship of accountability to procedures, processes, and programs such as quality control, quality assurance, continuous quality improvement, total quality management, evaluation, and to the new emphasis on health care outcomes.

Accountability to Whom?

To whom is the parish nurse accountable? In addition to yourself, the covenant is with the persons cared for by you in this role: the congregation taken in the entirety as the population served, as well as individuals and groups of parishioners when they become the direct recipients of your care. You are accountable to the nursing profession and to the body of scientifically based knowledge for nursing practice. When you agree to take on the role and the title of parish nurse, this accountability differentiates your services from others who may also care but who do not bring your education, experience, and expertise to their caring. You are accountable to other interdisciplinary colleagues with whom you interact while in the parish nurse role: physicians, social workers, physical therapists, and other nurse colleagues, most especially those in case or care management roles.

Who are the directly responsible parties to whom you are accountable (referred to in the Matek definition cited above)? They are your employers, however defined in your particular situation: the sponsoring institution, the director of pastoral care, the director of nursing, the congregation, the pastor, and/or the health cabinet or committee. Who are the indirectly responsible parties, and who might you nominate to be among the properly interested parties? First and foremost, as more openly established in this position than some others you may have held, you are responsible to your God! Is not the parish nurse role an extension of the covenanting God, the God who exchanges embraces with us, cares and loves us?

Accountability Rationale: For What?

We are accountable for adherence to standards that are related to structure, processes, and outcomes. In the parish nurse role, as professional nurses, we are subject to the American Nurses Association (ANA) Standards of Clinical Nursing Practice (ANA, 1991). Lack of dues-paying membership in the association does not exempt you from adherence to the standards set by this officially recognized professional organization. The association's Social Policy Statement (ANA, 1980), its Committee on Ethics: Code for Nurses (ANA, 1985), and its Standards of Parish Nursing Practice (ANA, 1998) are also worthy of your consideration and should be consulted. In addition, the International Parish Nurse Resource Center has developed a set of standards (Djupe, Olson, Ryan, & Lantz, 1994). Adherence to your state's Nurse Practice Act, a legal description of professional practice, is expected, as well as adherence to institutional and congregational standards that might exist (Djupe et al., 1994).

The parish nurse should also be familiar with documents pertaining to patient rights as promulgated by the National League for Nursing, the American Nurses Association, and the American Hospital Association. Some specific religious denominations have also developed related materials that can be consulted. Use of and adherence to these standards will serve as an oasis for many judgments made by the nurse and will assist in both day-to-day, pragmatic problem solving and in more complex ethical decision making. A parish nurse position description, as referred to earlier and to which the nurse is also accountable, will be fundamental to the parish nurse's performance evaluation.

Accountability to or Disclosure of What?

The formal nature of a parish nurse program, rather than being a very fine but informal and incidental health ministry, is distinguishable in part from this classification by a public disclosure of purposes that might include a mission and vision statement as well as goals and objectives for the program. Principles such as might be found in a statement of philosophy, a set of assumptions, and an acknowledgment of the specific congregational values that will be addressed in this program should be publicized at the outset and then reviewed periodically for relevance. A detailed outline of program services, based on a well-documented needs and strengths assessment, should be distributed. Procedural matters, such as how and when to make a referral of self or a neighbor to the nurse and who is eligible for the services, should be shared. Congregations have the right to know relevant relationships: where the resources (financial, material, and human) are coming from, how this program and staff person relates to other program and staff of the congregation, and, if relevant, how both relate to a sponsoring institution. Will referrals to health care professionals, agencies, and institutions be made solely within the sponsoring institution's network? This point needs to be well understood by the nurse as well as the congregation. Is the parish nurse program an arm for marketing as well as mission in the sponsoring institution? Accountability includes the disclosure of outcomes and budget matters, described regularly and specifically to the directly responsible parties and, more likely, in monthly, quarterly, or annual global or summary reports to indirectly responsible parties and to other properly interested parties.

Program Accountability

The purpose of program accountability is decision making. The acknowledged framework for professional nursing practice is, currently, the nursing process. Not unlike traditional problem solving, but certainly less linear, and cognizant of systems theory, the nursing process (assessment, inference, diagnosis, planning, implementation-intervention, evaluation-outcomes, and a feedback loop) provides a structure for both thinking about and carrying out the work of nursing and sets the stage for program accountability. Chapter 19 discusses the nursing process in some detail. The immediate objective of program accountability is information, and the method is appropriate communication. The first consideration of most nurses will be for record keeping, data collection, and documentation. This will mean selection and decisions about charting methodologies and forms: how much, how often, and in what format. The confidentiality of the records will be of paramount importance. See Chapter 21 for more on documentation.

Other communication decisions related to program accountability are (a) performance evaluation, both formative and summative, based on a mutually agreed-upon position description as well as appropriate and consistent measurement of performance protocols; (b) collection and reporting tools and instruments, which might include community or congregational needs and strengths assessments, descriptive brochures, parish bulletin or newsletter entries, annual reports, parishioner and staff satisfaction surveys (written or oral), and one tool that is often formally neglected but of which I am quite fond—an archival collection (photographs, anecdotal notes, journal entries, program flyers, meeting minutes, letters of appreciation); (c) concurrent as well as retrospective peer review and audit(s) of documentation or charts, with written feedback; (d) the monitoring of integrated system effectiveness (appropriate to institutional sponsorship); (e) quality improvement techniques to be implemented; and (f) the identification of adequate and appropriate legal, ethical, financial, and administrative support systems.

Disincentives and Challenges to Accountability

Parish nurses and clergy alike speak to the seemingly exorbitant amounts of resources devoted to accountability that are inherent in parish nursing. The cost, in both time and energy, of carrying out professional accountability is indeed great. Reports, performance evaluations, and record keeping take time. Nurses are more familiar with the necessity, having worked in health care institutions where payment mechanisms demand detailed documentation, than are the clergy, but they are by no means any more enthusiastic. This is particularly true as parish nurses explore the use of computers in record keeping. The learning time for those unfamiliar with the technology can be excessive.

Will the hoped-for outcomes, including better data for decision making and demonstrating program worth to interested parties, be realized? One certainly prays that this expectation will come to fruition. Accountability in all the many ways we have outlined has the potential to be problematic. It generates questions from all those involved. It has the potential to weaken credibility, effectiveness, and the prestige of the parish nurse program and/or the parish nurse. These are risks we must take at this point in this developing practice.

Other present and future challenges affecting accountability include the many "trickle down" effects of health care reform. Will sponsoring organizations, be they a health care organization, congregation, or religious-sponsored educational institution, initiate or continue to support a ministry that is, by design, congruent with their main mission but a call on capital when margins will certainly only continue to decrease? As an opportunity for reform, will we see new investments made for health promotion and disease prevention as hospitals look for ways to improve the health status of communities and form with congregations a healthier community network of services, one in which parish nursing will be an integral and major player?

Will the parish nurse role of health promotion and disease prevention be threatened and see substituted for it an expectation for a home care nurse surrogate in the congregation for the too-early discharges of those insured ("covered lives") within the sponsoring organization? Will the ever-increasing use and expectations about emerging new technology, especially information technologies, be a help or a hindrance to the parish nurse? Emphasis on and expectations of outcome data by those "invested" in health care could be a great boon to parish nursing—if only we can identify and agree on what those outcomes are for a healthy population and find acceptable ways to document these still rather ambiguous outcomes. The ethical dilemmas ahead for parish nursing practice in congregations that professes gospel values that speak to the dignity and worth of all individuals will, no doubt, be among the nurse's greatest and most important challenges.

I have adapted the format for my conclusion from a speech attributed to Wilfred Smith (Wallot, 1988), National Archivist of Canada (retired), which he wrote many years ago about the value of an archival collection.

Accountability, and thus Documentation, is:

The mirror of our experience,
A collective parish nurse ministry memory,
The origin of a future continuity of care heritage,
The source of our history.
A rich database from which nursing decision making
    can be optimized,
The record of victories and defeats, minimal
    achievements as well as enormous failures,
    pause for thanksgiving and a moment for petition,
The product as well as the process of individual and
    collective endeavors (parish nurse, parish staff,
    health cabinet, pastor, and parishioners) in the
    promotion of health and wholeness in the life
    of the congregation and, thus, the community,
One means to ensure professional and personal
    accountability
In His Name!

References

American Nurses Association. (1980). *Nursing: A social policy statement.* Kansas City, MO: Author.

American Nurses Association. (1985). *Code for nurses with interpretive statements.* Kansas City, MO: Author.

American Nurses Association. (1991). *Standards of clinical nursing practice.* Kansas City, MO: Author.

American Nurses Association. (1998). *Scope and standards of parish nursing practice.* Washington, DC: Author.

Djupe, A. M., Olson, H., Ryan, J., & Lantz, J. (1994) *Reaching out: Parish nursing services* (2nd ed.). Park Ridge, IL: Lutheran General Health System.

Huber, D. (1996). *Leadership and nursing care management.* Philadelphia: W. B. Saunders.

Lieberman, M. (1972). *Accountability: Review of literature and recommendations for implementation.* Raleigh: North Carolina Department of Public Instruction.

Matek, S. (1977). *Accountability: Its meaning and its relevance to the health care field* (DHEW Pub. No. [HRA] 77-72 HRP-0500101). Hyattsville, MD: U.S. Department of Health, Education and Welfare.

Wallot, J. P. (1988, January-February). *The Archivist, 15*(1), 2.

Additional Reading

Callahan, C., & Wall, L. (1987). Participative management: A contingency approach. *Nursing Journal of Administration, 17*(9), 9-15.

Dean-Baar, S. (1994). Standards and guidelines: How do they assure quality? In J. McCloskey & H. Grace (Eds.), *Current issues in nursing* (4th ed., pp. 316-320). St. Louis, MO: Mosby.

Donabedian, A. (1980). *Explorations in quality assessment and monitoring: The definition of quality and approaches to its assessment* (Vol. 1). Ann Arbor, MI: Health Administration.

Hammer, M., & Champy, J. (1993). *Reengineering the corporation: A manifesto for business revolution.* New York: HarperCollins.

Manthey, M. (1989). Control over practice: Who owns it? *Nursing Management, 20*(7), 14-16.

McDermott, M. A. (1990). Accountability: The rationale for documentation. In P. A. Solari-Twadell, A. M. Djupe, & M. A. McDermott (Eds.), *Parish nursing: The developing practice.* Park Ridge, IL: National Parish Nurse Resource Center.

McDermott, M. A., & Burke, J. (1993). When the population is a congregation: The emerging role of the parish nurse. *Journal of Community Health Nursing, 10*(3), 179-190.

Roberts, H., & Sergesketter, B. (1993). *Quality is personal.* New York: Free Press.

21

Documenting the Practice

Bethany Johnson
Patti Ludwig-Beymer
Wendy Tuzik Micek

Why Nurses Document

Documentation is an age-old issue that confronts the more than 30 nursing specialties, including parish nursing. In the very early 1900s, Florence Nightingale observed
that despite the level of a nurse's devotion, it is useless if the observations are not noted
(Nightingale, 1946).

The primary purpose of charting in the patient record is to chronologically document
the care administered to the patient. Documentation is necessary for informational
purposes. It serves as a vehicle for communicating (to exchange written or verbal
thoughts, messages, or information), from one professional to another, the status and
needs of the patient. Efforts to define the nursing profession's scope of practice have
intensified the need for documentation.

The basic questions regarding the contributions of nurses remain: What is it that
nurses do? Do the actions of nurses make a difference to the quality of care received?
As nurses function in multiple roles and settings, they must be able to present evidence
that what they do makes a difference.

Nursing Documentation

A framework is needed to document nursing actions. The foundation of the framework is the nursing process. There are many different types of nursing documentation
systems that incorporate checklists, logs, graphs, and other forms of abbreviated charting. Table 21.1 provides a summary of the different systems that exist in the nursing
arena, with the strengths and weaknesses highlighted for these evolving systems.

In addition to these formalized documentation systems, there are also a number of
hybrid systems that have been "homegrown" independently by sites of care. Some
examples include the CORE (Concise Organized Responsive and Evaluate) documenta-

TABLE 21.1 Summary of Documentation Systems

Documentation System	Description	Strengths	Weaknesses
1. Narrative charting (Burke & Murphy, 1988)	A traditional documentation method that requires all assessment findings, nursing interventions, and patient responses to therapy be charted in the order in which they occur.	Very complete.	Not the most effective way to track specific problems or evaluate trends. Not objective. Creates many pages of notes, making data extraction difficult.
2. SOAP/SOAPIER (Reilly, 1981)	One problem per SOAP. Acronym means: Subjective data, Objective data, Assessment and conclusion, Plan of care, Interventions, Evaluation of the outcome, Revisions of the plan of care. The addition of I, E, R completes the nursing process.	Easier to identify pertinent documentation by specific problem.	Documentation may become time-consuming and lengthy. Data must be extracted from notes.
3. Problem Oriented Record (Weed, 1969)	A traditional method that includes four parts: database, problem list, initial plans, and narrative progress notes. Organizes charting into categories under specific problems.	Eliminates the documentation of nonessential data. Promotes documentation of the nursing process.	Does not allow for wellness-oriented documentation. Trend evaluation becomes difficult.
4. Problem Centered (Kerr, 1992)	Incorporates the use of comprehensive checklists for assessment and supplements progress notes to document interventions.	Allows for easy retrieval of data and decreases the length of narrative notes. Incorporates evaluation into the progress notes.	Does not allow for wellness-oriented documentation.
5. PIE (Siegrist, Dettor, & Stocks, 1985)	Acronym means: Problem, Intervention, Evaluation. Care is recorded in the progress notes. Checklists are also used for assessments.	Makes for easy data retrieval. Eliminates the traditional care plan.	Lengthens progress notes. Does not allow for wellness-oriented documentation.
6. FOCUS (Lampe, 1993a)	Reflects a patient concern, a nursing diagnosis, or a significant event in the patient's care. Progress notes are organized according to data, action, and response.	Very flexible. Uses a word or phrase that most clearly communicates the patient information.	Narrative notes may become longer.

TABLE 21.1 Continued

Documentation System	Description	Strengths	Weaknesses
7. Charting by Exception (Murphy, Beglinger, & Johnson, 1988)	Only significant findings or exceptions to norms are documented. A problem list is developed from the assessment.	Enhances the documentation of interventions. Trends in the patient's status can be seen immediately through flow charts. Abnormal data are easily retrieved. Documentation of routine care is eliminated through the implementation of standards of nursing practice.	Care plans become very lengthy. Major changes to forms are required.
8. Critical Paths (Zander, 1988)	Paths replace nursing care plans. Show standards of care and standards of practice. Care may be individualized by analyzing and acting upon variances.	Provides a database for continuous quality improvement. Describes the contributions of every department.	Requires interdisciplinary cooperation. May require multiple critical paths for each patient. Requires development of critical paths for numerous diagnoses.

tion system (Montemuro, 1988), the FACT (Flow Sheets Assessment Concise Narrative Notes Timely) charting system (Warne & McWeeny, 1991), and the diary documentation system (Rydholm, 1997). In general, nursing is beginning to put a greater emphasis on alternatives to care plans with such things as standardized care plans, protocols, critical paths, flow sheets, evaluation of patient responses to treatments, teaching and preventive care, documenting the outcome, and point-of-care charting.

The documentation systems enumerated have been modified throughout the years and have become more streamlined while maintaining quality. The lesson is that there is no single right, or best, way to chart. However, "good patient care deserves good documentation" (DiMotto, 1994, p. 17). It is expected that the nursing profession will continue to look for new ways of charting to address the changes in health care and overcome the challenges in nursing.

Parish Nursing Documentation

Parish nurses recognize that documentation is a professional responsibility. However, parish nurses often struggle with the perceived value of documentation versus the legal need. Many parish nurses feel documentation is constraining and takes time away from the service they have been called to provide to parishioners. They keep minimal records, primarily for legal purposes as required by their sponsoring institution. As a result, most documentation systems used by parish nurses are homegrown. Monthly statistical reports, required by most sponsoring institutions, have become a link in the chain that requires parish nurses to set aside time for record keeping.

Complicating the situation is the parish nurse's schedule. Most parish nurses work or volunteer part-time within their congregation (Lloyd & Solari-Twadell, 1994), creating an incredible time management issue for most nurses: How can they best serve parishioners in the limited time they have when they need to take time to document?

One of the joys of parish nursing is the blending of the humanities and sciences, the powerful ability to nurture the spirit while tending the body. This unique role within a congregation can complicate documentation. Many pastors and parish workers have not been expected to keep records. As a consequence, the parish nurse steps into an environment that does not see the necessity of charting as part of accountability. Although some pastors and pastoral care workers have come to recognize the legal and professional need for record keeping, many congregations still do not understand why nurses must take time away from their practice to document their activities. Ultimately the differences result in a culture conflict: the professional responsibility to document versus congregational and even parish leadership perceptions and needs.

A grant from the W. K. Kellogg Foundation was awarded to Lutheran General Health System, in collaboration with Trinity Regional HealthSystem, in 1994 to develop the infrastructure for parish nursing, which included a documentation system. Parish Nursing Services at Advocate Health Care is the product of two separate parish nurse programs that combined when Lutheran General HealthSystem and Evangelical Health System merged in 1995. The parish nurse program at Advocate consists of 23 parish nurses working in 30 congregations. These parish nurses are salaried employees of Advocate and the congregations they serve. The parish nurses serve the inner city and the suburbs, in congregations ranging in size from 50 to 17,000 members. Trinity Regional HealthSystem is located in Moline, Illinois, and serves the Quad Cities and the surrounding rural population. Trinity has supported salaried and volunteer parish nurses since 1990; their program has grown to include 54 parish nurses. The "Partners in Health and Healing" grant has been an excellent vehicle by which to learn about what is needed in a documentation system for parish nursing and how to achieve this goal.

Documentation Requirements

To meet the needs of all stakeholders, such as pastors, congregational leaders, parishioners, the health care system, and parish nurses themselves, data must be collected in many ways. Documentation of parish nursing practice to date has included qualitative and quantitative elements as well as evaluative components. Each component is described below.

Qualitative Documentation Elements

To describe parish nursing, stories are often used. Some individuals, such as pastors, congregational leaders, and parishioners, appreciate and require this qualitative documentation. They like the details of parish nurse-parishioner interactions. They want to read vignettes: complete stories of people served by parish nurses, including why the need existed and how the parish nurse functioned with the individual and family. This type of documentation has been found to be very effective when describing the parish nurse program to groups of people who ask the question "How does this program benefit specific parishioners?"

Qualitative documentation is captured by parish nurses in multiple ways. First, nurses may use narrative notes as part of their formal documentation system. In addition, parish nurses share narratives with other nurses and with church staff. At Advocate Health Care, for example, time is devoted at each biweekly parish nurse meeting to allow a parish nurse to summarize an actual client interaction for a small group of parish nurses. Using a Verbatim format (a theological reflection methodology), the parish nurse provides case details, as well as descriptions of her interventions and her feelings about the interaction. Parish nurses then provide support, verification, and suggestions to alter or improve future interactions.

Quantitative Documentation Elements

On the other hand, some institutions require quantitative documentation. They deal with aggregate data such as how many people were served in a given time period and what services those people received. This type of documentation is critical when attempting to answer the question "What parish nursing services do parishioners typically use?"

Many parish nurses use their own system for record keeping. They document, using paper and pencil, on parishioner encounter forms that they have created or have adapted from elsewhere. To ensure confidentiality, documentation is stored in locked files by each parish nurse in her church. In addition, parish nurses may complete monthly statistical forms and submit them to their church or sponsoring health care agency. Parish nurses use these forms to aggregate their monthly service data based on parishioner demographics (e.g., age, gender, race or ethnicity), previous visits, and reason for contact. This activity is not always viewed as meaningful by parish nurses. One of the intentions of the parish nurse documentation system developed as part of the W. K. Kellogg grant is to streamline the process. Parish nurses will document individual and group client encounters. These encounters will populate a database that will then be used to run monthly statistical reports. In addition to this new process saving time, it will also increase accuracy because aggregated results will not depend on the parish nurse's recall of the month.

Documentation for Evaluation Purposes

In addition to collecting both qualitative and quantitative data, some individuals seek to compare the scope and impact of services provided by parish nurses to those provided by other community based-programs. Program evaluators want to know the numbers of people reached by parish nursing services and, most important, the relationship between the services provided by parish nurses and the overall health status of the defined population. They want to calculate a cost-benefit ratio. There is an opportunity for program evaluators to inform and shape public policy based on these data.

Such an analysis requires a heavy dependence on at least two facets of outcomes: (a) measurement of the outcomes of specific nursing interventions and (b) additional planned outcomes measures. Advocate's parish nurse documentation system will include

TABLE 21.2 Additional Aspects of Documentation for Parish Nurses

Issues	Goals
Time constraints	Documentation system balances time spent in documentation with consequences and benefits of documentation.
	Parish nurses view documentation as valuable use of their time.
Fit within a continuum of care	Documentation system allows parish nurses to communicate more effectively with practitioners in various sites of care.
	Documentation system uses existing nursing language.
Link with existing documentation systems	Documentation system links with existing electronic databases.
Documents the spiritual component	Documentation system captures the spiritual essence of parish nursing.

the nursing-sensitive outcomes being developed as part of the Nursing Outcomes Classification (NOC) study at the University of Iowa (Johnson & Maas, 1997).

Even with the addition of NOC, however, the documentation system will not completely meet the need for overall aggregate outcome measures. Large-scale studies are needed. One such set of studies is being conducted using the population served by the congregational health program (Solari-Twadell, Truty, Ludwig-Beymer, See, & Yang, 1995; Solari-Twadell, Truty, & See, 1994; Truty, Solari-Twadell, Ludwig-Beymer, Yang, & Dunn, 1996). These studies examine changes in health status using the Health Status Questionnaire (HSQ) and physical parameters such as weight, blood pressure, and cholesterol level. Additional research is needed to examine the outcomes of all aspects of parish nursing practice.

Qualitative, quantitative, and evaluative data collection are important to consider in a documentation system. Documentation will be used to evaluate the impact of parish nursing, and data elements must be carefully selected based on that knowledge. In addition, as summarized by the authors in Table 21.2, a documentation system for parish nurses must be time efficient, must fit within the continuum of care and existing documentation systems, and must capture the spiritual aspects of the parish nurse's work.

Process for Developing a Documentation System

This section describes the process used at Advocate and Trinity, with the assistance of the W. K. Kellogg Foundation, to move forward in client record documentation for the parish nurses. The Advocate experience may prove helpful to parish nurses practicing in a variety of sites, but the process and the products will need to be modified and adapted as needed. Key components of the process included (a) standardizing paperwork, (b) conducting an analysis of existing nursing languages, (c) conducting national research to identify typical parish nurse interventions, (d) forming documentation subgroups, (e) providing education to parish nurses, and (f) conducting an analysis for computer software. Each step is detailed below.

Standardizing Paperwork

Parish nurses at Advocate and Trinity were accustomed to completing monthly report forms. When Advocate began the move toward standard client encounter documentation, the monthly form was revised to be consistent with the Omaha documentation system. Later, however, the monthly report was reformatted to reflect the North American Nursing Diagnosis Association (NANDA) and Nursing Intervention Classification (NIC) languages. As the NANDA and NIC languages become available on the computerized system at Advocate, the forms will be phased out. At Trinity Regional HealthSystem, the forms will be computerized, and most of the parish nurses will enter their own data. Some parish nurse programs, however, may wish to continue the use of paper forms and use data entry operators to compile the data.

Analysis of Existing Nursing Languages

To develop an appropriate and consistent documentation system, a standard nursing intervention language must be clearly delineated and used. Based on the literature, the authors identified four potential nursing languages appropriate for the documentation system: NANDA, the Omaha system, Saba's (1992) Home Health Classification, and NIC. Each of these four nursing nomenclatures are included in the National Liary of Medicine. A description and identification of strengths and weaknesses for their use in documentation by parish nurses are summarized in Table 21.3. After comparing these nursing languages, a decision was reached and endorsed by the Kellogg Grant Advisory Committee to base the Advocate and Trinity parish nurse documentation on NANDA and NIC.

National Survey of Parish Nurse Interventions

To understand the practice of parish nursing nationally, a modified NIC survey was distributed to 509 known parish nurses and parish nurse program coordinators, based on a mailing list provided by the International Parish Nurse Resource Center (Ludwig-Beymer, Micek, & Johnson, 1997; Ludwig-Beymer, Yang, & Johnson, 1996). A total of 220 surveys were returned, for a 43% response rate. Respondents tended to be female (99%), middle-aged (mean age = 51), part-time (mean number of hours worked = 16.3 per week), and volunteer (53%).

The most frequently performed interventions were presence (95.8%), emotional support (95.3%), active listening (94.8%), and spiritual support (94.0%). Least commonly reported interventions were those in the physiological domains. Additionally, 139 nurses suggested interventions not yet classified within the NIC system. Based on their responses, one major theme was identified: A prime role of parish nurses is to provide spiritual care to members of their community. This spiritual care is provided through the

TABLE 21.3 Analysis of Nursing Language

Language	Description	Strengths	Weaknesses
North American Nursing Diagnosis Association (NANDA) (1994)	Identifies, develops and classifies nursing diagnoses. Each diagnosis contains a label (name), definition, defining characteristics, related factors, and risk factors. Currently contains 128 nursing diagnoses.	New diagnoses may be incorporated into the system through a formal review process. Language is well known in nursing and used in many sites of care.	Language is viewed as cumbersome by some nurses.
Omaha System (Martin & Scheet, 1992)	Problem classification scheme includes domains, problems, modifiers, signs, and symptoms. Domains are Environmental, Psychosocial, Physiological, and Health Related Behaviors. Contains 40 nursing diagnoses. Includes outcomes for knowledge, behaviors, and status.	Useful for individuals, families and groups. Emphasizes environmental and health-related behaviors. Self-contained system, with diagnoses, interventions, and outcomes included.	Used primarily in community health settings. No formal mechanism in place for incorporating modifications to diagnoses, interventions, and outcomes.
Saba (1992) Home Health Classification	Twenty home health care components provide the framework for the classification and coding of nursing diagnoses and interventions.	Includes both diagnoses and interventions.	In use primarily within home health. No formal mechanism in place for revising the system.
Nursing Intervention Classification (NIC) system (McCloskey & Bulechek, 1992)	Contains six domains, 27 classes, and 433 interventions. Domains are Physiological: Basic; Physiological: Complex; Behavioral; Safety; Family; and Health System. Interventions include a definition and a list of specific activities.	List of interventions is fairly comprehensive. Standard approach in place for incorporating additional interventions.	Only one spiritual intervention included.

promotion of faith, spirituality, and wholeness and the provision and promotion of prayer, ritual, and ministry.

The results of this study proved helpful as the documentation team identified a list of core parish nurse interventions. The authors have shared the results with the NIC Project Team at the University of Iowa. This process is in keeping with the policies currently in place for modifying the NIC system (McCloskey & Bulechek, 1992). A list of the core parish nurse interventions is included in Table 21.4.

TABLE 21.4 Core Parish Nurse Interventions

1. Abuse protection	47. Multidisciplinary care conference
2. Abuse protection: Spiritual[a]	48. Mutual goal setting
3. Active listening	49. Networking: Community[a]
4. Activity therapy	50. Nutritional counseling
5. Advocacy: Community[a]	51. Oral health promotion
6. Advocacy: Individual[a]	52. Pain management
7. Anticipatory guidance	53. Patient rights protection
8. Anxiety reduction	54. Preceptor: Parish nurse[a]
9. Bibliotherapy	55. Preparatory sensory information
10. Caregiver support	56. Presence
11. Communication enhancement[a]	57. Reality orientation
12. Complex relationship building	58. Recreation therapy
13. Coping enhancement	59. Referral
14. Counseling	60. Religious addiction prevention[a]
15. Crisis intervention	61. Religious brokerage[a]
16. Culture brokerage	62. Reminiscence therapy
17. Decision-making support	63. Risk identification
18. Discharge planning	64. Role enhancement
19. Dying care	65. Security enhancement
20. Emergency care	66. Self-esteem enhancement
21. Emotional support	67. Self-responsibility facilitation
22. Energy management	68. Simple guided imagery
23. Exercise promotion	69. Simple relaxation therapy
24. Faith and health enhancement[a]	70. Skin surveillance
25. Family integrity promotion	71. Smoking cessation assistance
26. Family involvement	72. Socialization enhancement
27. Family mobilization	73. Spiritual care[a]
28. Family process maintenance	74. Spiritual ritual enhancement[a]
29. Family support	75. Spiritual support
30. First aid	76. Support group
31. Forgiveness facilitation[a]	77. Support system enhancement
32. Grief work facilitation	78. Surveillance
33. Guilt work facilitation	79. Surveillance: Safety
34. Health education	80. Sustenance support
35. Health screening	81. Teaching: Group
36. Health system guidance	82. Teaching: Individual
37. Home maintenance assistance	83. Telephone consultation
38. Hope instillation	84. Touch
39. Humor	85. Truth telling
40. Learning facilitation	86. Values clarification
41. Learning readiness enhancement	87. Visitation facilitation
42. Limit setting	88. Volunteer coordination[a]
43. Medication management	89. Volunteer support[a]
44. Meditation	90. Weight reduction assistance
45. Memory training	91. Wholeness enhancement[a]
46. Milieu therapy	

SOURCE: Based on the work of the Diagnosis and Intervention subgroup: JoAnn Boss, R.N., M.S.N., M.A.; Bethany Johnson, B.A.; Cindy Johnson, R.N.; Patricia Kellen, R.N., B.S.N.; Michelle Knapp, R.N.; Patti Ludwig-Beymer, R.N., Ph.D.; Wendy Tuzik Micek, R.N., D.N.Sc.; Harriet Olson, R.N., B.S.N., M.S.N.; Linda Robb, R.N.; Mary Slutz, R.N., B.S.; and Mary Vann, R.N., B.S.N., M.P.H.

a. Proposed interventions.

TABLE 21.5 Subgroup Structure

Diagnosis and Intervention subgroup	Reviewed and critiqued NANDA diagnosis and NIC interventions. Identified core nursing diagnoses and nursing interventions. Identified and defined additional diagnoses and interventions. Worked with Education subgroup to implement education.
Forms subgroup	Developed paper-and-pencil forms, including a demographic form, an assessment form, an initial encounter form, and a brief encounter form.
Education subgroup	Planned and implemented education for parish nurses at AHC. Presented basic information on nursing process and language. Provided formal education at each biweekly parish nurse meeting. Used case studies to work through documentation process. Provided one-to-one mentorship to apply learning in the parish setting.
Work Flow subgroup	Created flow charts to capture the flow of the parish nurse's work.

Formation of Documentation Subgroups

The subgroup structure used at Advocate and Trinity is described in Table 21.5. Again, this format may be revised as needed at other sites. Every Advocate parish nurse participated in one of the documentation subgroups.

Analysis for Computer Software

Because Advocate had reached a decision to automate documentation, the final step was to conduct a market analysis for computer software. When the project began in 1994, no vendor for a documentation system using NANDA and NIC language could be located. Fortunately, with the passage of time, vendors have begun to develop the type of documentation system required: one that combines NANDA with NIC, will incorporate NOC when available, and is flexible enough to meet the needs of nurses practicing in nontraditional settings. A Request for Proposals was issued, and negotiations were made with Ergo Systems in Kansas City to purchase their documentation system, Care Manager NDx. Trinity Regional HealthSystem, on the other hand, will use NANDA and NIC languages to develop their own homegrown documentation system, using the Microsoft Access database.

Lessons Learned

As underscored throughout this chapter, documentation is a vital link in sharing the stories of parish nurses. The "Partners in Health and Healing" grant awarded by the W. K. Kellogg Foundation to Advocate Health Care allowed its Parish Nursing Services to complete an enormous amount of work in a relatively short period of time. During the grant period, project staff, parish nurses at Advocate and Trinity, parish pastors, and management have learned many lessons, which are detailed in Table 21.6. The development and implementation of a documentation system for parish nurses is a process. By recognizing this, the key stakeholders (parish nurses, pastors, congregational leaders, and sponsoring institutions) can celebrate more than a successful documentation system—they can contribute to the ongoing development of parish nursing.

Adapting Documentation for Specific Parish Nurse Situations

Each parish nurse program or site will need to identify its particular needs and answer its own questions about how it wishes to document. Modifications may be made to the documentation system to meet the needs of individual practices. However, the authors suggest that critical elements be retained.

Key decision points exist, and these are outlined below:

- Is there recognition of the benefits of parish nurse documentation by the key stakeholders, such as pastors, congregational leaders, parishioners, the sponsoring health care organizations, and parish nurses themselves?
- How do the perceived benefits differ within the constituencies, and what are the conflicts?
- Is there commitment to use a standardized nursing language?
- Is there a desire to use all NANDA diagnoses, NIC interventions, and NOC outcomes in the documentation system, or is there a preference for using only the identified core parish nurse diagnoses, interventions, and outcomes?
- Can an individual parish nurse work with other parish nurses to develop a documentation system?
- Has the parish nurse or group consulted with the International Parish Nurse Resource Center?
- Can personnel, financial, and time resources be committed to redesigning and implementing a documentation system?
- Will the parish nurse have access to self-education, external assistance, printed or on-line training materials, and other documentation resources?
- Does the site prefer a computerized documentation system or a paper-and-pencil system?
- If a computerized system is preferable, will it be developed on-site or purchased?
- Are ongoing resources available to sustain the documentation system, be it computerized or paper-and-pencil?

The Advocate and Trinity parish nurse documentation project has contributed to an increased understanding of the role of parish nursing and has positioned parish nursing as an integral part of the nursing profession, a continuum of care, and an integrated delivery network. The ongoing documentation and resultant studies will continue to contribute to the knowledge base of nursing science. The documentation journey continues!

TABLE 21.6 Lessons Learned

Understanding	The stakeholders of the project need to answer the following questions: 1. What are the long-range goals of the project? 2. What will be the benefit of this documentation system to parishioners, parish nurses, congregations, and other health care providers? 3. With whom do we want to link (share records)? 4. How can we best accomplish this linkage? 5. How will health care reform affect our decisions? 6. Who will be responsible for ongoing documentation costs? 7. With whom do we need to communicate to accomplish these goals? 8. Who needs to be involved in the decision making? 9. What impact will documentation have on the parish nurse's time and energy?
Assumptions	All assumptions should be identified, even those that may be implicit. Assumptions may include: • All parish nurses will use this system of documentation. • This project will consume a large portion of the parish nurses' time and energy. • The learning curve for various components may be steep. • Support from the parish pastors and congregational leaders is vital. • The development process is ongoing. • There will be multiple opportunities for feedback from the users. • Everyone has a voice in decision making.
Team building and trust building	Trust is the basis of any healthy relationship and is necessary for stable co-operation and effective communication. Cultivate a trusting environment through activities such as: • Meeting reviews: Share "did wells" and "could improves." • Open dialogue sessions with parish nurses: Allow group members to share their feelings honestly and openly. • Biannual meetings with parish pastors: Share feedback and individual learnings.
Time constraints	Do not underestimate the amount of time and energy necessary to succeed. For many parish nurses, diagnosis, intervention, and outcome languages will be challenging. Make use of the following activities to minimize the time necessary and to communicate honestly the investment that will need to be made: • Information-gathering meetings • Educational sessions for parish nurses and pastors • Computer training on an ongoing basis • Ongoing dialogue • Continued support for parish nurses through theological reflection and retreat days
Identification of resources needed	All resources need to be identified from the outset of the documentation project. Some of the resources include: • Nursing expertise: Ongoing communication with nursing organizations is vital to understanding the climate of documentation within the field of nursing and the health care arena. • Information systems (IS) expertise: Technology is changing rapidly. A contact within IS can help the staff make decisions about equipment and software that will be compatible with existing systems. • Project management expertise: Careful planning, coordination of many components, and ongoing communication with key individuals is vital to the success of a documentation project. A good project manager will provide the skills necessary. • Financial resources: Monies need to be budgeted for consultation, development of forms, educational tools, software development, equipment needs, travel costs, and personnel needs. Time contributed by parish nurses over and above their regular hours needs to be valued.

References

Burke, L. J., & Murphy, J. (1988). *Charting by exception: A cost-effective, quality approach.* Media, PA: Harwal.

DiMotto, J. W. (1994). Documentation pitfalls and strategies to overcome them. *Nursing Dynamics, 3*(1), 17-20.

Johnson, M., & Maas, M. (Eds.). (1997). *Nursing outcomes classification (NOC).* St. Louis, MO: Mosby-Year Book.

Kerr, S. D. (1992, January/February). A comparison of four nursing documentation systems. *Journal of Nursing Staff Development,* pp. 26-31.

Lampe, S. (1993a, October). *Focus charting.* Paper presented at the Innovative Nursing Documentation Meeting, Marquette University, Marquette, WI.

Lampe, S. (1993b, October). *Innovations in planning care.* Paper presented at the Innovative Nursing Documentation Meeting, Marquette University, Marquette, WI.

Lloyd, R., & Solari-Twadell, A. (1994). Organizational framework, functions and education preparation of parish nurses: National survey 1991 and 1994. In P. A. Twadell (Ed.), *Eighth Annual Westberg Symposium: Ethics and values: A Framework for parish nursing practice* (pp. 105-115). Park Ridge, IL: National Parish Nurse Resource Center.

Ludwig-Beymer, P., Micek, W., & Johnson, B. (1997, May). *Spiritual themes in parish nursing practice: A national study.* Poster presented at the Fifth Annual Naurice M. Nesset Research Forum, Park Ridge, IL.

Ludwig-Beymer, P., Yang, J. J., & Johnson, B. (1996, May). *Interventions used by parish nurses nationally.* Poster presented at the Fourth Annual Naurice M. Nesset Research Forum, Park Ridge, IL.

Martin, K. S., & Scheet, N. J. (1992). *The Omaha system: A pocket guide for community health nursing.* Philadelphia, PA: W. E. B. Sanders.

McCloskey, J. C., & Bulechek, G. M. (Eds.). (1992). *Nursing interventions classification (NIC).* St. Louis, MO: Mosby-Year Book.

Montemuro, M. (1988). CORE documentation: A complete system for charting nursing care. *Nursing Management, 19*(8), 28-32.

Murphy, J., Beglinger, J. E., & Johnson, B. (1988). Charting by exception: Meeting the challenge of cost containment. *Nursing Economics, 19*(2), 56-58, 62, 64, 68-72.

Nightingale, F. (1946). *Notes on nursing: What it is and what it is not.* Philadelphia: J. B. Lippincott.

North American Nursing Diagnosis Association. (1994). *Nursing diagnoses: Definitions and classification.* Philadelphia: Author.

Reilly, M. M. (1981). Charting your patient's progress: How to use the problem-oriented system. In J. Robinson (Ed.), *Documenting patient care responsibility.* Springhouse, PA: Intermed Communications.

Rydholm, L. (1997). Patient-focused care in parish nursing. *Holistic Nursing Practice, 11*(2), 47-60.

Saba, V. (1992). The classification of home health care nursing. *Caring, 11*(3), 50-57.

Siegrist, L. M., Dettor, R. E., & Stocks, B. (1985). The PIE System: Complete planning and documentation of nursing care. *Quality Review Bulletin, 11,* 186-189.

Solari-Twadell, P. A., Truty, L., Ludwig-Beymer, P., See, C., & Yang, J. J. (1995, May). *Congregational health services: A one year perspective.* Poster session presented at the Third Annual Naurice M. Nesset Research Forum, Park Ridge, IL.

Solari-Twadell, A., Truty, L., & See, C. (1994, May). *Congregational health services: Age, gender and self-care issues.* Poster session presented at the Second Annual Naurice M. Nesset Research Forum, Park Ridge, IL.

Truty, L., Solari-Twadell, A., Ludwig-Beymer, P., Yang, J. J., & Dunn, B. (1996, May). *Congregational health services database: Self-reported health using the health status questionnaire 2.0.* Poster session presented at the Fourth Annual Naurice M. Nesset Research Forum, Park Ridge, IL.

Warne, M. A., & McWeeny, M. C. (1991). Managing the cost of documentation: The FACT charting system. *Nursing Economics, 9*(3), 181-187.

Weed, L. L. (1969). *Medical records, medical education and patient care.* Cleveland, OH: Case Western Reserve University Press.

Zander, K. (1988). Nursing case management—Resolving the DRG paradox. *Nursing Clinics of North America, 23,* 503-519.

IV

PARISH NURSING

Challenges to the Practice

22

Nurses in Churches

Differentiation of the Practice

Phyllis Ann Solari-Twadell

Hildegard Peplau, nurse theorist and expert in psychiatric nursing, stated that the psychiatric nurse was a "registered nurse who has completed a program of study in psychiatric nursing in a university setting and who, therefore, holds a master's or a doctoral degree" (quoted in Church, 1991, p. 402). Thus the definition of the psychiatric nurse would be determined by virtue of the nurse's educational credentials and competency. In other words, the nurse who happened to be working in a psychiatric setting did not automatically qualify for the role of psychiatric nurse. This reference is presented as an example of a nurse's practice having the potential to be defined by the setting rather than education, experience, and competency. A work setting can be a significant determinant in creating the need for a particular type of practitioner, but it is not the defining element for the set of knowledge, experience, and competencies needed by the nurse. Every nurse who works in the context of a congregation is not a parish nurse. For example, there are nurse practitioners and nurse case managers who can also work in the setting of the congregation and not be parish nurses. Nurses with differing education bring different capabilities to their nursing role in the church, and they must be able to practice according to these differences. Diversity in the application of parish nurse functions is present in the practice. The positive side is that this allows for development of the parish nurse role according to the needs of the congregation and the skills of the nurse. However, at the same time, great disparity in the functioning of the parish nurse has the capability of producing confusion over what really is the role of the parish nurse.

Parish nursing cannot be all things to all people. Perhaps it is time to begin to explore the differentiation of nursing practice in the context of the faith community. This exploration may more clearly define who the parish nurse is and how this nursing role differs from other nursing roles working in this setting. For some, this idea of exploring differentiated nursing practice in a congregational setting may produce irritation. After all, is parish nursing not ministry? If this is so, then why is this exploration necessary? Parish nursing is not one or the other; it is not *either* ministry *or* professional practice, it is both. Parish nursing is a professional model of health ministry. The nurse working in the capacity of a parish nurse is a registered professional nurse practicing under the Nurse Practice Act of the state in which she resides; this nurse is also functioning as a minister of health. Not all ministers of health need to be registered nurses, but a parish nurse does. This nursing role is a professional one, whether the nurse is paid or unpaid.

Differentiated Nursing Practice— What Is It?

Differentiated practice is referred to as a philosophy that focuses on the structuring of roles and functions of nurses according to education, experience, and competence. It establishes that the domain of professional nursing is broad, with multiple roles and responsibilities of various degrees and complexities. It assumes that nurses with different educational preparation, expertise, and background bring different competencies to the role in which they practice. Differentiated practice recognizes the contribution of all nursing personnel to patient care delivery as unique and valuable (Koerner & Karpiuk, 1994, p. 10). Each nurse practicing in a congregation has unique dimensions to offer to the faith community being served. However, is it not critical to be able to inform the faith community as to what to expect from a nurse who is functioning in the parish nurse role? For example, if a nurse is in an unpaid position in which she can commit 2 to 5 hours a week to providing services to the congregation, is it not important to be able to detail what services the faith community might expect? This could mean that the nurse's role is limited to providing blood pressure screenings on Sunday morning in conjunction with worship services. This is an important service to offer. It might save someone's life if they were unaware of an elevated, life-threatening blood pressure. However, is it parish nursing? Is the nurse functioning out of a health-promotion-disease-prevention mind-set, or the traditional medical model? Is the nurse in a position to address the well-being of the whole person, or does her knowledge base, past experience, and time restraint allow her only to address the physical dimension? Does the nurse have the capability to actually follow up with the person who has the elevated blood pressure? Or is the blood pressure screening merely an opportunity for identification of health risks, not the beginning of following up and coaching someone into new, healthier response patterns? If the nurse providing this service is not a parish nurse, what is an appropriate way to indicate the contribution of this nursing professional? Is there another title that may differentiate this level of activity and competency from that of the parish nurse who is prepared to educate, counsel, refer, advocate, and follow up, integrating the spiritual care appropriate for making the necessary lifestyle changes to decrease the likelihood of a hypertensive crisis? Is this even an issue of concern for the development of parish nursing? A review of collected data on the growth and development of the movement may help in responding to this question.

TABLE 22.1 Respondent Profile: Respondent Characteristics

	1992	1994	1996
Number of respondents	293	509	536
Number of states represented	34	48	43
Gender (%)	F-99	F-98	F-99
	M-1	M-2	M-1
Practicing parish nurses (%)	78	74	78
Parish nurse coordinator (%)	8	11	8
Both practicing parish nursing and coordinating parish nurses (%)	14	15	14
Average age (years)	49	51	51

Tracking the Diversity:
Results of National Surveys on Parish Nursing

The International Parish Nurse Resource Center at Advocate Health Care has, over the past 6 years, done three national surveys looking at the organizational framework, functions, and educational preparation of parish nurses. The survey time frames were 1992, 1994, and 1996. Although these data are not generalizable as a convenience sample was used, the surveys did begin to provide some baseline information about this specialty practice.

Respondent Profile

The profile of the respondents can be found in Table 22.1. Although the number of respondents continues to increase, the percentage of increase from year 1994 to year 1996 decreased—both in the number of respondents and the number of states represented. This raises the question of whether some parish nurse programs are able to sustain themselves over long periods of time. When a program is dependent on either a particular nurse or pastor or when one or the other leaves, the sustainability of a parish nurse program may be jeopardized. The data relating to age is similar for each year, giving a strong profile of the parish nurse as being a mature practitioner.

Type of Organizational Framework

The data reflect that if an institution is going to invest in a parish nurse partnership, it will usually be an institutional paid model. In contrast, it appears that congregations, although they support both paid and unpaid models, are not as frequently offering paid parish nurse positions. This is understandable, due to the eagerness of nurses to provide this ministry for their faith community even though many churches do not have the resources to provide payment for these services. The congregational unpaid model was the most frequent response to the question about type of organizational framework (Table 22.2).

TABLE 22.2 Type of Model or Organizational Framework (in percentages)

Model	1992 (n = 293)	1994 (n = 509)	1996 (n = 536)
Institutional paid	23	23	29
Institutional unpaid	8	9	13
Congregational paid	22	18	11
Congregational unpaid	47	50	47

Denominational Affiliation of Congregations With Parish Nurse Programs

Parish nursing has been ecumenical from its inception (Djupe, Olson, & Ryan, 1994). The responses from the surveys reflect that today parish nursing represents Christian as well as non-Christian faith traditions (Table 22.3). The Lutheran denomination maintained the largest response over the 6-year surveying period. This is not a surprise when one notes that the originator of the concept was a Lutheran clergyman, Rev. Granger Westberg, and the first institution to sponsor a parish nurse program was Lutheran.

Services Provided

The survey addressed five out of the seven functions of the parish nurse. The functions surveyed were *health educator, personal health counselor, referral source, developer of support groups,* and *facilitator and teacher of volunteers.* The respondents were not asked about the functions of *integrator of faith and health* and *health advocate.* Overall, the general pattern of providing these services did not change over the three survey periods (Table 22.4). Most parish nurses were consistently providing health education, personal health counseling, and referral resourcing. It is understandable that the developing of support groups and training of volunteers are functions that are not as well developed, as the largest organizational framework response was the unpaid model. How would the nurse have sufficient time to provide for all of these functions?

TABLE 22.3 Denominational Affiliation of Congregations Served (in percentages)*

Denomination	1992 (n = 293)	1994 (n = 509)	1996 (n = 536)
Baptist	5	9	11
Episcopal	6	8	9
Jewish	1	2	2
Lutheran	44	45	35
Methodist	20	21	23
Presbyterian	9	14	14
Roman Catholic	28	30	31
United Church of Christ	9	11	9
Other	13	10	19

NOTE: *Parish nurse respondants in several instances serve more than one denomination.

TABLE 22.4 Functions Provided by Parish Nurse Respondents (in percentages)

Functions	1992 (n = 293)	1994 (n = 509)	1996 (n = 536)
Health educator	81.2	80.4	80
Personal health counselor	77.6	74	71
Referral agent	55.5	58.1	46
Developer of support groups	15.5	16.6	18
Trainer of volunteers	13.8	16.2	21

Educational Levels

The educational preparation of the respondents fluctuates over the survey periods (Table 22.5). What is consistent, however, is the diversity in the highest level of preparation. These results emphasize one of the key considerations in differentiating nursing practice—the educational preparation of the nurse. If each of the different educational preparation levels results in a practitioner that has a different nursing skill mix, then attention needs to be given to discriminating between the different levels of experience, knowledge, and competencies present within parish nursing practice.

Time

It is unclear what role time plays in dictating the delivery of parish nursing services. However, it is known that the predominance of nurses working in the unpaid model are contributing 5 hours or less a week (Lloyd & Solari-Twadell, 1994). This is quite different than a nurse who is paid, through an institutionally paid model, to serve 16 to 20 hours a week or more. Corresponding to this is the ability to implement the seven primary functions of the parish nurse role, given the limitation exercised by the amount of available time. When Rev. Granger Westberg conceived the parish nurse role, he projected that it would be a half-time, paid position. A nurse working 20 hours a week could address the seven functions of the parish nurse role. How is the nursing role identified and the functions implemented when the time available and service provided are severely diminished?

TABLE 22.5 Highest Education Levels of Parish Nurse Respondents (in percentages)

Education	1992 (n = 293)	1994 (n = 509)	1996 (n = 536)
L.P.N.	2	1	1
Diploma degree in nursing	7	11	11
Associate degree in nursing	40	27	27
Nursing B.S.	21	29	29
Non-nursing B.S.	11	10	9
Nursing M.S.	18	20	11
Non-nursing M.S.	—	—	11
Doctorate	1	2	1

Discussions

These studies reflect that the overall patterns of response were quite similar over the three survey periods. What is described are the characteristics of those who identify themselves as parish nurses. The studies have begun the establishment of a comprehensive database that can serve as a baseline for others who are interested in further exploration of this congregationally based nursing role. They also raise additional questions. Is there a need to identify the competencies that are present and being used by parish nurses? Is the parish nurse's level of educational preparation making a difference in the nature and quality of the services offered? Is there a differentiation of practice that can be identified within the parish nurse community? If so, is there a need for additional position titles that would reflect implementation of different functions and their value? The place to begin in addressing these questions is with the identification of the diversity of nursing roles related to parish nursing today.

Identification of Diverse Nursing Roles Related to Parish Nursing

As the awareness of the congregation as a health place has continued to grow nationally and internationally, there are different nursing roles that are or could be developed. The following descriptions are intended to provide information and stimulate thinking.

Director/Coordinator of Parish Nursing Services

This position is found in institutions that have an established infrastructure to support the growth and development of parish nursing services. The nature of the role is administrative. This individual has the accountability and responsibility for the growth, development, and supervision of parish nursing services. This is traditionally a nursing role, with the nurse having experience in management and parish nursing. The educational preparation for this person is a master's degree in nursing or some related area of study, along with attendance at an endorsed basic preparation course for parish nurse coordinators.

Coordinator of a Parish Nurse Program

This role may or may not be held by a nurse. It may be another professional such as a clergyperson, nutritionist, or social worker. This title may be used by an individual at the congregation who is responsible for coordinating the nurses affiliated with the institution or participating in a team parish nurse model (Conrad, 1995). If this role is held by a nurse, the recommended educational preparation is, minimally, a bachelor's degree in nursing. Attendance at an endorsed basic preparation course for parish nurse coordinators is optional.

Parish Nurse Practitioner

Nurse practitioners are those registered nurses who have completed advanced preparation as a nurse practitioner. A parish nurse practitioner uses the competencies, education, and experience of a nurse practitioner but has expanded the care to include the spiritual care that is the hallmark of parish nursing. In addition, this nurse practitioner has a focus on the aggregate faith community, as well as the individual. This distinguishes her from the nurse practitioner who cares for the individual or family, basing her practice out of the traditional medical model. The parish nurse practitioner may operate a nurse-managed center in a congregation.

Care Manager Working in a Congregational Setting

This nursing role operates within a managed care framework and has a focus of working with the individual in the congregation rather than through the corporate whole or the aggregate. The aim is to reduce incidences of illnesses that require costly levels of intervention. This role is occupied by a registered professional nurse employed by a managed care organization. It relates primarily to high-risk individuals documenting whole person and health-promoting interventions intended to sustain a current level of wellness. The preparation for this role would be a master's degree in nursing, with course work in case management. Is this a derivation of the present parish nurse role?

Parish Nurse

Introduced by Rev. Granger Westberg in 1984, this nursing role has as its primary client the faith community (McDermott & Burke, 1993). This may be one congregation or several located in close proximity to each other. The emphasis of this nursing role is health promotion, disease prevention from a whole person perspective. The hallmark is spiritual care. The primary functions of this role are integrator of faith and health, health educator, personal health counselor, referral agent, developer of support groups, trainer of volunteers, and health advocate. The nature of this role does not include any invasive types of care such as drawing blood. This role was envisioned as a half-time nursing role consisting of approximately 20 hours a week in one or more congregations. The preferred educational preparation for this role is a bachelor's degree in nursing, with basic preparation in parish nursing as endorsed by the International Parish Nurse Resource Center.

Parish Nurse Associate

This is a registered licensed professional nurse who is functioning within the context of a faith community and is providing a specific service, such as blood pressure screening. This nurse may be working under the direction of a parish nurse or parish nurse coordinator, assisting in the delivery of specific programming such as health education or personal health counseling. The individual in this role is not able to

incorporate all the functions of the parish nurse role, either because of time or competence. The educational preparation for this role can be at the doctoral, master's, bachelor's, associate, or diploma level in nursing.

Parish Health Advocate

Some institutions are interested in providing health promotion services to many
congregations in a geographic area. This is an opportunity for congregations that do not
have the resources to have their own parish nurse or are not interested in having a parish
nurse as part of the staff of their congregation. The parish health advocate position allows
a nurse from the institution to be available to respond to requests from multiple
congregations for such services as health promotion programming, to answer health-
related questions, to provide needed referrals, and to act as a liaison between a health
care facility and a member of a faith community during an episode of illness. The
educational preparation preferred for this role is a master's degree in nursing.

Summary

For some, the idea of examining the emerging possibilities of nursing within the
congregational setting as described here will be frustrating. The thought that there might
be change that would benefit nursing in congregations and congregation members is
difficult. However, as they say, "Keep changing. When you're through changing, you're
through." Parish nursing is important to these times. Those interested in seeing that the
role of the nurse in a congregation continues to be of importance need to be willing to
be part of the ongoing dialogue that will shape the future of parish nursing. This means
being willing to be open minded, to listen carefully, and to grace-fully be the conscience
for the other.

References

Church, O. M. (1991). Parallels and paradoxes: Differentiated nursing practice in psychiatric care. In I. E.
    Goertzen (Ed.), *Differentiating nursing practice into the twenty-first century.* Washington, DC: American
    Nurses Association.
Conrad, D. M. (1995). Team nursing in parish nurse ministry—even Jesus had 12 apostles. In *Proceedings from
    the Ninth Annual Westberg Symposium: Parish nursing: Ministering through the arts.* Park Ridge, IL:
    International Parish Nurse Resource Center.
Djupe, A. M., Olson, H., & Ryan, J. A. (1994). *Reaching out: Parish nursing services.* Park Ridge, IL: Lutheran
    General HealthSystem.
Koerner, J. E., & Karpiuk, K. L. (1994). *Implementing differentiated nursing practice: Transformation by
    design.* Gaithersberg, MD: Aspen.
Lloyd, R. C., & Solari-Twadell, A. (1994). Organizational framework, functions and educational preparation
    of parish nurses: A comparison of national survey results. In *Proceedings of the Eighth Annual Westberg
    Symposium: Ethics and values: A framework for parish nursing practice.* Park Ridge, IL: International
    Parish Nurse Resource Center.
McDermott, M. A., & Burke, J. (1993). When the population is a congregation: The emerging role of the parish
    nurse. *Journal of Community Health Nursing, 10*(3), 179-190.

23

Proposed Diagnoses and Interventions

Lisa Burkhart
Patricia Kellen

In this health care environment of increasing computer automation and financial accountability, parish nurses are being asked to document their practice within an automated environment that describes how their practice affects patient outcomes. One way to do this is by using standardized nursing languages. Currently, there are four nursing languages accepted by the Library of Medicine. However, the only languages that were designed to cover all nursing specialties are the North American Nursing Diagnosis Association (NANDA) (1994) system, used to describe nursing-sensitive diagnoses, and the Iowa Nursing Intervention Classification (NIC) system, used to describe nursing interventions (McCloskey & Bulechek, 1996).

Even though these languages are intended to be inclusive, both NANDA and NIC have some limitations when applied to parish nursing practice. The primary limitation is their application to spiritual and religious situations. For example, the only two NANDA spiritual diagnoses are "Spiritual Distress" and "Spiritual Well-Being, Potential for Enhanced." Therefore, the only two situations related to spiritual issues are one in which there is a generic spiritual problem and the other in which the nurse can enhance a spiritual connection. NIC only includes one intervention specifically related to spirituality (i.e., "spiritual support"). However, parish nurses can apply other interventions that relate to spiritual and religious practice; for example, "presence" and "emotional support." Parish nurses practice within a spiritual domain, and they need to be able to choose from a language system that includes terminology that describes their practice.

AUTHORS' NOTE: These diagnoses were developed, as part of a Kellogg grant, by a committee of parish nurses from Advocate Health Care and Trinity Medical Center, including the following parish nurses: JoAnn Gragnani Boss; Cynthia Johnson; Patricia Kellen; Michelle Knapp; Harriet S. Olson; Linda Robb; Mary Slutz; and Mary Vann. Assistance was provided by the following staff members: Lisa Burkhart and Bethany Johnson.

Both NANDA and NIC also lack diagnoses and interventions related to community-based practice, including population-focused care, wellness diagnoses, and individual problems related to community factors. In many situations, nurses are concerned about the health of a community, the congregation, or a family—not only an individual.

NANDA and NIC also lack labels related to interpersonal issues that are more common and relevant to parish nurse-client relationships. Many parish nurses develop long-term relationships with parishioners and require additional labels to better reflect their practice. Because NANDA and NIC lack enough spiritual, religious, community, and interpersonal descriptors, parish nurses have difficulty in describing their practice using these systems as they currently exist.

Acknowledging these limitations, a committee of parish nurses, with the financial assistance of a Kellogg grant, developed new diagnoses and interventions to be used with NANDA and NIC to better describe their whole person, community-based practice. The following diagnoses and interventions are preliminary and are currently being developed, further researched, and analyzed to meet the standards for possible inclusion in NANDA and NIC. The diagnoses are being refined as part of a relationship with the University of Iowa's Nursing Diagnosis Extension Classification (NDEC) team and the North American Nursing Diagnosis Association. The interventions are being reviewed and revised with the assistance of the University of Iowa's Nursing Intervention Classification team. Therefore, many of the labels and definitions as they appear in this book will probably differ from their final form.

The diagnoses and interventions that follow reflect and are organized based on three areas of practice: spiritual or religious, community, and interpersonal issues. Although the diagnoses are organized based on these categories, the labels have blurred boundaries and could fall into more than one category. For example, "depression" can be considered a medical diagnosis, an interpersonal or psychosocial issue, or a spiritual issue; for the purposes of this chapter, it will be considered an interpersonal issue.

Because some of the nursing diagnoses reflect complicated cases, examples and possible interventions are provided within the description to better clarify the meaning of the diagnosis. Also, although intervention labels follow diagnosis labels in each spiritual or religious, community, and interpersonal section, they are not necessarily linked. Parish nurses should choose the appropriate diagnoses and interventions that reflect their practice.

Spiritual or Religious Nursing Diagnoses

Acceptance, Potential for Enhanced: The emotional, intellectual, and spiritual journey that an individual experiences in the process of modifying his or her perception of actual or potential loss or change.

In the process of coming to terms with life-altering events or circumstances, an individual or family may experience denial, anger, depression, and isolation. It is to be hoped that at some time the individual or family will be able to integrate the change or loss, achieving some sense of peace. All people who are on this journey will need support to remain in a healthful place.

In her work, a parish nurse will encounter people at various places along the wellness continuum. She will meet those who have just learned of their cancer diagnosis, infertility, job loss, or death of a loved one or who have been confronted by addictive behavior and are still in denial. The parish nurse can be an influence in aiding the patient or family to maintain or move toward acceptance, a positive stage of growth.

Hope, Potential for Enhanced: A subjective state in which an individual expresses belief in an anticipated or an expectation for a positive future outcome or event.

Hope is fundamental to life. It is positively oriented to the future; its opposite, hopelessness, views the future with suspicion, anxiety, or apathy. There are dynamic differences between the two states in the way they affect thinking about *what comes next?* "Hope is a thing longed for . . . something not known, but you anticipate it. It is something good, and it keeps you going when things get really difficult, or sad, or bad. If you have hope, you keep on keeping on" (Gaskins & Forte, 1995, p. 22). A person with hope may speak in positive terms about seeing a future and verbalize a desire to seek a positive outcome. This individual may be involved with family and friends, be energetic, and display a bright affect. Having a person maintain him- or herself in this state would be a desirable outcome.

Image of God, Disabling: The state in which the individual or group is unable to modify (perception and) understanding of the life principle (higher power, deity) in a manner consistent with spiritual growth and development.

Membership and participation in a community of faith does not assure a mature understanding of or relationship with one's deity or higher power. The way an individual perceives God, or the higher power, affects his or her relationships with others. Individuals who have a disabled image of God may have a view of God that is immature and limited by or incompatible with a physically, psychosocially, and spiritually healthy lifestyle. Such individuals may be socially withdrawn or isolated and may passively resign themselves to the circumstances of life. They are, perhaps, noncollegial in their work and relationships. Others with this image may present as perfectionists, may be impatient with others' weaknesses, or may stereotype and devalue others. Their anger may be destructive, and they may view God as nonaccepting and nonforgiving.

The parish nurse's efforts may be directed along various plans of action. Establishing a basic trust in and a gracious acceptance of the individual, even at this most challenging or distancing time, is paramount in supporting this individual in becoming spiritually mature and able to engage in healthy relationships.

Image of God, Potential for Growth: Symbolic patterns of perceiving that reveal our fundamental understanding of and relationship with a higher power and lead us further into the unfolding mystery of our lives.

Some individuals, by nature or through maturing as spiritual beings, examine their relationship with their higher power. They may seek to explore images, symbols, and signs of faith as well as their own dreams, feelings, and projections.

The parish nurse may support the person's spiritual journey by putting him or her in touch with clergy, spiritual companions, or groups that share similar maturity, interests, and goals. A sense of understanding and acceptance, as well as allowing the person to share his or her perceptions, may encourage movement in this fluid state of spiritual health and growth.

Spiritual Concern: The ability and desire to cope with spiritual problems without additional resources.

Parishioners who experience a concern in the spiritual realm may be experiencing a disillusionment with traditional social structures, perhaps even questioning the meaning and value of their own existence. These feelings of uneasiness, mild discontent, or emptiness are a motivator to search for fulfillment and spiritual growth. This can encourage them to improve relationships that meet their own needs or to return to or enhance their spiritual rituals. The concern does not indicate a crisis but is a question. However, unresolved or unsupported, the problem could lead to Altered Spiritual Development or Spiritual Distress.

Spiritual Development, Altered: The inability to identify, manage, or seek out help to maintain spiritual connectedness.

On the continuum of spiritual health, this diagnosis is appropriate for an individual who has not resolved a spiritual concern. Individuals experience more diminishment of their spiritual "life-support," begin to distance themselves from others, and experience emptiness in the rituals and spiritual practices that once provided nourishment and meaning.

The challenge to the spirit, whether occasioned by situational or maturational crisis, is more serious than that experienced in a spiritual concern. Such an alteration requires "care of the soul," without which spiritual distress can evolve.

Spiritual Development, Potential for Growth: The individual identifies a need to manage or seek out help to increase or sustain his or her spiritual connectedness.

This individual recognizes the need to sustain or increase his or her spiritual connectedness. There is movement toward resolving the question. Such clients may request information regarding other belief systems or seek experiences that will enhance their sense of meaning and value. The need for fulfillment in marriage, family, or other relationships, as well as work and worship, have brought them to a turning point—a conscious choice to "press on."

The parish nurse can assist the individual by providing spiritual support, moving the individual toward self-responsibility, or by using spiritual resources available within or outside the faith community.

Spiritual Isolation: A state of separation from God, a higher power, or a related faith tradition as experienced by the individual; perceived as being imposed by others.

Spiritual isolation is complex, with numerous factors affecting this feeling of separation from God, a higher power, or a faith tradition. A person may be religiously isolated but still have a connection with a higher power. When diagnosing spiritual isolation, it is important to uncover grudges, repressed anger, resentment, and hurt feelings. Assessment should consider effects from physical disabilities as well as from emotional concerns and life-principle beliefs. Individuals who are spiritually isolated may state feelings of abandonment; may avoid members of their faith community; may have a sad, dull affect; may seek inappropriate solitude; may be hostile; or may show behavior unacceptable to the faith community.

Spiritual Ritual Patterns, Altered: Disruption of a meaningful act conducted in relation to one's spiritual or religious values and/or faith traditions.

Rituals express the truths, relationships, and beliefs by which people live. Ritual is an important way to provide a structure that allows people to express their emotions. Rituals tend to unite people emotionally. They establish and maintain various kinds of social and cosmic order. The need for rituals is intensified in situations that threaten meaning or coherence. In many cases, the desire for rituals may grow most urgent when people feel a prolonged or acute absence of moral guidance. Individuals who have this diagnosis express the need to participate in ritual patterns but may be unable to participate due to barriers. These barriers include hospitalization; being homebound; and experiencing a lack of access to religious artifacts, sacred objects, or a community of believers.

Spiritual or Religious Nursing Interventions

Faith and Health Enhancement: Facilitation of integration for individuals and groups towards healthier lifestyles, wholeness, and salvation.

To promote the highest level of well-being, the parish nurse supports individuals and congregations in integrating faith and health activities. One of the activities of a parish nurse is to promote an understanding of the relationship between values, beliefs, behaviors, and well-being. This intervention includes performing a physical, psychosocial, and spiritual assessment; teaching the connection between spiritual well-being, physical, and psychosocial well-being; coordinating services with appropriate medical, allied health, and pastoral professionals; and promoting the concept of the church as a health place in the community.

Religious Addiction Prevention: Prevention of a religious addiction lifestyle.

Some individuals depend on the church in an unhealthy way by being excessively dependent upon religion, religious leaders, and/or religious practices. Parish nurses can attempt to discourage this from occurring by identifying those at risk, assisting parishioners in maintaining balanced lives, referring clients to self-help groups, and making available other resources and counseling services. Prevention activities include education about faith development and the dangers of using religion to control others.

> Cultural Brokerage, Religious: Bridging, negotiating, or linking the faith or religious beliefs and traditions of an individual and/or family of a particular culture or faith tradition with the health care system and/or community.

Cultures can differ among individuals, groups, communities, and systems. In addition, religious beliefs and faith traditions can also be different. The nurse needs to be aware of these diversities because such beliefs and practices can positively and/or negatively affect care, relationships, and outcomes. When systems clash, the parish nurse can act as an interpreter, educator, or mediator to facilitate understanding, cooperation, and acceptance. For example, the parish nurse can interpret, for the health team or community, the connection between the belief system and the importance of the family in caring for the patient. In addition, the parish nurse may be the advocate for the patient in acknowledging the importance of certain rituals, dietary practices, rules of conduct, male/female interactions, privacy, modesty, and prayer.

> Spiritual Care: Facilitation of spiritual growth toward becoming self-actualized and transcendent.

Spiritual care relates to other incorporeal needs of the person. Although similar to *presence* and *spiritual support,* this intervention supports the individual toward a new appreciation of spirituality. Presence assumes involvement in times of need only, while spiritual support "assists the patient to feel balance and connection with a greater power" (McCloskey & Bulechek, 1996, p. 529). Spiritual care acknowledges that the client is a spiritual being with spiritual needs.

Activities speak to the assistance needed to sort out spiritual concerns. Clients may need education on the process of spiritual growth and development as well as referral to other appropriate spiritual- and religious-based resources.

Community Nursing Diagnosis

> Access Limitations Related to Health Care: Difficulty in independently obtaining needed services due to life circumstances, conditions, or environment.

A significant segment of the population may have limited access to health care or other community resources due to disability, decreased awareness of resources in the area, living in an underserved geographic location (rural, inner city area, or lower economic), or limited ability to seek and obtain necessary resources.

Disability includes not only physical limitations—for example, wheelchair access and transportation deficits—but inappropriate educational materials, social isolation, and community prejudicesFor example, disabled individuals may wish to participate in community activities, but physical barriers (e.g., wheelchair access or lack of adequate transportation), educational barriers (e.g., excluding disabled persons from marketing campaigns or providing educational material at an inappropriate cognitive level), or community prejudices (e.g., negative communication fostering lack of acceptance of disabled persons in a group) may prevent them from participating. This diagnosis also includes issues related to both the client and the provider. From the client perspective, deficits include insufficient transportation to health care facilities, inadequate financial or insurance coverage, lack of knowledge of resources, and not recognizing their own health care need. From the provider side, deficits include lack of or insufficient number of providers (generalists and specialists) and inadequate hours of operation.

> Communication Pattern Deficit, Ineffective Literacy: The state in which an individual is unable to process information due to a lack of or inefficient ability to read, write, and/or interpret needed information for one's well-being.

Certain educational and lifetime experiences or opportunities may have a negative impact on a client's communication skills. The result may be an inability or limited ability to read, write, or comprehend these modes of communication. Such individuals may have coped adequately with this deficit, but a crisis may bring its existence to the forefront.

The parish nurse needs to be aware of the existence of these deficits among congregants and will have to adjust activities to cope with these limitations. An individual's noncompliance with health maintenance behaviors may stem from a lack of ability to read the discharge instructions. Yet another person's fifth-grade education may prevent him or her from advocating for a part in health care decisions due to possible exposure of the educational deficit or to being overpowered by the system. Young, poorly educated parents who hope to better provide for their growing family may feel trapped because their limitation keeps better jobs beyond their reach.

The parish nurse may respond to such individuals by referring them to a literacy program, helping them navigate the health care system, or amending teaching plans by using graphics to reinforce desired behaviors.

> Cultural Incongruity, Risk For: A deviation from the cultural norm or value of an individual or group that negatively affects health and well-being.

Societies consist of many different cultures and subcultures, many of which will define health and care differently. Nurses need to promote the concept of caring that is compatible with the client's culture. This includes enabling and empowering actions or decision-making processes that preserve and maintain the client's cultural care. Parish nurses must accommodate or negotiate restructuring or repatterning activities to maximize health within a cultural context. If this does not occur when a client from one culture seeks health care from a provider system of a different culture, the client can be at risk for cultural incongruity. For example, certain chronic illnesses require changes in lifestyle (e.g., diet) that are not compatible with the client's culture. This incompatibility can manifest as noncompliance, spiritual distress, or unwillingness to jointly develop a plan of care.

Homelessness: A state in which the individual experiences the inability to manage and/or seek out help to maintain a safe, meaningful, viable, permanent, and intact dwelling place.

Parish nurses encounter individuals or families who are homeless or who are at risk for becoming homeless. Individuals are considered homeless if they are sheltered or unsheltered, are living with several families in one home, or are migrant workers. For these individuals, entry into the parish nurse caseload usually is very slow, often due to trust issues. Homeless clients require high-intensity care and complex relationship building, along with interagency networking and health care collaboration.

Community Nursing Interventions

Community Empowerment: Actions at the local, state, and national level to promote citizen quality of life and to encourage the community to advocate for itself.

As a health advocate, the parish nurse is able to represent those who cannot speak for themselves. This includes being able to articulate client needs to those in power. This intervention is appropriate when representing groups on local, state, or national committees, at meetings, or at other events. Activities include identifying and researching community health and safety risks, gaining support for the chosen position, articulating the position in speech and writing, and seeking funding to support a position or program.

Volunteer Coordination: The development of a volunteer program for performing select activities.

The church has many resources to help faith communities. One of its richest resources is its parishioners. Part of the parish nurse's role may be to engage, manage, and coordinate parishioner volunteer activities. Volunteer coordination includes identifying volunteers, maintaining a spirit of volunteerism, and providing ongoing support and continuing education. Management functions may include developing program needs, goals, objectives, budgets, and resources; communicating through publications; and networking while integrating the program into other church functions.

Volunteer Support: The use of volunteers to enhance an individual's health.

Many individuals provide for spiritual fulfillment through volunteering. The parish nurse facilitates the instruction needed for the volunteer role, encourages the volunteer's participation in educational programs, and helps the volunteer understand the scope and limitations of the position.

Interpersonal Nursing Diagnoses

> Authoritarian Role Conflict: The state in which a person experiences role confusion and a conflicting response to perceived or actual authority.

A person's attitude, beliefs, and feelings may predispose a response to another person or event. A common assumption is that a person's attitude and actions are interconnected. An important aspect of self-concept pertains to whether we learn to see ourselves as in control or being controlled. Behavior is affected by whether a person perceives the control of their life as internal (within themselves) or external (at the mercy of the outside world). This diagnosis is appropriate when there is a problem associated with internal control and external control imposed by others, be it individuals, family members, or community-focused organizations or agencies. Authoritarian role conflict can be manifested by outward anger, guilt, passivity, withdrawal, inability to perform social roles, or lowered self-esteem. For example, such conflict can occur in the work place between formal or informal leaders, in a family between parents and children, in a church between the pastor and parishioners, or in a community agency between those individuals working in the agency and the public for whom they serve.

> Depression: A subjective state in which an individual experiences a lowering of mood that is beginning to negatively interfere with normal activities of daily living.

Many individuals experience a lowering of mood in response to life events. It is when this alteration begins to have a negative impact on areas of a person's life, including sleep and eating habits, energy level, concentration, and sociability, that steps need to be taken to interrupt the process. Gone unchecked, depression can affect compliance, health-seeking behaviors, relationships, employment, and financial integrity.

Depression can appear as withdrawal from social or service groups, anger, agitation, or inattention to self-care. In extreme cases, clients may express a preoccupation with death or suicide. The parish nurse may initiate a referral to a self-help or support group while providing emotional support through active presence.

> Individual Coping, Potential for Growth: The positive adaptation and management of an individual's problem-solving abilities and tasks as related to health issues and concerns when demands regarding the individual's welfare have a potential for improvement as life's issues change and evolve.

Interactions with others are not limited to those who "need" us to advocate, validate decisions, or problem solve. In the face of challenges and choices, there are individuals who are able to function appropriately in the presence of actual or potential stressors. Clients who exhibit this or some degree of coping, faith, and hope can benefit from the parish nurse's encouragement and support. The nurse's intervention is to support these individuals along the positive end of the wellness continuum. This may be done through various functions—as a personal health counselor, health educator, referral source, interpreter of the relationship between faith and health, or health advocate.

Ineffective Boundaries: Inability to identify and/or preserve self and integrity.

Boundaries define space. Boundaries are invisible, symbolic fences that keep others from entering an individual's personal space and disrupting his or her ability to discriminate. Personal boundaries give each individual a way to embody a sense of identity. The ability to set limits provides a feeling of self-respect and freedom. This enhances energy and the ability to relate to others. An inability to maintain boundaries may cause self-esteem disturbances, anger, and resistance to accepting help.

Interpersonal Nursing Interventions

Communication Enhancement: Using principles of effective and therapeutic communication in gathering information and providing care to patients, significant others, and communities in a more effective manner, recognizing cultural, developmental, intellectual, physical, psychosocial, and spiritual differences.

Communication enhancement is more than interventions used for hearing, speech, or visual deficits. It is more basic than active listening or complex relationship building, although the activities may be similar. Communication enhancement refers to behaviors that maximize an interaction.

Activities include tailoring the model of interaction to the situation and needs of those involved. This includes using nontechnical language or explaining information in terms more easily understood by clients, avoiding unnecessary repetition of questions, and obtaining or reviewing existing records prior to the beginning of the interaction.

Mediation Skills, Ineffective: The act of intervening between two parties who are in conflict or disagreement, with the goal of a mutually satisfactory resolution.

Clients in any setting may be in the midst of conflict management or creating conflict in dealing with emotional, physical, or spiritual health. Individuals who experience ineffective mediation may show hostility, anxiety, or disagreement. Nurses may deal with conflict in various situations requiring third-party facilitation before effective health care can be provided. The parties involved hold mutually exclusive ideas, attitudes, feelings, or goals. They may have inaccurate information or hold different values or cultural beliefs.

Summary

To communicate the practice of parish nursing—be it in documentation or professional communications—parish nurses need to define concepts that relate to this practice. These proposed diagnoses and interventions can help in that process. The Parish Nurse Committee of Advocate Health Care, through its work with the University of Iowa's NDEC and NIC teams, will continue to refine these diagnoses and interventions so that the concepts underlying them will be accepted for inclusion in the respective national classification systems. Additional interventions have already been accepted by the Iowa NIC team.

References

Gaskins, S., & Forte, L. (1995, March). The meaning of hope—Implications for nursing practice and research. *Journal of Gerontological Nursing, 21*(3), 17-24.

McCloskey, J. C., & Bulechek, G. M. (1996). *Iowa Intervention Project: Nursing interventions classification (NIC).* St. Louis, MO: Mosby.

North American Nursing Diagnosis Association. (1994). *Nursing diagnoses: Definitions and classification.* Philadelphia: Author.

24

Educational Preparation

Mary Ann McDermott
Phyllis Ann Solari-Twadell
Rosemarie Matheus

Historical Overview

More than a decade has passed since 1984, when Granger Westberg approached Lutheran General Hospital about the idea of piloting his concept of parish nursing. Granger, in his charismatic way, subsequently traveled as a "Johnny Appleseed" not only around the Chicagoland area but across the nation, talking about this exciting opportunity for nursing and churches. Listeners wanted additional information and were curious to learn more about this innovative role. There was no formal education available on parish nursing. Interested individuals began to seek out the original six nurses in the northwest Chicago area in attempts to hear more about their experiences and to explore how they could apply these learnings to their own settings. These inquiries began to create a burden for this small group of pioneering nurses, as they themselves were learning day by day what it meant to be a parish nurse.

In an attempt to relieve the nurse pioneers and yet funnel their learnings to other faith communities, the Parish Nurse Resource Center ("the Resource Center") was formed out of the office of Church Relations, Lutheran General Health Care System, in Park Ridge, Illinois. A director for the Resource Center, Phyllis Ann Solari-Twadell, was appointed. An advisory board was established, with local and national nursing and clergy representation. Interestingly, it was this group that recommended that a membership organization be formed outside the Resource Center's purview, which later (in September 1988) gave birth to the Health Ministries Association. The purpose of the Resource Center, as it was articulated at that time and as it continues to be, is to promote the development of quality parish nurse programs and to study the organizational models, functions, educational preparation, and denominational affiliations of the nurses (Lloyd & Solari-Twadell, 1994). From its inception, the aim of the Resource Center has been to provide resources essential to catalyze the development of quality parish nurse programs through education, research, publishing, and consulting and also to serve a clearinghouse function.

The Resource Center offered the first continuing education program on parish nursing in September 1987. Over the years, this evolved into the Annual Westberg Symposium on Parish Nursing. A major theme is established (i.e., "Ethics and Values," 1994; "Ministering Through the Arts," 1995; "A Celebration of Health, Healing and Wholeness," 1996; "Documenting the Journey" 1997; "Valuing the Lived Experience," 1998; "Journey in Wisdom," 1999), a nurse keynote speaker is selected as well as a major clergy presenter, preconference workshops on specific topics of current interest are held, abstracts for presentations and posters are solicited internationally from practicing parish nurses, worship is celebrated, networking is facilitated, and a book of proceedings is distributed to all participants. Attendance has grown from 74 in 1987 to approximately 930 in 1998, and the conference itself has grown from a local offering to an international event, with participants from Australia, Korea, Canada, England, and Ireland.

Consultation on parish nursing is a service that the Resource Center provides to health care facilities, universities, and religious denominations as well as to individuals. In the late 1980s and early 1990s, the Resource Center provided consultation to George-town University and Marquette University relating to the development of both credit-bearing coursework and continuing education offerings. In 1991, the Resource Center also served as the convener and catalyst for four nursing programs in Chicago—St. Xavier, North Park, Rush, and Loyola—and these, with several seminaries, came to-gether to explore educational preparation for the joint competency needed for those in parish nursing and other health ministries. A consortium was formed to offer a series of three courses in health ministries and consequently to develop a prototype of a combined M.Div. and M.S.N. degree program. This consortium has persisted, and two other nurs-ing programs at Lewis University and the University of Illinois have joined the group.

In 1989, the Resource Center began to offer an "Orientation to Parish Nursing." This was a 2½-day continuing education program that gave nurses basic information on the concept, how to get a program started, and a discussion of issues such as legal concerns and accountability. The program included a half-day accompaniment with one of the Lutheran General-sponsored parish nurses. The orientation sessions were discontinued by the Resource Center in 1996, as many interested individuals confused this offering with what the Resource Center considered more preferable: "Basic Preparation," a lengthier, more in-depth program. It was developed by educational institutions across the country and regional parish nurse networks.

Questions and Issues Pertinent to the
Education of Parish Nurses

What are the basic educational requirements for the nurse called to parish nursing practice? How best is the individual prepared for the seven functions and the varied activities unique to this role? What type of continuing education is most appropriate? Is there a body of core content for parish nursing, for parish nurse program coordinators? What strategies and expanding technologies can be used to make this education effective, available, and accessible throughout the world? Can ongoing professional development be mandated for a parish nurse who serves in an unpaid, voluntary position? Is there a need for advanced formal academic preparation? What should the educational and experiential qualifications be of those who teach parish nurses? Where does the education take place? Who will sponsor and finance this education? What type of collaborative and cooperative arrangement should be encouraged for addressing educational needs? Is preparation for the existing functions of the parish nurse sufficient for role development as envisioned by some for the not-too-distant future? What is the role of the Advocate Health Care System (successor organization to Lutheran General Health Care System in 1995)-sponsored International Parish Nurse Resource Center (the name was changed in 1996) in addressing these questions and issues as we approach the next millennium?

Current Preparation of the Parish Nurse

Studies conducted periodically over the past 10 years suggest that individuals practicing in the parish nurse role have a variety of educational backgrounds, from a diploma through the doctoral degree. Although the level of preparation has continued to increase, not all parish nurses with baccalaureate and higher degrees necessarily have them in nursing. Some have additional formal theology or pastoral care preparation (Lloyd & Solari-Twadell, 1994).

Since the advent of continuing education efforts for parish nursing under the sponsorship of Lutheran General and the Resource Center in 1987 (noted earlier), over 60 different parish nursing educational programs available nationally have become known to the Resource Center. These programs are sponsored primarily by health care institutions. Schools of nursing, other related schools in university settings, seminaries, church bodies, associations, regional parish nurse networks, and educational entrepreneurs are also engaged in this endeavor. Programs included 1-day and week-long orientations, continuing education workshops, seminars, distance learning, and ongoing cousework over weeks and months, as well as credit-bearing coursework in B.S.N., M.S.N., and M.Div. programs offered over the course of a semester or, for some, over several years.

This growth and diversity in offerings is in response to the demands of individual nurses, of professional organizations, and of congregations. All are swept up by the massive health care changes and are seeking alternative ways to deliver health and healing to the whole person. There is a desire on the part of the authors to eagerly embrace this growth and diversity as a positive sign of society's readiness for parish nursing. The differences, however, in curricular content, prioritization of content, faculty background, perspectives on content, number of course hours, and allotment of credit and noncredit that provide for a richness in these diverse offerings also present a number of challenges that we believe need to be acknowledged and addressed (McDermott, Solari-Twadell, & Matheus, 1998). Wide ranges in the preparation and consequent implementation of this still-new role could, it was felt, lead to confusion in the recipients of the services as well as in the professional health care community and program sponsors.

Development of Guidelines for
Parish Nurse Education Programs

In response to this growing concern, and at the recommendation of several parish nurse leaders and educators (Ruth Stoll, D.N.Sc. Messiah College, Grantham, PA; Norma Small, Ph.D. Georgetown University, Washington, DC, and Joan Zetterlund, Ph.D. North Park College, Chicago, IL), the Resource Center sponsored an invitational colloquium on the development of guidelines for parish nurse education in June 1994. The aim of the project was to assure the educational foundation for the future of parish nursing practice. Those invited to this $2\frac{1}{2}$-day meeting were 26 parish nurses, parish nurse educators, and clergy currently involved in parish nurse education from across the country. Types of programs represented by the educators included orientation, continuing professional education, and credit-bearing nursing coursework at the baccalaureate and master's level; one representative was from a Master's in Divinity program.

Colloquium conveners were convinced that guidelines must be developed to assure that the parish nurse role would continue to fit into emerging community networks of care and to assure the future viability of parish nurse education rather than to standardize or incrementally improve then current educational offerings. Colloquium participants were, therefore, given a prereading assignment and requested to think critically about what changes in health care delivery could mean for the future of parish nursing and parish nurse educational programs. Senge's (1990) work on dialogue guided the group's inquiry. The resulting publication, "Assuring Viability for the Future: Guideline Development for Parish Nurse Education Programs" (Solari-Twadell, McDermott, Ryan, & Djupe, 1994), has served as a valuable document to parish nurse educators.

During the same year, a workshop for 37 self-selected parish nurse coordinators was conducted prior to the Eighth Annual Westberg Symposium. Activities, skills needed, and preparatory knowledge and experience of these nurses in the managerial role were examined. Participants were asked to submit in advance to the workshop coordinator (a contributing author of this chapter), a copy of their position description, résumé, and a form titled "Parish Nurse Manager's Week-at-a-Glance." Requested to select 3 days of a recent work week, the coordinators were asked to reflect on the five activities each day that commanded most of their time. In addition, they were asked to identify the skills and the prerequisite knowledge and experience needed for implementation of those activities. Last, coordinators were asked: "If you could reorder your day, which activities would you include and in what priority? These may or may not be already on your lists." The discussion and findings from this workshop served as an additional springboard to the curriculum work described below.

Basic Preparation for Parish Nurses and
Parish Nurse Coordinators

It is the responsibility of a profession to monitor its own practice. The profession of nursing is ethically responsible for the quality of care that is delivered to the public in the name of parish nursing. One method of attaining quality is to define educational standards for the practice. The public deserves the assurance that when the title *parish nurse* is used, the nurse has received the necessary preparation to function in this specialized role. For this purpose, the International Parish Nurse Resource Center has led the development of a standardized core curriculum for parish nurses, as well as one for parish nurse coordinators.

Process of Creating a Standardized Curriculum

An educational programming needs assessment was begun in June 1996, using a convenience sample of 50 parish nurse coordinators known to the International Parish Nurse Resource Center. They were queried regarding the content of their own basic parish nurse educational preparation, as well as about additional education they had experienced to prepare for the coordinator role. These nurses were also asked to identify content they would rate as most helpful to them in their role. Additionally, the coordinators were requested to comment on the specifics of such a program offering in terms of site, length, and cost of such a program and indicate if they would participate or encourage a new coordinator to attend.

The findings from the needs assessment have served as the basis for a 3-year collaborative curriculum development and implementation venture between Marquette University, Loyola University Chicago, and the International Parish Nurse Resource Center. The first year focused on identifying core content for curriculum models for the basic preparation of the parish nurse, as well as for the coordinator role (see Appendix A). A format for the course was established. Three thousand readers of *Perspectives in Parish Nursing Practice,* a publication of the International Parish Nurse Resource Center, were solicited to submit the names of content experts who could develop curriculum modules on the queried coordinator-identified content topics. Content experts were then invited to create detailed syllabi for specific course content areas.

The completed work of the identified experts was peer-reviewed by the entire group of other content experts prior to their coming together for an invitational colloquium in April 1997. At that time, with the assistance of a panel of external, nationally recognized nurse and ministerial leaders and educators (including representatives of the American Nurses Association and the National League for Nursing, three nursing school deans or dean representatives, and reviewers from Canada and Australia), a critical review of all submitted materials was made and subsequently endorsed by the group. After piloting and further refinement (in 1997 and 1998), the curricula both for basic parish nurse preparation and for the coordinator role is being distributed through the Resource Center to those participating in a faculty preparation program.

Core Curriculum Content for Parish Nurses

The International Parish Nurse Resource Center recommends that any nurse practicing under the title *parish nurse* should have completed a course of specialized instruction that includes but is not limited to the core curriculum for parish nursing. Detailed syllabi of the required content with specific objectives, sequencing, and time allotments have been developed for the following:

- The Role of the Church in Health
- Theology of Health
- History of Parish Nursing
- Philosophy of Parish Nursing
- Models of Parish Nursing Practice
- Function of the Parish Nurse: Teacher
- Function of the Parish Nurse: Counselor
- Function of the Parish Nurse: Referral Agent
- Function of the Parish Nurse: Trainer of Volunteers
- Function of the Parish Nurse: Integrator of Faith and Health
- Community Assessment
- Health Promotion and Maintenance
- Faith Community and Family as Client
- Self-Care for the Parish Nurse
- Working With Churches
- Functioning Within a Ministerial Team
- Accountability
- Documentation
- Legal Considerations
- Ethical Issues
- Prayer
- Worship Leadership
- Getting Started

Process as a Mode of Learning

Although the content of the curricula is considered necessary and appears as the essence of the educational experience for the novice parish nurse, it is the process of the educational experience that has paramount importance. The practice of parish nursing is more than a new work role, it is a call to ministry. This requires that the preparation be more than attaining new knowledge.

The structure of the curricular offering, in a setting that encourages intimate sharing when possible, spiritual inspiration and challenges, positive reinforcement of vision, play, and peer interaction, creates a learning experience that affects the learner in subtle yet impressionable ways. The ideal setting is apart from the learner's usual environment, creating a break from the demands of family and work. This enables the learner to focus on self and to attend to personal needs for understanding and responding to the new role and call to ministry. The sense of being cared for by others during this learning experience nurtures the learner's spirit and mental well-being.

Opportunity for play, structured and spontaneous, will facilitate the desired inter-action of the group and foster deeper relationships. Humor integrated into the experience will demonstrate a healthy mode of self-care and ease the intensity of some of the sessions.

Time should be built into the total experience for public and private worship, including a healing worship service when possible. Devotional time at meals and/or at the beginning and end of sessions are important opportunities for the participants during which they can prepare devotions and share their spiritual lives and thoughts with the group. Scriptural passages, readings, and written inspirational messages may be distributed unexpectedly and privately among the group. A final celebratory closure of the experience is essential to the process. This may take the form of a worship service, a dedication ceremony, a festive meal, or a ritual. When appropriate, family, clergy, and others may be included in these events to emphasize the value of the parish nurse ministry to both the nurse and those who will support the new ministry.

The Core Curriculum Content for
Parish Nurse Coordinators

The core curriculum for parish nurse coordinators consists of these content areas:

- The Role of the Parish Nurse Coordinator
- Working With Churches
- Trends in Health Care
- Infrastructure for Parish Nurse Programs
- Accountability
- Documentation Systems
- Human Resource Management
- Budgeting
- Grant Writing
- Orientation of the New Parish Nurse
- Planning for the Ongoing Development of the Parish Nurse
- Continuing Education Experiential Sharing Exercise
- Spiritual Development of the Parish Nurse

A prerequisite to coordinator education is completion of the basic parish nurse core curriculum. Content deficits in the basic parish nurse preparation education of coordinators will be offered in an abbreviated coordinator preconference as needed. It should be noted that not all parish nurse coordinators have a background in parish nursing and, in fact, may not be nurses. Recommendations made above about process as a mode of learning are also applicable to the preparation of parish nurse coordinators.

Other and Future Considerations

Mentoring

Merriam-Webster's Collegiate Dictionary (10th edition) defines *mentor* as a wise and trusted teacher and counselor. Many parish nurse educators deem it essential that newly prepared parish nurses experience a period of time during which they are in a mentoring relationship with an experienced parish nurse. During this time, the mentor has regular contact with the new parish nurse. The mentor is available to advise appropriately, nurture an emerging identity as a parish nurse, support and encourage continued spiritual development, and facilitate adjustment to the new environment. Preferably, these contacts would be in-person meetings, but realistically, more will be done by telephone or in written correspondence, using fax and e-mail technology.

Both the availability and willingness of sufficient numbers of experienced parish nurses and the financial considerations inherent in this well-recognized but very time-consuming teaching and learning strategy have impeded widespread implementation. Accessibility to one another is key!

Ongoing Network of Support

The basic educational experience will lay the foundation of a necessary network of peers that is essential as the parish nurse weans herself from the group learning experience. When the parish nurse is part of an institutional program, this network may be ready-made. When practicing outside an institutional program, the parish nurse needs to locate or create a network of support. This can be done locally or regionally; however, the contingency plan often used is to mobilize peers from the educational program.

There are many other considerations that emerge from the list of questions and issues pertinent to the education of parish nurses posed earlier. The Resource Center, regional networks, and educational institutions working collaboratively or alone have begun or are about to begin to address a number of these. Others are on hold until adequate resources (human, time, or financial) can be identified or until an urgency mandates a shift of priority.

Future considerations include the development of appropriate and cost-effective distance-learning opportunities for the basic preparation and continuing education of both parish nurses and coordinators. Credentialing and/or certification of parish nurses has been proposed; however, no action regarding this issue has been taken by the Resource Center at the time of this writing.

References

Lloyd, R., & Solari-Twadell, A. (1994). Organizational framework, functions and educational preparation of parish nurses: National survey 1991 and 1994. In *Proceedings of the Eighth Annual Westberg Parish Nurse Symposium: "Ethics and values: A framework for parish nursing practice"* (pp. 105-115). Park Ridge, IL: National Parish Nurse Resource Center.

McDermott, M. A., Solari-Twadell, P. A., & Matheus, R. (1998). Promoting quality education for the parish nurse and the parish nurse coordinator. *Nursing and Health Care Perspective, 19*(4), 4-6.

Senge, P. (1990). *The fifth discipline: The art and practice of the learning organization.* New York: Currency/Doubleday.

Solari-Twadell, A., McDermott, M. A., Ryan, J., & Djupe, A. M. (1994). *Assuring viability for the future: Guideline development for parish nurse education programs.* Park Ridge, IL: National Parish Nurse Resource Center.

25

The Canadian Experience

Joanne K. Olson
Margaret B. Clark
Jane A. Simington

Although parish nursing practice in Canada shares elements common to parish nursing in other countries, this specialized area of community nursing practice is evolving somewhat uniquely within the Canadian context. Built on principles of health promotion and values of autonomy and equity, the Canadian health care system serves as a rich background upon which parish nursing can develop. This chapter includes a discussion of the uniqueness of Canada, the Canadian health care system, the development of parish nursing within this system, and initial Canadian parish nursing initiatives. Emphasis is placed upon the development of parish nursing education at the University of Alberta Faculty of Nursing, to provide an example of program development that could serve as a model in other locations.

The Uniqueness of the Canadian Context

The promotion of equality and multicultural diversity are themes central to Canadian life, and in many ways they dictate how health care in Canada is delivered. Although the Battle on the Plains of Abraham established British dominance in 1759, the French maintained their language, culture, religion, and legal system. And although the Canadian system of government flowed from the British model, French religious orders established the first hospitals in what is now Quebec and moved steadily westward, bringing health, education, and social services to the fur traders, local aboriginals, and new settlers (Kerr & McPhail, 1996). The goal of early Christian missionaries was to convert the Indian and Métis (originating from the union of Indian and French ancestry), but there is now a renewed respect for the interconnectedness between spirituality and health so deeply rooted in the First Nations people's traditional beliefs and ceremonies (Bopp, 1985).

Discovery of Canada's vast natural resources led to large waves of European immigration. Like their predecessors, the newcomers were encouraged to contribute from the diversity of their cultures. Most newcomers now arrive from Asia and South America, and they too are invited to maintain, and to share with pride, their heritage. This "cultural mosaic" approach of honoring diversity differs from the "melting pot" assimilation model in the United States and has influenced how parish nursing was introduced and will continue to develop in this country. People from non-Christian backgrounds, for example, may be unfamiliar with the Christian term *parish*. They can identify value in the concept of parish nursing, but they question the appropriateness of the word parish when used in a Canadian context.

Canada as a Leader in Health Promotion

Canadian policymakers have demonstrated world leadership with their broad approach to health promotion and disease prevention. *A New Perspective on the Health of Canadians* (Lalonde, 1974) noted that "the traditional view of equating the levels of health . . . with the availability of physicians and hospitals is inadequate" (p. 18). Yeo (1993) suggested that whereas helping, curing, and caring for ill people is important, these activities often occur to the relative neglect of the deeper determinants of ill health: individual, biological, and environmental factors. He defined health promotion as "a reform movement advocating a shift of priorities and resources in alignment with a broader way of thinking about health, and advocating new and broader social interventions in order to protect, maintain and promote health" (p. 225).

At a conference in Alma Ata, USSR, the World Health Organization (1978) identified primary health care (which includes health promotion), as the favored strategy to achieve *Health for All by the Year 2000*. Awareness that health is influenced by a wide range of factors, including biological, physical, social, spiritual, and environmental, was strengthened again in Canada's Epp Report (Epp, 1986), *Achieving Health for All: A Framework for Health Promotion*. This document emphasized that the key to successful health services is to ensure, through regular evaluation, that services meet the real needs of people in a way that is readily accessible, empowering, culturally appropriate, gender sensitive, and cost effective. Principles that guide health-promoting activities have also taken into account the notion of self-responsibility for health, adopted from the internationally accepted definition of health promotion given in the *Ottawa Charter for Health Promotion* (1986).This document emphasized that health promotion "is the process of enabling people to increasing control over, and to improve, their health . . . it is not just the responsibility of the health sector, but goes beyond healthy lifestyles to well-being" (p. 426).

The Canadian Health Care System

Models of health care delivery range from private health insurance systems, governed by a market orientation in which government plays a residual role, to the opposite extreme of socialized health care in which government defines health care as an essential service (Najman & Western, 1984). Preserving the autonomy of the individual, the physician, and the health institution takes priority in private health insurance systems. The fact that a substantial minority of people might be without health care is unfortunate but unavoidable. In socialized health systems, decreased autonomy is accepted because the goal is to preserve the collective good. If the United States system of health care delivery is an example of a private system and the United Kingdom is typical of a socialized system, the National Health Insurance System in Canada can be viewed as a blend of these two systems. By encouraging health professional and health agency autonomy and ensuring relatively easy access to health care for all individuals regardless of their ability to pay, important Canadian values are protected. Developed from the belief that health is a right, not a privilege, and in an attempt to preserve autonomy and equity, the Canadian health care system has been built upon five main principles: universality, accessibility, comprehensiveness, portability, and public administration, as spelled out in the 1984 Canada Health Act. Although the phrase "Canadian health care system" is commonly used, Canada does not have a federal health care system; it has 10 provincial, plus 2 territorial, health care systems (Deber & Vayda, 1992).

Funding Canadian Health Care

Even though the roots of Canadian health care are closely tied to the spread of Christianity across the country, a post-World War II desire to have health care costs covered by tax revenue led to the relinquishing of private health care agencies and the need for private health care insurance. Provincial tax revenues and federal transfer payments now fund Canadian health care. The acceptance of parish nursing in Canada has been influenced by the method used to pay for Canadian health care. Many churches recognize that government-funded health care has been less than effective in meeting the total needs of people and are attempting to regain their health and healing mission, but they must face the issue of financing these reclaimed endeavors. Canadians are not accustomed to paying for nursing or other health or social services. In this time of fiscal restraint and health care reform, some suspect that programs such as parish nursing are a way to "download" the responsibility of government onto alternative providers, who will take responsibility for administering quality health care but without government funding. Others question whether such initiatives violate the Canada Health Act, insisting that some Canadians will have access to health services not available to all.

Health Care Reform in Canada

By the mid-1990s, it was recognized that in spite of Canada's leadership in health promotion, a discrepancy existed between what was known about determinants of health and how health care was being delivered. A call for health care reform across Canada came from a recognition that (a) governmental funding could no longer match escalating costs, (b) the bulk of spending was on the most expensive acute care services, (c) the majority of conditions being treated could have been prevented, (d) chronic conditions such as cancer and social concerns such as alcoholism and family violence were increasing, (e) there are many determinants of health, (f) individuals could take more responsibility for maintaining wellness, and (g) health care services did not address the deeper needs of people.

With health care reform came rapid change in the delivery of health care services. Canadians were encouraged to assume more responsibility in decisions regarding their health and were invited to propose new models for delivery of health promotion services. The door was now opening for creative and innovative strategies in achieving the vision, goals, and objectives of a reformed health system. Parish nursing was beginning to emerge as a promising new model, offering affordable, high-quality, community-based care, delivered in a more holistic way (Simington, Olson, & Douglass, 1996). As community-based health educators, health counselors, advocates, referral agents, coordinators of volunteers, and integrators of faith and health, parish nurses offered an innovative model for community-based health promotion efforts.

Early Development of Parish Nursing in Canada

The first formal introduction of parish nursing in Canada was in September, 1993, when the International Parish Nurse Resource Center exhibited at the International Conference on Community Health Nursing Research in Edmonton, Alberta. Following in 1994 and 1995, Lutheran Health Care Association, under the direction of Rev. Henry Fischer, contacted the Parish Nurse Resource Center to provide a series of introductory workshops on parish nursing in nine different cities in Canada. In 1994, a University of Alberta ad hoc Committee on Parish Nursing conducted a feasibility study. The results led to the decision to place the thrust of initial parish nursing activities in Alberta on education (Olson, Simington, & Douglass, 1995). A pilot project, funded by the Ontario Ministry of Health and directed by Rev. Henry Fischer, placed parish nurses in six southern Ontario faith communities in 1996. Initial efforts in British Columbia focused on introducing nurses, clergy, and congregations to the practice of nursing in the church (Martin, 1996). Although a great deal can be said of each of these initiatives, emphasis in this chapter is given to the Alberta experience, with which the authors are most familiar.

Alberta Parish Nursing Feasibility Study

To determine the feasibility of parish nursing in Alberta, face-to-face, semistructured interviews were conducted with clergy from six Christian denominational groups. The following questions were asked: (a) Does your denomination view its mission as including responsiveness to the health and healing needs of people? (b) Do you as a representative of your denomination believe that the clergy play a role in meeting the health needs of people? (c) Do you see value in adding another professional to the pastoral team to assist in meeting the total needs of congregational members? (d) Do you believe that a nurse would be the appropriate professional to fill such a role?

Results indicated that clergy were involved in health-related issues. They regularly assisted people during life transitions and recognized that these times of transition affect the total health of people. They felt prepared to address spiritual and psychosocial needs but were less able to deal with physical health issues. Clergy saw value in having another professional on the pastoral team and readily saw nurses as the appropriate professionals. Nurses had demonstrated the ability to view people holistically, seeing the interconnectedness of all dimensions of each person.

Members of Alberta's 17 newly formed regional health boards were informed about parish nursing and the feasibility study. They were invited to talk with faculty about the possibilities for parish nursing within their particular regions. The study indicated that both government and faith communities were interested in developing partnerships.

While government and health promotion documents were calling for increased community-based care, a whole person health promotion focus, and intersectoral cooperation, churches were asking how they could more fully carry out their healing missions. Leaders in faith communities suggested that they were already involved in activities that promote the health and well-being of parishioners as well as of the greater community. They further suggested that although the health care system was providing much in the way of illness care, the real issues that affect health and overall well-being were frequently not being addressed. Faith communities were willing to play an expanded role in promoting well-being, and they saw parish nursing as one way to accomplish this goal.

Parish Nursing Education at
the University of Alberta

Encouraged by the findings of the feasibility study, and accepting the responsibility of universities to provide education relevant to changing social needs, faculty at the University of Alberta in Edmonton initiated the first Canadian university education in parish nursing. With a vision that parish nursing in Alberta would reflect an interdisciplinary approach and its Canadian setting, nursing and pastoral care faculty embarked on a journey of designing and delivering two six-credit courses that would retool experienced nurses for promoting health in faith communities.

Developing Faculty Expertise and Creating Networks

Building upon strong academic and practice backgrounds, nursing and pastoral care faculty began an in-depth exploration of parish nursing. An extensive literature review was conducted, and international networking was initiated through the Parish Nurse Resource Center in Park Ridge, Illinois. In May 1995, faculty participated in the Edmonton parish nursing conference, sponsored by the Lutheran Health Care Association of Canada. One member of the faculty team attended a parish nurse preparation institute at Marquette University, Milwaukee, Wisconsin. These experiences resulted in establishing and strengthening both academic and professional practice connections. Responding to community interest, the faculty team organized a working conference. At this conference, held in Edmonton over 2 days in October 1995, Rosemarie Matheus of Marquette University further informed nurses, clergy, lay leaders, health care leaders, and government leaders about parish nursing.

Community Interest Grows

Through publication and conference presentations, the Alberta faculty team's concept of parish nursing in a Canadian context was disseminated (Clark, 1995; Douglass, 1995; Olson & Simington, 1995; Olson et al., 1995; Simington, 1996; Simington & Olson, 1995; Simington et al., 1996). The sharing of knowledge and experiences led to numerous requests for further information and resulted in presentations to Christian and non-Christian faith communities and in health care settings as well as local, provincial, and national media interviews. These contacts resulted in making connections with individuals and groups ready to join in pursuing the development of parish nursing in Canada.

Formation of a parish nursing program advisory committee provided visible community support for parish nursing and made tangible the growing partnership between the university, pastoral care leadership at two health care agencies, and the greater Edmonton community. Clergy and lay leaders from congregations expressing interest in parish nursing were invited to provide input to faculty about how parish nursing education could respond to needs within their faith community settings.

Interdisciplinary Approach to Course Development

Drawing forth the spiritual care dimension of the nurse for purposes of cultivating health promotion activities within faith communities required expertise from both nurse educators and clinical pastoral theological educators. Initial planning sessions were marked with frustrations and conflicting expectations regarding content and teaching methods. These tensions were connected to role stereotyping. Role stereotyping, if left unbridled, can lead to the collusion of dominance and subordination (Pierce & Page, 1986). Nursing faculty needed to become aware of the skill and expertise with which pastoral care professionals provide spiritual care, and pastoral care faculty needed to understand that the full scope of nursing practice includes spiritual care. Faculty had to come to realize that stereotyping would limit the potential for parish nurses to link faith and health, promote health and wholeness, and respond to the whole person needs of faith community members.

Determination to move from role stereotyping toward "mutuality in ministry" (Fenhagen, 1977) required a "decision to learn" (Pierce & Page, 1986). Faculty progressed through two distinct stages: (a) recognizing the scope and boundaries of their own discipline as well as determining the areas of overlap and (b) making a decision to learn. With each discipline's identity solidly established, both were ready to sort out the ambiguity and to listen and share. As interprofessional dialogue increased, mutuality was fostered and stereotyping replaced with respect, collaboration, and partnership.

When interdisciplinary faculty members made a conscious choice to learn from one another, creativity deepened, resulting in a decision to educate for partnership (Russell, 1981). Based upon this choice, neither a nurse-designed course with pastoral care input nor a pastoral education-designed course with nursing application resulted. A true interdisciplinary approach to course development and teaching was used to provide students with the best of both disciplines and to model interdisciplinary partnership that could develop between students and spiritual leaders in faith communities.

Theoretical Underpinnings for Health Promotion in Faith Communities

Thirty-nine students from five Canadian provinces or territories enrolled in the first course offered at the University of Alberta in the spring term of 1996. This six-credit course covered the theoretical foundations of nursing practice within a faith community. Students were required to be registered nurses or to be in the final year of a 4-year baccalaureate degree nursing program.

The McGill Nursing Model (Gottlieb & Rowat, 1987), which developed out of the Canadian focus on health promotion, was selected to provide the theoretical underpinnings of the course. In this model, the goal of nursing is to maintain, strengthen, and develop health in others by actively engaging them in a learning process. Clients learn to take greater responsibility for their own health. Nurses accompany and empower clients through health-promoting interventions. The outcome of this process is improved health and greater client autonomy.

Parish nursing has its roots in Christian tradition, but this course was developed to prepare nurses for practice in both Christian and non-Christian faith communities. Emphasis was placed on the Canadian value of respect for diversity. Students were encouraged to consider that all people possess a spiritual dimension whether or not they express their spirituality through an organized religion. Faculty modeled respect for students' individual religious beliefs and encouraged them to discover, with openness, the views and beliefs of others.

Course objectives were (a) to acquire the knowledge and skills needed to begin nursing practice within a faith community, (b) to enhance personal growth and professional development to fulfill the parish nursing role, and (c) to establish an ongoing network of interdisciplinary colleagues to foster continuing professional development for promoting well-being in faith communities. The course included four units: (a) health, healing, and wholeness; (b) nurses as facilitators of healing; (c) promoting health in times of transition; and (d) nursing within a faith community.

Two assignments were required. In the first, students, working in small groups, were asked to discover the collective story of a local faith community. They were to examine how this community understands and fulfills its healing mission. They met with congregational staff, leaders, and volunteers; attended committee meetings and worship services; and reviewed church documents and membership lists. Each group of students presented its findings to classmates, faculty, and representatives of the assigned faith communities. For the second assignment, students submitted a scholarly paper in which they identified a population within a faith community to whom they could deliver nursing services. Focusing on the role of a parish nurse, they identified health promotion activities appropriate for this population. The course ended with a commissioning service. Over 200 students, family members, clergy, and friends attended to celebrate course completion and the beginning of parish nurse ministries in various Canadian settings.

Partnership in Guiding a Parish Nurse Practicum

A 9-month clinical practicum also carrying six credits was offered to build upon the theory course. Thirteen students responded to an opportunity to practice parish nursing for at least 8 hours per week. They were guided by a preceptor in the faith community and supervised by a member of the faculty team. In collaboration with the parish nursing advisory committee, faculty established a process that made it possible for students to apply to congregations that seemed to fit their talents and interests and for faith communities to interview student interns. Congregations sanctioned the student intern of their choice and the learning process in a commissioning service. Each service emphasized the congregation's commitment to the support of the nurse's healing ministry. Participation by faculty members in the commissioning services formalized congregation and university partnership.

The development of clinical preceptors within the faith communities was an important component of the clinical course. The primary role of the preceptor was to assist the parish nurse intern in gaining entry to the faith community so that learning objectives could be achieved. Preceptors had been selected by the health committee of the faith community and included clergy, nurses, or lay members of the congregation. Preceptors maintained ongoing contact with faculty, providing feedback on the student's progress. They provided input at advisory committee meetings on their perspective of the clinical aspect of the course. They collaborated with faculty and other advisory committee members to determine future course direction. Advisory committee meetings were held prior to the five student weekend seminars. Seminars offered students the opportunity to share their learning, to gain from the experience of their peers, to obtain peer support, and to receive feedback and direction from faculty.

Students were evaluated on a learning contract, demonstrating their ability to conduct a community assessment and an assessment of the strengths and concerns of the faith community where they were practicing. This assessment provided a foundation upon which to develop the parish nursing roles of health educator, health counselor, advocate, referral agent, coordinator of volunteers, and integrator of faith and health. A second assignment involved a presentation in which the student focused upon an important aspect of her specific parish internship, demonstrating how theory was applied in practice. A worship service to conclude the practicum was conducted by a precepting clergyperson and took place in a placement-site parish. This time of worship, designed to pay tribute to students, clergy, congregations, preceptors, and faculty, also fostered community visibility for parish nursing education and practice.

Future Challenges

As discussed throughout this chapter, the greatest focus for faculty at the University of Alberta has been on educating the nurse for parish practice. The challenges of connecting education to ongoing practice development now need to be addressed. As faith communities begin to offer employment to newly educated parish nurses, questions emerge as to their ongoing supervision, coordination, and future education. Faculty are investigating linkages between the university and the community that would support ongoing parish nursing practice. Faculty continue to network and are becoming increasingly involved in providing consultation to faith communities, both in Alberta and in other regions of the country. As parish nursing becomes more grounded in Alberta, new questions will emerge, stimulating the development of further research.

Conclusion

As faculty at the University of Alberta provide parish nursing education to nurses from across Canada and as parish nursing practice is fostered in multiple Canadian settings, it is recognized that this work is a small part of something that will bear new life in faith communities for years to come. The model used to develop parish nursing in Alberta should provide a useful framework for others intending to implement new parish nursing endeavors. This model reflects beliefs that a solid educational foundation is essential to parish nursing practice and that both education and practice must be sensitive to the specific social and cultural context in which that practice takes place. Cultivating parish nursing in a new setting takes considerable time, effort, energy, commitment, and skill. It requires developing awareness within the larger community and readiness within each participating faith community for this new professional role. It has been a challenging, yet rewarding, experience for each member of the parish nursing faculty team at the University of Alberta. It is hoped that the steps taken here will be imprinted upon the sands of time and that the progress made in this setting will guide leaders in other locations as they embark upon similar journeys.

References

Bopp, J. (1985). *Taking time to listen: Using community-based research to build programs.* Lethbridge, AB: Four Worlds Development Press.

Clark, M. (1995, March). *The nurse and the church: An active partnership.* Paper presented at the Ninth Annual Margaret Scott Wright Research Day, Faculty of Nursing, University of Alberta and Mu Sigma Chapter, Sigma Theta Tau, Edmonton.

Deber, R., & Vayda, E. (1992). The political and health care systems of Canada and Ontario. In R. Deber (Ed.), *Case studies in Canadian health care policy and management* (Vol. 1, pp. 1-6). Ottawa: Canada Hospital Association.

Douglass, L. (1995). Parish nursing symposium. *AARN Newsletter, 51*(8), 17-18.

Epp, J. (1986). *Achieving health for all: A framework for health promotion.* Ottawa: Minister of Supply and Services.

Fenhagen, J. C. (1977). *Mutual ministry: New vitality for the local church.* New York: Seabury.

Gottlieb, L., & Rowat, K. (1987). The McGill model of nursing: A practice derived model. *Advances in Nursing Science, 9*(4), 51-61.

Kerr, J. R., & MacPhail, J. (1996). *Canadian nursing: Issues and perspectives.* Toronto: Mosby.

Lalonde, M. (1974). *A new perspective on the health of Canadians.* Ottawa: Minister of Supply and Services.

Martin, L. B. (1996). Parish nursing: Keeping body and soul together. *The Canadian Nurse, 92*(1), 25-28.

Najman, J. M., & Western, J. S. (1984). A comparative analysis of Australian health policy in the 1970's. *Social Science and Medicine, 18*(10), 949-958.

Olson, J., & Simington, J. (1995, March). *An investigation of the feasibility of parish nursing.* Paper presented at the Ninth Annual Margaret Scott Wright Research Day, Faculty of Nursing, University of Alberta and Mu Sigma Chapter, Sigma Theta Tau, Edmonton.

Olson, J., Simington, J., & Douglass, L. (1995, November). *The feasibility of parish nursing in a reformed health care system.* Paper presented at Sigma Theta Tau International Biennial Convention, Detroit, MI.

Ottawa Charter for Health Promotion. (1986). *Canadian Journal of Public Health, 77,* 425-430.

Pierce, C., & Page, B. (1986). *A male/female continuum: Paths to colleagueship.* Laconia, NH: New Dynamics.

Russell, L. (1981). *Growth in partnership.* Philadelphia: Westminster.

Simington, J. (1996, Fall). Parish nursing: Reclaiming the church's healing mission. *Catholic Health Review,* pp. 19-20.

Simington, J., & Olson, J. (1995). Parish nursing in Alberta. *AARN Newsletter, 51*(8), 16.

Simington, J., Olson, J., & Douglass, L. (1996). Promoting well-being within a parish. *Canadian Nurse, 92*(1), 20-24.

World Health Organization. (1978). *Report of the International Conference on Primary Health Care in Alma Ata, USSR.* Geneva, Switzerland: Author.

Yeo, M. (1993). Toward an ethic of empowerment for health promotion. *Health Promotion International, 8*(3), 225-235.

26

The Australian Concept
of Faith Community

Antonia Margaretha Van Loon

The Social Context

South Australia is one of seven states or territories in Australia. It has a large land mass with a population of 1.4 million, most of whom reside in urban centers, with 73% living in the capital city, Adelaide (Australian Bureau of Statistics, 1991; Gardner, 1993). As is the case with most of Australia, the population is consolidated around coastal areas and a few regional centers. The arid interior is sparsely populated and contains many small and isolated towns, with very few inhabitants.

The rural and remote areas of Australia have undergone significant social changes, due to the government's cutting back on resources to towns with small populations in favor of rationalizing and regionalizing services. This social change has been compounded by declining commodity prices in primary produce due to global market forces such as the agriculturally subsidized competition from Europe and North America. This rural downturn has led to spiraling rural unemployment, poverty, and inequality of resources. Many smaller towns have effectively been wiped off the map.

In Australia, our composite health statistics have been steadily improving over the past century. This is in part due to effective health interventions in material conditions for good health such as quality food production, water and sanitation, housing, immunization, child health programs, and so on. Australia has no civil war. It experiences a secure welfare system that creates supportive conditions for good health. Yet, despite these improvements, there is a significant problem of unequal access to the social and cultural determinants for good health, especially among specific population groups within our community. Statistics concerning the health of indigenous Australians certainly do not reflect the general improved trends in morbidity and mortality. This developing gap is being rapidly exacerbated by current political, economic, and social movements. Church authorities have attempted to warn policymakers of the ensuing social problems, with little effect.

Large policy issues, such as labor market deregulation to improve international competitiveness, are contributing to an escalation of unemployment and underemployment, leading to growing numbers of families living in poverty. The increase of gambling as a means of raising government revenue is having major social costs, particularly within the vulnerable group of the unemployed. The morality of these methods of boosting revenue continues to be brought up in church, but the economic gain appears to blind policymakers to the social plan. The commodified health dollar now linked to output-based funding in the "case-mix" model has moved the community health dollar away from its community development focus to programs supporting acute care within the community. The policies of rationalist economics are leading many people to despair over the future quality of the Australian health system.

Funding Health Care in Australia

Australia has a nationally funded public health care system accessible to all people. This universal approach encourages social unity and egalitarian distribution of services. The health care system is governed by federal, state, and local governments and sourced by contributions such as the medicare levy. A medium-sized, not-for-profit and private sector parallels the government-funded "Medicare" system and contributes largely to the tertiary hospital setting and the aged-care sector. The major issues that currently affect Australian health care include decreasing resources, increasing need, increasing uptake of resources, and equal access for people within unequal situations. Universal access to health care is untenable because it offers services to all people regardless of their social and financial circumstances, leading to an increasing tax burden on a declining tax base. The government response has been to employ "cost-sharing" and "user pays" principles. The insured user applies for reimbursement from the private health fund. Reimbursement is generally linked to government-scheduled fees. If services charge more than the scheduled fee, the consumer pays the gap. As a direct consequence, many health consumers with private insurance perceive limited benefit for spiraling premiums and are voting with their feet, creating a mass exodus out of private health insurance. This situation has led to health insurance funds carrying mainly high-risk clients, with their increased needs, which in turn causes premiums to escalate and fuels the departure from private insurance. The declining insured membership has led to a crisis of usage within some private and not-for-profit sectors and an increased burden on the public sector health services.

The faith community in Australia has always provided care for the frail, sick, and disabled. Church-based hospitals, aged- and complex-care facilities, and community welfare agencies are indicative of a meaningful presence of the faith community in the provision of tertiary and secondary health care. However, the church has been largely absent from the primary health care setting. This may be due to the lack of structural opportunities for funding such care within Australia. These structures are the result of the medicalization of health care and its illness-focused, intervention-based strategy for health. This fragmented approach to health care, exacerbated by disease-centered payment systems, has ensured that church-based health care will also be focused on disease and disability. The spiraling human and economic costs of an illness locus have led to government recognition of the need for a paradigmatic shift to an approach encouraging prevention and early intervention rather than crisis management. This includes refocusing structures and payment systems to provide and fund prevention and community management programs.

David Legge (1997), the director of the Centre for Development in Health at LaTrobe University (Victoria, Australia), points out that health outcomes often do not match community needs. Society is a complex and dynamic concept, and a simplistic dollar-based outcome may in fact fall far from the mark of a desirable health outcome. Australian society is more likely to achieve health for all if we think of health promotion programs in terms of social development investments rather than in terms of the purchasing of outcomes. The faith community needs to take such a position because the debate concerning where the health dollar is placed is a social justice and advocacy issue that requires vigorous engagement from the churches.

Legge (1997) summarizes four social and cultural conditions for health that are verified repeatedly in research studies. They are the following:

- Mutual support and discipline (the norms by which we live)
- Opportunities for contribution and being valued for the contribution we make
- Recognition and respect in ourselves and our contribution
- Control, autonomy, and security in our lives

It is not difficult to see how being part of a faith community can provide a person with the social and cultural preconditions for good health. Religious faith provides the guiding principles and framework upon which congregation members build their lives. These principles provide a sense of meaning and purpose for our lives. In a faith community, people are supported in gaining standards to live by and through mutual networks of support, instruction, and worship. People in the faith community are able to provide a creative contribution that should be affirmed; the contributor should be recognized for his or her offering. Having a secure relationship with God and with others in the faith community provides a sense of purpose, the freedom and independence to grow and become within those relationships. It is a tragedy that these preconditions for good health, so freely available within a faith community, are not accessed by the wider community—a community so obviously in need. The time is right for the faith community to enter its place within primary health care, providing an ethical and socially just network of community support and an environment for sustainable and equitable health promotion programs grounded within the worldview of the local community. Commencement of the faith community nursing program seeks to do this.

A Brief Overview of South Australia's Community Health Program

The early 1970s in Australia saw a groundswell of public discontent over the inability of the traditional hospital-based health services to meet the health needs and changing illness patterns of the population. In 1973, a report titled *A Community Health*

Program for Australia (Hospital and Health Services Commission, 1973) was tabled by the newly elected federal government led by Prime Minister Whitlam. The report provided a blueprint for the integration and development of community health services. Although the report fell short in its ability to deliver what was required for the Australian health system, it did succeed in shifting funding into community health projects, and the new role of the *community health nurse,* based in a community health center, emerged by 1975. However, the focus of these early programs continued to be on individual treatment and service provision (Raftery, 1995, p. 25).

After the Ottawa Charter for Health Promotion was published by the World Health Organization (WHO, 1986), a review of community health care in Australia saw a shift in focus to include a more concentrated examination of intersectoral collaboration, community support, and effective policy making. This reorientation was stimulated by the earlier WHO (1978) Declaration of Alma Ata, which used as its policy framework the philosophy of "Health for All by the Year 2000" to develop strategic direction. Favorable state government financial and policy support, under the leadership of Dr. John Cornwall (the Minister of Health and Community Welfare, 1985-1988, of the South Australian government's Labour Party), was rendered to the community health program. There has been some departure from that exciting focus of the 1980s, induced by the new economic rationalism and fiscal constraints of the 1990s. The successful multi-disciplinary programs, with their population health focus, are being replaced by fee-for-service programs directed at groups of individuals, with a disease or developmental focus. These programs now tend to be conducted by general practitioners, not community health workers. Within this context, South Australia has achieved worldwide recognition for its high-functioning and successful community health program. In the midst of great changes, there remains a culture of commitment to community health within the Australian health care bureaucracy and by health care professionals. This includes a steady challenge to the dominant biomedical paradigm and the introduction of university preparation in public health, primary health care, and community health nursing. It is into this setting that the concept of faith community nursing is being introduced.

The Situation of Faith Communities Within Australia

The 1991 census indicates the spread of nominal religious affiliation in Australia. From this data, we know that 74.2% of Australians state that they are affiliated with a Christian religion. Of this group, 27.3% are Roman Catholic and 23.9% are Anglican, with the remainder being made up of other Christian denominations. Non-Christian religious affiliations were indicated by 2.6% of the Australian population. These include Islam, 0.9%; Buddhism, 0.8%; Judaism, 0.4%; and other religions, 0.5%. The non-Christian group is rising with each census, as new migration within Australia is generally from the Middle Eastern and Asian countries. Religious affiliation certainly does not correspond with the level of church attendance and active congregational participation, which is on average 40%-70% lower than the nominal affiliation figures supplied by the census (Hughes, 1993). However, it does demonstrate the potential number of people within the community who could have direct access to a congregational health ministry through the faith community nurse.

A recent National Church Life Survey (NCLS) found that 80% of those who attend church were positive about their involvement in their church, but only 29% wanted their congregations to keep going the way they were (Kaldor, 1994, p. vii). This means the majority of people want their church to be dynamic. Kaldor goes on to point out that the two most valued aspects of congregational life were spiritual nurture and caring (p. 195), with 44% of all people surveyed stating that they most value the care and nurture they received in the church (p. 186). Newcomers to the faith community valued being part of a caring congregation higher than any other aspect (p. 190). A nurse working in the context of the faith community is all about caring and spiritual nuture; therefore, it may be predicted that such a program will benefit church growth as well as improving the nurture and support activities of the community members.

It is important to realize that data from the NCLS indicated that 27% of church-going people are motivated to become involved within their faith community by the sense of family or community they experience, with a further 27% motivated by being able to care for and share with others (Kaldor, 1994, p. 192). A faith community nursing program can provide opportunities to contribute and to feel valued and supported within the faith community.

A Pilot Demonstration Project of
Faith Community Nursing

Evidence from the successful parish nursing programs commenced by Granger Westberg in the United States (Djupe, Olson, Ryan, & Lantz, 1994; Westberg & Westberg-McNamara, 1990) was examined thoroughly. The experiences in their entirety could not be replicated within this country due to fundamental variations, evident in several key areas in expanded below. An ongoing relationship was established in 1995 with the International Parish Nurse Resource Center, resulting in on-site consultation in the United States and Australia.

Framework

Information was advertised widely to government and nursing bodies about the concept of faith community nursing. All faith communities received an invitation to be involved in the pilot demonstration project, but after 12 months of disseminating information, the only faith communities to respond were from a Judeo-Christian world-view. After considerable discussion, the choice was made to use a Christian worldview as the organizing principle for the development of the framework for faith community nursing practice.

In such a worldview, the person is perceived as made in the image of God, as an integrated whole, and as part of the world God created. Through sin, the relationship between the creation, humanity, and God was disrupted, but through Jesus Christ there is salvation, healing, wholeness, and hope for the complete restoration of these relationships. The person is dynamic, always in the process of becoming, growing toward wholeness in Christ. The person is a synthesis of physical, psychosocial, and spiritual dimensions, with the spirit animating the person and enabling relationships with others, the environment, and God. Disorganization and disruption in this synthesis lead to disease and illness.

In this context, health is the experience of healing, leading to a sense of well-being. It involves internal harmony that leads to inner peace and growth toward wholeness, enabling an individual to freely adapt to the changing environment within and without. Thus health involves harmony in relationships between the person and God, the person and others, the person and their environment.

Purpose of the Faith Community Nurse Pilot Project

The project, developed and coordinated by Anne van Loon, was designed to demonstrate to faith communities, the nursing profession, the community, and the government the unique position that nurses can play in developing the congregational ministry of stewardship and service within the health and healing context of the faith community. The project demonstrates how the faith community can be a healing community, with human resources and meaningful support services for the wider community to access that can assist them in the growth of healthy relationships.

Christians have two major roles in life: first, to love God, and second, to love their neighbors as themselves (Matthew 22:37-40). These two roles are largely summarized in the three ministries of worship, stewardship, and service. In the Australian model of faith community nursing, these three functions provide the original organizing framework on which models of practice are being developed. The purpose of the faith community nurse role is to provide health promotion and illness prevention activities within the faith community, which may be described as *stewardship* endeavors. The other key purpose is to provide supportive care activities for the congregation and the wider community, which may be described as *service* endeavors. *All* aspects of the faith community nurse's life and practice are to the worship and glory of God.

Infrastructure

Information was widely disseminated to key individuals in the major religious denominations and through the popular and religious media. This process was backed up through prayer and active work such as speaking, writing, and lobbying. Those faith communities who felt God wanted them to partake in such a ministry have independently proceeded toward implementation. This was done according to the denominational structures of operation, accountability, and decision making pertinent to that faith community's worldview. For some congregations, this involved appointment and implementation directed by the priest and the parish council. In other congregations, committee structures were commenced to investigate proposals, study feasibility, make recommendations, adopt and plan for implementation of the program, and, finally, appoint the nurse. In other faith communities, the decision was made after individuals saw the faith community nurse ministry as an answer to their prayers concerning their mission and/or the specific needs within their faith community.

No directives were put into place on how this ministry should be conducted. When people want information, a variety of approaches are offered and the group is counseled to prayerfully inform itself and select or develop a method that most suits its cultural group and adheres to the tenets and traditions of its worldview. The management and accountability structures of each faith community nurse program is the responsibility of that faith community. The nurses were selected or appointed to the position by the leadership of the faith community. In all cases to date, the nurses have had a sense of vocational calling to this role as a form of combining their faith, professional knowledge, and skills to benefit the faith community and the wider collective. Some faith communities choose to appoint the nurse first, followed by a committee of support; others have a committee first and then appoint the nurse. Again, there are no directives given because this process must unfold in a culturally appropriate manner for each particular faith community. All faith communities in the demonstration project understand that the laws governing nursing practice must be adhered to. (Of note is the current change to Australian legislation that states that anyone applying to themselves the term *nurse* must hold current authorized nursing registration.)

A second aspect of the demonstration project has included the development of an association titled the Australian Faith Community Nurses Association (AFCNA). Its mandate is to act as a conduit and support network for faith community nursing, providing ecumenical education on religion and health issues; peer support; continuing education in nursing; resource development, procurement, and distribution; consultancy; political action and lobbying; and promotion of and publicity for the faith community nurse role. This association is open to all nurses, clergy, health professionals, pastoral care workers, and laity. The first basic preparation course, "Introduction to Faith Community Nursing" (30 hours), was held in July 1997. Continuing education occurs through the production and dissemination of newsletters, resource materials, and bi-monthly workshops and seminars. All educational enterprises are aimed at increasing opportunities for skill and knowledge development pertinent to the role and providing occasions for theological reflection and spiritual nurture. The association is working alongside colleagues nationally and internationally to further the faith community nursing role and assure that a quality standard of community health care is provided by the faith community.

Funding

Australian churches are generally quite small, with more than half having fewer than 50 members (Kaldor, 1994, p. ix). Most churches experience difficulties financing their programs and salaried workers. This is due to declining congregation size; lower disposable incomes; declining real salaries; and the fact that donations, tithes, and offerings to the church are not tax-deductible. These factors make funding a faith community nurse a major challenge.

There are 10 congregations that started faith community nurse programs in 1997 from the Anglican, Roman Catholic, and Lutheran churches. (Several other denominations are examining the possibility of commencing in the near future.) These congregations vary in size from less than 100 members to a parish of 3,000 members. All the nurses are volunteering their time; the maximum number of hours is 8 to 12 hours per week. One church is providing some remuneration to the parish nurse coordinator. Three congregations have received small establishment grants from local government; these grants are defraying some of their costs, such as telephone, mileage, and equipment.

Negotiations are ongoing between the AFCNA and government health departments, which administer general health care funding. There is an attempt to allow appropriately educated and qualified nurses working within faith communities to be reimbursed for care coordination activities that take place within the continuum of care. These discussions are in the early stages, but the restructuring of Australia's health service is set to provide the faith community with a unique opportunity to situate faith community nursing in the domain of primary health care within the continuum of care, giving the faith community a presence at primary, secondary, and tertiary levels of care.

The Faith Community Nurse Role

The faith community nursing role focuses on clarifying health values, guiding choices, and increasing possibilities for the individual and the community (Parse, 1981); caring, nurturing, and sustaining the whole person to maximize health and well-being (Leininger, 1985; Watson, 1985); and establishing and cultivating healing relationships (Travelbee, 1971) within the faith community and the wider community.

The purpose of the nursing role is stewardship, service, and a life of worship. This is carried out through both personal and group education and counseling activities that provide health promotion and illness prevention information. Opportunities for transformation and growth are offered from the philosophical and theological perspective of the faith community. Supportive care activities for individuals, the congregation, and the wider community include assistance in navigating the complex health care system; the establishment and nurture of care and support structures within the faith community; training volunteers; acting as a resource and referral agent between the client, congregation, and private and community services; assisting clients to maintain their optimal level of wellness; and nurturing their growth toward wholeness within the context of the faith community. The faith community nurse role is similar to the community health nurse role in Australia. The major difference is the specific population with which each faith community nurse works and the philosophy and faith community structure that undergird this nurse's work.

One of the key issues requiring continued focus in health programs conducted by faith community nurses is the vexing question: "How do we best generate structural change while sustaining and nurturing personal growth?" To effect change at a societal level, the congregation needs to challenge the wider social and economic inequalities within the community and also seek to sustain individuals, thus preventing the health problems that occur due to social injustice.

Future Implications

Long-term growth and viability of the faith community nurse program will depend on securing permanent mechanisms of funding and developing sound frameworks and infrastructures to support the educational and professional development of the nurses. Public policy has a direct impact on the shaping of faith community nursing. Rapidly changing health and social policy, such as the guidelines of community health and primary health care developed within frameworks such as the Ottawa Charter and the Alma Ata Declaration, provides a blueprint for the development of health promotion programs within the faith community. Similarly, restructuring the health service provides a new challenge and opportunity for the faith community to place itself as a viable service provider within the continuum of health care.

Baum (1995) points out that the way forward is through intersectoral collaboration and true participation within the health care continuum. Australian faith community nursing programs are establishing links between existing government and private sector services. Successful partnerships across sectors depend on all parties defining the needs, planning the process to meet these needs, and seeing the value of their joint venture. There are preliminary discussions with government, but much thought needs to go into how a "win/win" situation can be achieved for all parties. Cost burdens must not be shifted to the faith community without government reimbursement. There must be equitable distribution of funding between illness care and primary health care. The congregation must remain autonomous and in control of its program, and the government must be assured of quality service available to its constituents.

There are precedents in Australia for this type of autonomy and self-regulation within quality-control parameters set by the government. These include Christian school movements, the aged-care housing and nursing home provision, and Christian social welfare agencies. These movements offer opportunities to attach faith community nurses to aged-care complexes, church-based schools, and other care agencies. Through refining denominational, regional, and ecumenical organizational structures, the possibilities are exciting and need to be embraced as an opportunity for churches to reach into the wider community.

Conclusion

Through faith community nursing and health ministry we are able to begin to provide the precursor social and cultural circumstances for good health and well-being by providing education, resources, counseling, and a network of support through which people can contribute their talents and receive assistance to manage life and health. As we head toward a new millennium, it is a continual challenge for faith communities to reach out to their community in love and service. The faith community is able to influence people at the microlevel, empowering individuals to take control of their life with boldness. They can encourage the community of support that shapes the way people grow and become, role modeling the full and abundant life experienced when the individual lives in harmony with self, others, and God.

References

Australian Bureau of Statistics. (1991). *Census of population and housing, 1911-1991*. Canberra: Author.

Baum, F. (1995). *Health for all: The South Australian experience*. Kent Town, South Australia: Wakefield.

Djupe, A. M., Olson, H., Ryan, A., & Lantz, J. C. (1994). *Reaching out: Parish nursing services* (2nd ed.). Park Ridge, IL: National Parish Nurse Resource Center.

Gardner, P. (1993). *Adelaide: A social atlas*. Adelaide: Australian Bureau of Statistics.

Hospital and Health Services Commission. (1973). *A community health program for Australia*. Canberra: Australian Government Publishing Service.

Hughes, P. (1993). *Religion: A view from the Australian census*. Victoria: Christian Research Association.

Kaldor, P. (1994). *Winds of change: The experience of church in a changing Australia*. New South Wales: ANZEA.

Legge, D. (1997, April 3). *Challenging broader social and economic inequalities*. Paper presented to the South Australian Community Health Research Unit Seminar, Adelaide, South Australia.

Leininger, M. (1985). Transcultural care, diversity and universality: A theory of nursing. *Nursing and Health Care, 6*(4), 209-212.

Nutbeam, D. (1986). Health promotion glossary, *Health promotion.* 1(1), [113-127.

Parse, R. R. (1981). *Man-living-health: A theory of nursing*. New York: John Wiley.

Raftery, J. (1995). The social and historical context. In F. Baum (Ed.), *Health for all: The South Australian experience* (pp. 19-37). Kent Town, South Australia: Wakefield.

Travelbee, J. (1971). *Interpersonal aspects of nursing* (2nd ed.). Philadelphia: Davis.

Watson, J. (1985). *Nursing: Human science and human care*. Norwalk, CT: Appleton-Century-Croft.

Westberg, G. E., & Westberg-McNamara, J. (1990). *The parish nurse: Providing a minister of health for your congregation*. Minneapolis, MN: Augsburg Fortress.

World Health Organization. (1978). *Primary health care* (Report of the International Conference on Primary Health Care, Alma Ata). Geneva, Switzerland: Author.

World Health Organization. (1986). Ottawa charter for health promotion. *Health Promotion International, 1*(4), i-v.

Postscript

Phyllis Ann Solari-Twadell

As the work of this text concludes, there are a few issues that need mention and comments. As parish nursing continues to be considered from the perspective of the health care institution, the church, and the client, differences can arise. These differences will continue to offer an opportunity to be in dialogue with each other. Dialogue will hopefully lead to new ways for those in our faith communities to experience health and wholeness.

As parish nursing is considered part of an integrated delivery system, the rhetoric, regulations, and time frames of the health care institution may impinge on the manner in which the congregation manages its affairs. For example, the documentation of services provided by a parish nurse results in the creation of a medical record. If the parish nurse is employed by the health care institution and contracted for by the church, that medical record is the property of the health care institution. All of a sudden the institution's regulations are framing the delivery of health promotion services in the faith community. This ongoing development of parish nursing cannot be lost in the differentiated perspective of health, institution, and congregation. Time, resources, and creative thinking will continue to be needed to address blocks and avert obstacles. There will be no quick fixes or easy solutions, for parish nursing will continue to push traditional thinking.

The financing of health promotion services in the community will also continue to nag at current policies for the payment of health services. Traditionally, health promotion services have been resourced. This continues to be the case for parish nursing. Nurses interested in serving in this role are most often underpaid or not paid at all, yet the services are provided by licensed health professionals. An answer to the continual question of what levels or kinds of services constitute unpaid services to a faith community versus what levels of services a professional nurse should expect to receive compensation for is yet unclear. Ministry does not mean receiving no compensation. Being in service to another does not mean there will be no compensation. These issues will require ongoing attention when the economics of parish nursing are addressed.

The economics of parish nursing are sometimes flavored by the feminist dimension of this role. Of all parish nurses, 98% are women. Historically, women in the context of church have often been the unspoken and least recognized contributors, particularly in traditions dominated largely by a male hierarchy. This thread runs deep within nursing, where, historically, male physicians have been the dominant figures. Do these perspectives continue to contribute to the giving of self in service with inadequate or no compensation? The most extreme example of this mind-set is the shifting of the cost of health care to the backs of the uncompensated. The shadows of economic injustice need to be examined when ongoing health services are expected to be made available by those who are already working another job in addition to attempting to serve their faith community.

If parish nursing is going to continue to grow and mature, the acquisition of grants, research, and publication of that research will need to be a part of the process. As more and more nurses who have skills in research are attracted to parish nursing, it can be hoped that the body of knowledge regarding this practice area will grow. Today, parish nursing is seen primarily in a Christian context. The editors of this text invite comments, information, and documentation of parish nurse experiences in other religious traditions as well as about the transportability of parish nursing to other countries and specific ethnic groups. It is only through documentation of experiences and knowledge that the universal application of this practice will be understood.

Index

About the Editors

Mary Ann McDermott, R.N., Ed.D., Professor of Maternal Child Health Nursing, Niehoff School of Nursing, Loyola University, Chicago, has her doctorate in curriculum and supervision. Her interest in nurses in churches began when she became a cofounder and served as the director of a Loyola University faculty nurse-managed center in a Roman Catholic congregation from 1981 through 1987. Accountability and, subsequently, documentation issues were a high priority and led to much debate and discussion among faculty peers and students regarding the necessity, format, and evaluation of record keeping in this nontraditional care site. She has been active with parish nursing and the Resource Center since being named to their Advisory Committee at Lutheran General Hospital in 1986. She serves as Chair of the system board of Advocate Health Care. Currently, she holds the title of Director for the Center of Faith and Mission for Loyola University of Chicago.

Phyllis Ann Solari-Twadell, R.N., B.S.N., M.P.A., M.S.N., received her Bachelor of Science degree in nursing and her Master of Science in nursing from Loyola University. She received her master's in public administration from Roosevelt University and is now enrolled in the doctoral program in nursing at Loyola University as a part-time student. She has been employed for 22 years at Lutheran General Hospital/Advocate Health Care in Park Ridge, Illinois: For 10 of those years she worked in addiction treatment, and for the last 6 of those 10 she held the position of Director of Nursing Services at Parkside Lutheran Hospital, a specialty hospital for addicted patients. From 1984 to 1988, she was president of the National Nurses Society on Addictions. Currently, she is Director of the International Parish Nurse Resource Center and Interim Director of Parish Nursing Services, Advocate Health Care. In that capacity, she is the editor of *Perspectives on Parish Nursing Practice,* a regular publication of the International Parish Nurse Resource Center. She has coedited and is a contributing author of the text *Parish Nursing: The Developing Practice.* As director of the resource center, she coordinates the Annual Granger Westberg Symposium on Parish Nursing.

About the Contributors

Patricia Benner, R.N., Ph.D., F.A.A.N., is Professor in the Department of Physiological Nursing in the School of Nursing at the University of California, San Francisco. She received her Ph.D. from the University of California, Berkeley in stress and coping and health under the direction of Hubert Dreyfus and Richard Lazarus. She is the author of eight books, including *From Novice to Expert: The Primacy of Caring,* coauthored with Judith Wrubel; *Interpretive Phenomenology: Embodiment, Caring and Ethics in Health and Illness* and *The Crisis of Care,* with Susan Phillips; *Expertise in Nursing Practice: Caring, Clinical Judgment, and Ethics,* with Christine Tanner and Catherine Chesla; and *Caregiving,* with Suzanne Gordon and Nel Noddings. She is an internationally noted researcher and lecturer on health, stress and coping, skill acquisition, and ethics. Her work has had wide influence on nursing both in the United States and internationally—for example, in providing the basis for new legislation and design for nursing practice and education for three states in Australia. She was recently elected an honorary fellow of the Royal College of Nursing. Her work has influence beyond nursing in the areas of clinical practice and clinical ethics.

JoAnn Gragnani Boss, R.N., M.S.N., M.S., is Parish Nurse Coordinator at Community Memorial Hospital, Menomonee Falls, Wisconsin, a suburb northwest of Milwaukee. She serves in a dual role that includes clinical practice and the management of a volunteer parish nurse network. Her clinical practice is partially funded by the cooperating churches of Sussex. Prior to this position, she practiced parish nursing in inner-city Chicago. She has had several articles on parish nursing printed in *Health and Development,* which is produced by the Christian Community Health Fellowship, and is a member of Sigma Theta Tau and the National Association of Catholic Chaplains. She is also on the CCHF Board of Directors.

Sandra Schmidt Bunkers, R.N., Ph.D., is Associate Professor and Chair of the Department of Nursing at Augustana College in Sioux Falls, South Dakota. She obtained her bachelor's in nursing from Augustana College, her master's in nursing from South

Dakota State University, and a Ph.D. in nursing from Loyola University, Chicago. She has practiced in a variety of settings, including psychiatric-mental health, community health, long-term care, and nursing education. Her focus of research is on lived experiences of health, using Parse's theory of human becoming and research methodology to guide such research as "Considering Tomorrow" for women who are homeless; "The Lived Experience of Hope" for those working with persons who are homeless; and "The Lived Experience of Feeling Cared For." She serves as a consultant to a variety of health care entities interested in developing nursing theory-based practice models.

Lisa Burkhart, R.N., M.P.H., is currently employed by Advocate Health Care Parish Nursing Services. Since May 1996, she has coordinated educational efforts (funded by a Kellogg grant) to automate parish nursing documentation, using nursing-standardized coding systems (NANDA and NIC) that are both practically and theoretically sound. She earned her bachelor's in nursing at the University of North Carolina–Chapel Hill in 1985 and a master's in public health at the University of Illinois–Chicago. She is currently a doctoral student at Loyola University, Chicago, Niehoff School of Nursing, studying nursing information systems as they relate to nursing-standardized languages. Her past positions include Director of Nursing Education, Regulation, and Legislation at the American Hospital Association, where she developed nursing policy, staffed national committees, and published articles related to nursing. Before that, she was Program Administrator for the American Medical Association, where she coordinated efforts in long-term care and managed care policy and was a member of the CPT editorial staff, which developed the coding system used for physician reimbursement.

Mary Chase-Ziolek, Ph.D., R.N., has been Coordinator of Geriatric Health Ministry at Northwestern Memorial Hospital in Chicago since 1991, working with churches and synagogues to develop health programs. She directs the Volunteer Congregational Health Program (VCHP), an interfaith, multiethnic network of 27 nurses volunteering in 21 churches that provides health promotion services. She is responsible for the training and ongoing support of the nurses who participate in the VCHP as well as for program development and evaluation. In addition to these responsibilities, she provides a weekly nurse drop-in center at a downtown parish. The VCHP began with a $231,000 grant from the Retirement Research Foundation in 1994 and is currently the recipient of a grant from the VNA Foundation.

Margaret B. Clark, M.C.Sp., is Coordinator of Pastoral Care Services and Supervised Pastoral Education Programs at the University of Alberta Hospital, Edmonton, Alberta. She holds a baccalaureate degree in sociology, master's degrees in Christian spirituality and theology, and is currently enrolled in a doctor of ministry program. She is certified as a teaching supervisor in clinical pastoral education (CPE) with the Canadian Association for Pastoral Practice and Education (CAAPE). She ministered for 12 years in Roman Catholic parishes in Montana and California. For the past 14 years, she has been doing hospital ministry in Montana, Utah, and Alberta. She codeveloped and has cotaught both theoretical and clinical parish nursing courses offered at the University of Alberta and has been involved in professional presentations and publications related to that effort.

Rev. Robert Cotton Fite, Ph.D., is an ordained pastor of the Episcopal Church, USA and a licensed psychologist. He is the director of the Pastoral Counseling Center at Lutheran General Hospital, Park Ridge, Illinois. He is also Adjunct Faculty at Garrett-Evangelical Theological Seminary in Evanston, Illinois, where he received his Ph.D. He serves on the parish nurse faculty at Lutheran General Hospital, part of Advocate Health Care. Together with Herbert Anderson, he published *Becoming Married.*

Marsha Fowler, Ph.D., M.Div., M.S., R.N., F.A.A.N., is Professor, Haggard Graduate School of Theology and Graduate Program, School of Nursing, at Azusa Pacific University in Azusa, California, and the director of the university's Parish Nurse and Health Ministries Master's Degree Program. She is also Interim Pastor, Trinity Presbyterian Church, Pasadena, California. She lectures and consults nationally and internationally and writes in the fields of ethics, spirituality, and theology.

Janet Griffin, R.N., M.S., is Director of the Parish Nurse Program at Trinity Regional Health System, Rock Island, Illinois. She is a graduate of St. Luke's Hospital School of Nursing, Davenport, Iowa; has a Master of Science degree in health education from Western Illinois University, Macomb; and has a certificate in health ministry from Iowa Lutheran Hospital, Des Moines. Her nursing practice includes clinical experience, teaching experience, and 4 years as a parish nurse for a large congregation in Davenport, Iowa. She was a coauthor of *The Child in the Congregation: A Resource Guide for Parish Nurses* (1995); the author of "Reminiscence: Enriching Life Through Memories," an article in the January 1996 *Home Health Focus* newsletter; and has written a module on professional development for the endorsed curriculum the International Parish Nurse Resource Center developed for coordinators of parish nurse programs.

Phyllis B. Heffron, R.N., M.S.N. is currently Research Associate at the University of Iowa College of Nursing, Iowa City. Her work is with the Family Involvement in Care research study, which involves the study of nursing home residents with a diagnosis of Alzheimer's disease and how family interventions and interaction with staff contribute to quality-of-life issues. She received a diploma in nursing from St. Luke's Hospital School of Nursing in Davenport, Iowa, her B.S.N. from the University of Maryland, Baltimore, and her M.S.N. from the Catholic University of America, Washington, DC. She has been a Faculty Facilitator with the R.N.-B.S.N. Program at the College of Nursing, University of Iowa, and is a member of the American Nurses' Association, the National League for Nursing, and the Gamma and Pi Chapters of Sigma Theta Tau International. She is a charter member of the Association of Nurses in AIDS Care.

Rev. Lawrence E. Holst has been affiliated with Lutheran General Hospital (Park Ridge, Illinois) for its entire history. In June 1959 he began there as a chaplain-resident and was named Chairman of the Department of Pastoral Care in July 1960. He held this position for 31 years. In 1991, he began a new position with the Lutheran General Health System as Senior Staff Associate to the Office of Mission/Church Relations. In 1996, he retired. He received a B.A. from St. Olaf College, Northfield, Minnesota, followed by a B.Th. from Luther Theological Seminar, St. Paul, Minnesota and was later ordained into the Evangelical Lutheran Church. He has edited two books, *Toward a Creative Chaplaincy* and *Hospital Ministry: The Role of the Chaplain Today* and coauthored another, *Ministry to Outpatients: A New Challenge in Pastoral Care*. He has written numerous articles and is a lecturer in the fields of pastoral care and clinical ethics.

Saralea Holstrom, R.N., has been a parish nurse at Our Saviour's Lutheran Church, Naperville, Illinois, of which she is a member, since May 1985. She graduated from Northwestern Memorial Hospital's School of Nursing and has had experience in medical-surgical and obstetric units in this hospital setting. Before she became a parish nurse, she was Medicare Charge Nurse and Assistant Director of Nursing at a convalescent-rehabilitation center in Naperville. As a parish nurse, she is a member of her church's pastoral care team, along with its four pastors and counselor, dedicated to providing whole person care of mind, body, and spirit to families of the congregation according to their needs. She and her husband Bruce have three grown children and have dealt with caregiving issues with their own aging parents.

Reverend Leroy Joesten is Vice President, Religion and Health of Lutheran General Hospital, Park Ridge, Illinois, Advocate Health Care in the Chicago area. An ordained minister in the Lutheran Church (Missouri Synod) since 1967, he has served as an institutional chaplain for the last 25 years and as an educator in the Association for Clinical Pastoral Education since 1974. Prior to becoming a hospital chaplain, he served a Lutheran congregation in rural Iowa. He has administered a parish nurse program at Lutheran General and has also served as a faculty member to Lutheran General's program.

Bethany Johnson, B.A., previously was with Parish Nursing Services, Advocate Health Care as office coordinator. In this position she managed the day-to-day functions of the Office of Parish Nursing Services. Historically, she had management responsibilities for Lutheran General Hospital's first W. K. Kellogg grant, "Parish Nursing Services Project." She also had management responsibilities for a second W. K. Kellogg grant, "Partners in Health and Healing," which had a major focus on the development and refinement of a documentation system for parish nursing. She has a B.A. in English from Augustana College, Rockford, Illinois. Currently, she is pursuing a master's degree in education at Loyola University in Chicago.

Patricia Kellen, R.N., B.S.N., serves as parish nurse at St. Isaac Jogues Church, Niles, Illinois, part of Advocate Health Care's parish nurse program. She has held this position since February 1994. After receiving her baccalaureate degree from Marycrest College, Davenport, Iowa, she served three years active duty in the Nurse Corps, U.S. Navy Reserves, at the National Naval Medical Center, Bethesda, Maryland. She has held staff and management positions in psychiatric nursing at Lutheran General Hospital in Park Ridge, Illinois and continued in that specialty at Sheridan Road Hospital, Chicago before changing to addictions nursing with a move to Alexian Brothers Medical Center, Elk Grove Village, Illinois. She is a member of the Documentation Committee, whose charge has been to develop nursing diagnoses and interventions specific to parish nurse practice.

Jean King, R.N., M.S., is the Faculty Facilitator for the University of Iowa College of Nursing R.N.-B.S.N. Satellite Program in Emmetsburg, Iowa. She received her diploma from Mercy Hospital School of Nursing in Des Moines, Iowa, her B.S. from Buena Vista College, Storm Lake, Iowa and her M.S. in nursing from South Dakota State University in Brookings. She has worked in medical-surgical and public health nursing and has served as a curriculum and evaluation consultant in parish nurse grant projects and in hospice program development. She is a member of the American Nurses' Association and the Phi Chapter of Sigma Theta Tau. She serves as Chairperson of the Advisory Committee for Hospice of Northwest Iowa and Vice-Chairperson for the Clay County Board of Health, Spencer, Iowa.

Greg Kirschner, M.D., M.P.H., is a family physician who attended medical school at Duke University and took his residency training at Lutheran General Hospital in Park Ridge, Illinois. He went on to become Associate Director of the Family Practice Residency Program there and develop an association with the Lutheran General Hospital parish nurse program as a physician advisor, faculty member, and steering committee member. Since 1995, he and his physician-wife, Carolyn, have served as medical missionaries in northern Nigeria.

Robert Lloyd, Ph.D., in his current role as Director of System Quality for Advocate Health Care in Oak Brook, Illinois, is responsible for the development of systemwide quality indicators, measurement of the voice of the customer, and CQI education. He also serves as liaison to external organizations interested in quality data and its use. Before joining Advocate, he served as Director of Quality Measurement for Lutheran General Hospital and directed the American Hospital Association's national demonstration project on quality, the Quality Measurement and Management Project. He is a frequent speaker at national conferences and seminars and has published numerous articles, reports, and books on a wide range of topics.

Patti Ludwig-Beymer, Ph.D., R.N., is currently employed as a clinical quality specialist at Advocate Health Care in Oakbrook, Illinois. As such, she serves as the project manager for systemwide clinical improvement projects on asthma, diabetes mellitus, and cardiac services. A nurse for over 20 years, she received her diploma in nursing from Mercy Hospital School of Nursing in Pittsburgh, her B.A.N. and M.S.Ed. from Duquesne University in Pittsburgh, and her doctorate in nursing from the University of Utah. She has practiced in a variety of settings, including acute care, community-based programs, and nursing education. She also conducts health services research and has published over 25 articles and book chapters on nursing and health care topics, including transcultural nursing, parish nursing, pathophysiology, cost accounting in nursing, advanced practice nursing, medication errors, patient satisfaction, and clinical quality improvement.

Rosemarie Matheus, R.N., M.S.N., received her Master of Science degree in nursing from Marquette University in Milwaukee, Wisconsin as well as a certificate in theology from that university. She currently holds several positions: faculty on the staff of Marquette College of Nursing and coordinator of placement and supervision for parish nurses in Milwaukee Churches at Sinai Samaritan Medical Center and St. Luke's

Medical Center. She has directed the Parish Nurse Preparation Institute, Phases I and II, and has consulted, published, and spoken extensively on a variety of aspects of parish nursing.

Wendy Tuzik Micek, D.N.Sc., R.N., received her bachelor's, master's, and doctorate degrees in nursing science from Rush University College of Nursing, Illinois. She has practiced in a variety of settings, including acute care, the operating room, ambulatory surgery, and health services research. She is a member of the Midwest Nursing Research Society, Sigma Theta Tau International, Sigma Xi, the American Academy of Ambulatory Care Nursing, Ambulatory Management Network-Metropolitan Chicago Health Care Council, Association of Managed Care Nurses, and Association for Health Services Research. She has twice served as president of the Gamma Phi Chapter of Sigma Theta Tau International and has authored and coauthored publications for journals and book chapters; she also reviews abstracts for the annual Midwest Nursing Research Society conferences. She has presented at many professional seminars and conferences on such topics as patient satisfaction, quality of life, patient-centered care, patient care outcomes, professional nursing documentation languages, project management, and various clinical process improvement projects. Currently she is employed as a Clinical Quality Specialist by Advocate Health Care, where she develops, implements, evaluates, and manages systemwide clinical improvement projects on topics such as total joint replacements, anticoagulation, and mother and baby services. In addition, she provides continuous quality improvement education and supports quality management and care management within Advocate. Before joining Advocate, she was a nurse researcher for Rush Presbyterian St. Luke's Medical Center, where she served as a coordinator for the Picker Commonwealth study on patient-centered care and various other special projects.

Rev. Gerald Nelson, M.Div., has been the Senior Pastor of Our Saviour's Lutheran Church in Naperville, Illinois, for the past 23 years. He is a Concordia College and Lutheran School of Theology graduate and has served congregations in Waterbury, Connecticut, and St. Claire Shore, Michigan. He leads seminars around the country on the theme "Making It Work in the Parish." Under his leadership, the congregation of Our Saviour's has grown to over 4,000 members and has added a Parish Nurse staff position and a Parish Counselor to its pastoral care team. Other ministry developments include a new mission led by his son, Michael, which is growing rapidly and has started a successful preschool. In addition, under Rev. Nelson, Our Saviour's has purchased a second facility where an Early Childhood Center (called "Celebration") is serving over 200 families and where additional worship services will be added.

Joanne K. Olson, R.N., Ph.D., holds a Ph.D. in nursing with a focus on nurse-client interaction. She has a master's degree in public health and a baccalaureate degree in nursing and has held positions as a clinician, supervisor, and educator in Minnesota, Missouri, Ontario, and Alberta. She has been a faculty member at Maryville University, St. Louis, Missouri, the University of Western Ontario, London, Ontario, and is presently Associate Professor on the Faculty of Nursing at the Univiersity of Alberta. Her teaching, research, and writing interests are in the areas of community and family health, nursing education, nurse-client interaction, and parish nursing. She has numerous professional publications, frequently presents her work at professional conferences, and serves on the Board of Directors of Sigma Theta Tau International Nursing Honor Society. She has codeveloped and cotaught both theoretical and clinical parish nursing courses offered at the University of Alberta.

H. Scott Sarran, M.D., M.M., at the time of this writing, was Vice President for Clinical Quality Improvement for Advocate Health Care, Oakbrook, Illinois, an integrated delivery system serving the entire Chicago area. In this capacity, he is responsible for clinical process improvement and care management initiatives, including practice guidelines, utilization management, and case management; medical leadership for Advocate Health Partners, the umbrella organization for Advocate's eight PHOs, with approximately 140,000 covered lives including Medicare and Medicaid full-risk capitation; system quality, including support of continuous quality improvement, patient satisfaction, clinical indicators, and infection control; and clinical information systems. He has been Medical Director for a 50,000-member PHO and Chairman and Residency Program Director for Family Practice at Lutheran General Hospital and continues to practice Family Medicine. He is Board-Certified in Family Practice with Certificates of added Qualifications in Geriatrics and Sports Medicine. He receive his master's in management from the J. L. Kellogg Graduate School of Management at Northwestern University and his M.D. from Northwestern University Medical School.

Marcia Schnorr, R.N., Ed.D., has been active in the practice, promotion, and education of parish nursing for many years. She is the parish nurse at St. Paul Lutheran Church in Rochelle, Illinois; National Parish Nurse Coordinator for the Lutheran Church Missouri Synod; Adjunct Professor in Parish Nursing for Concordia University, Wisconsin; and on the nursing faculty at Kishwaukee College in Malta, Illinois. She has a diploma in nursing from the Swedish-American Hospital School of Nursing in Rockford, Illinois, a B.S. and M.S. (with majors in nursing), and an Ed.D. (adult education) from Northern Illinois University. She has presented at numerous regional, national, and international parish nurse conferences and has been a regular contributor to newsletters, journals, and other publications. She has completed the requirements to become certified by the Lutheran Church Missouri Synod as a lay church worker and has a Solemn Appointment to St. Paul Lutheran Church in Rochelle, Illinois.

Jane A. Simington, R.N., Ph.D., holds a Ph.D. in health sciences with a focus in mental health and program planning. She has a master's degree in nursing with a clinical specialization in gerontology and a baccalaureate degree in both nursing and psychology. She has held positions as a clinician, supervisor, counselor, researcher, and educator. She has been a faculty member at the college and university level, including Hawaii Pacific University, and is presently a sessional lecturer on the Faculty of Nursing at the University of Alberta. Her teaching, research and writing interests are in the areas of gerontology, mental health, and complementary methods of healing and spiritual well-being. She has numerous professional publications and frequently presents her work at seminars, workshops, and conferences. She has an independent practice that focuses on life transition management and has codeveloped and cotaught both theoretical and clinical parish nursing courses at the University of Alberta.

Antonia Margaretha Van Loon, R.N. DipAppsScCHN, B.N., M.N., Ph.D.(cand.), is a doctoral candidate at Flinders University of South Australia. Her research project involves designing and developing conceptual models of faith community nursing within the Australian context. She is the founder and chairperson of the Australian Faith Community Nurses Association, which provides nurses working in Australian faith communities with support, basic educational preparation, networks, continuing education, resources, and consultancy for this new role. She holds a degree in nursing, postgraduate qualifications in community health nursing, and a master's by research degree from Flinders University. Her research focus is on spiritual care and primary health care in nursing practice. She continues to practice as a registered nurse at Flinders Medical Centre, where her clinical focus is on emergency nursing. She was a Lecturer in Nursing at the University of South Australia from 1988 to 1997 when she began full-time doctoral studies to introduce faith community nursing to Australia.

Rev. Granger Westberg, author of the best-seller *Good Grief* and many other articles and texts, is best known for his work with the Wholistic Health Centers and his work in conceptualizing, developing, and telling the story of parish nursing. He has been a parish pastor; hospital chaplain at Augustana Hospital in Chicago; Professor at the University of Chicago; the first Dean of the Institute of Religion at Texas Medical Center in Houston; Professor of Practical Theology at Wittenberg University in Springfield, Ohio; consultant; and well-known public speaker and writer, advocating the church's role in preventive medicine since the early 1940s. He is now retired and remains in a consultative capacity to the International Parish Nurse Resource Center, Advocate Health Care.

Rev. L. James Wylie assumed his present responsibility as Senior Vice President, Religion and Health, Advocate Health Care in 1995. He has been associated with Lutheran General Hospital from its opening on Christmas Eve, 1959, to the present. From 1963 to 1967 he served at Lutheran Medical Center in Brooklyn, New York, which was then an affiliate of the HealthSystem. In the late 1960s, his involvement with the Corporate Board and management in the areas of health strategy and global health interests resulted in the development of the early strains of what is called today Congregational Health Partners. During the 1970s, he served as Vice President of Human Resources; in the early 1980s, he was involved in the formation of what is now the Park Ridge Center, a HealthSystem affiliate which has gained national renown as the Center for Health, Faith and Ethics. In addition, he has maintained corporate responsibility for parish nursing since its inception. This includes supporting the ongoing development of the International Parish Nurse Resource Center.